Invertebrate Blood Cells

Invertebrate Blood Cells

Volume 2

Arthropods to urochordates, invertebrates and vertebrates compared

Edited by

N. A. Ratcliffe and A. F. Rowley

Department of Zoology
University College of Swansea
Singleton Park
Swansea SA2 8PP
Wales

1981

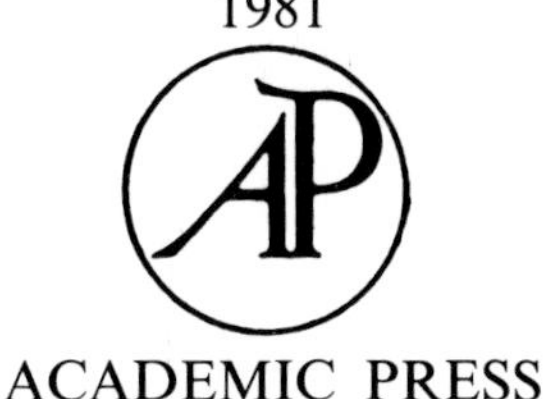

ACADEMIC PRESS
A Subsidiary of Harcourt Brace Jovanovich, Publishers

London · New York · Toronto · Sydney · San Francisco

ACADEMIC PRESS INC. (LONDON) LTD.
24—28 Oval Road
London NW1 7DX

U.S. Edition published by
ACADEMIC PRESS INC.
111 Fifth Avenue
New York, New York 10003

British Library Cataloguing in Publication Data

Invertebrate blood cells.
1. Invertebrates—physiology
2. Blood cells
I. Ratcliffe, N A II. Rowley, A F
592′.01′13 QL364 80-41248

ISBN 0-12-582102-6

LCCCN 80-41248

Filmset in 'Monophoto' Times New Roman by
Eta Services (Typesetters) Ltd, Beccles, Suffolk
Printed in Great Britain by
Galliard (Printers) Ltd, Great Yarmouth

List of contributors

ANDERSON, R. S. *Sloan-Kettering Institute for Cancer Research, Donald S. Walker Laboratory, 145 Boston Post Road, Rye, New York 10580, U.S.A.*

BAUCHAU, A. G. *Departement de Biologie Animale, Facultes Universitaires de Namur, Belgium.*

CHENG, T. C. *Marine Biomedical Research Program and Department of Anatomy (Cell Biology), Medical University of South Carolina, Charleston, South Carolina 29412, U.S.A.*

COOPER, E. L. *Department of Anatomy, School of Medicine, University of California, Los Angeles, California 90024, U.S.A.*

COWDEN, R. R. *Department of Anatomy and Program in Biophysics, College of Medicine, East Tennessee State University, Johnson City, Tennessee 37601, U.S.A.*

CURTIS, S. K. *Department of Anatomy and Program in Biophysics, College of Medicine, East Tennessee State University, Johnson City, Tennessee 37614, U.S.A.*

DALES, R. P. *Department of Zoology, Bedford College, University of London, Regent's Park, London NW1 4NS, England.*

DIXON, L. R. J. *Department of Zoology, Bedford College, University of London, Regent's Park, London NW1 4NS, England.*

DYBAS, L. *Department of Biology, Knox College, Galesburg, Illinois 61401, U.S.A.*

FITZGERALD, S. W. *Department of Zoology, University College of Swansea, Singleton Park, Swansea SA2 8PP, U.K.*

HAYWARD, P. J. *Department of Zoology, University College of Swansea, Singleton Park, Swansea SA2 8PP, U.K.*

RATCLIFFE, N. A. *Department of Zoology, University College of Swansea, Singleton Park, Swansea, SA2 8PP, U.K.*

RAVINDRANATH, M. N. *Department of Zoology, University of Madras, Chepauk, Tamil Nadu 600 005, India.*

ROWLEY, A. F. *Department of Zoology, University College of Swansea, Singleton Park, Swansea, SA2 8PP, U.K.*

SAWYER, R. T. *Department of Molecular Biology, University of California, Berkeley, California 94720, U.S.A.*

SHERMAN, R. G. *Department of Zoology, Miami University, Oxford, Ohio 45056, U.S.A.*

SMINIA, T. *Vrije Universiteit, Biologisch Laboratorium, Amsterdam 1007mc, The Netherlands.*

SMITH, V. J. *University Marine Biological Station, Millport, Isle of Cumbrae, Scotland.*

STEIN, E. A. *Department of Anatomy, School of Medicine, University of California, Los Angeles, California 90024, U.S.A.*

VAN DE VYVER, G. *Université Libre De Bruxelles, Faculte des Sciences, Laboratoire de Biologie, Animale et Cellulaire, Ave. F. D. Roosevelt, 50, 1050 Bruxelles, Belgium.*

WRIGHT, R. K. *Department of Anatomy, School of Medicine, Center for the Health Services, University of California, Los Angeles, California 90024, U.S.A.*

Preface

Renewed interest in invertebrate "blood cells" has developed for a number of reasons. First, there has been a recent escalation in research into comparative immunology, including many studies on invertebrates. These animals provide relatively simple experimental models, they may supply clues to the ancestry of the lymphoid system, and they may have novel defence reactions not yet discovered in the more complex immune systems of vertebrates. Secondly, many invertebrates, but especially the molluscs and crustaceans, are now being extensively farmed to augment the food resources of man. Clearly, a better understanding of the host defence reactions of such species would help to avoid and overcome disastrous outbreaks of disease which are likely to occur under the artificial and potentially stressful conditions of commercial culture. Thirdly, many invertebrates act as vectors of parasitic organisms which are the scourge of mankind. The insects and molluscs, in particular, include species responsible for the transmission of malaria, sleeping sickness, filariasis, onchocerciasis and schistosomiasis. The means by which these parasites invade and multiply in their hosts and yet fail to elicit an effective "immune" response is now the subject of intensive research. Fourthly, with the increasing resistance of invertebrate pests to chemical pesticides, and the accumulation of these noxious substances at higher levels in the food chains, greater efforts are being made to develop and utilize biological control agents such as the viruses, bacteria, fungi, nematodes and parasitoids. The potentially immense practical value of such agents has provided yet a further stimulus for researches into the host defence reactions of invertebrates. Finally, many biologists are beginning to realize that invertebrate blood cells not only function in "immune" or host defence reactions but also serve, at least in some species, to store, transport and/or synthesize food, waste products and hormones and are thus involved in many other vital life processes. Our lack of knowledge of the role of invertebrate blood cells in these basic functions provides a major area for future research utilizing modern biochemical techniques.

Much of the recent work on invertebrate blood cells, particularly in the fields of comparative immunology and cellular defence reactions, has been summarized in a number of excellent volumes including *Contemporary*

Topics in Immunobiology, Vol. 4, Invertebrate Immunology (E. L. Cooper, Ed., Plenum Press, 1974); *Invertebrate Immunity* (K. Maramorosch and R. E. Shope, Eds, Academic Press, 1975); *Comparative Immunology* (J. J. Marchalonis, Ed., Blackwell Scientific, 1976); *Comparative Immunobiology* by M. J. Manning and R. J. Turner (Blackie, 1976); and *Insect Hemocytes* (A. P. Gupta, Ed., Cambridge University Press, 1979). However, not since the publication of Warren Andrews *Comparative Hematology* (Grune and Stratton, 1965) has an attempt been made to summarize comprehensively our knowledge of the structure and function of invertebrate blood cells. Such a synopsis is urgently required in the light of current research interests and the many advances which have been made utilizing sophisticated modern techniques.

Volumes 1 and 2 of *Invertebrate Blood Cells* have been prepared specifically to bridge the gap since the publication of *Comparative Hematology*, with each chapter written by an expert in his or her particular group of animals. We have attempted to present information on as many invertebrate groups as possible and to this end have included much unpublished material, some of which was researched specifically for these books, e.g. Chapters 5, 14 and 15 on the leeches, lophophorates and echinoderms, respectively. We hope these volumes will generate further interest in many areas of invertebrate haematology and provide a source of comparative data for those workers already researching into particular aspects of invertebrate blood cells.

February, 1981 N. A. Ratcliffe and A. F. Rowley

Contents of Volume 2

Section IX: Comparative Aspects of the Structure and Function of Invertebrate and Vertebrate Leucocytes

Contents of Volume 1

Section V

Arthropods

10. Onychophorans and myriapods

M. H. RAVINDRANATH

Department of Zoology, University of Madras, Chepauk, Tamil Nadu 600005, India

CONTENTS

I. Introduction

The close affinity of onychophorans and myriapods with insects, and a lack of affinity between them and the other arthropods are suggested by their embryonic development, uniramous limbs and terminal functioning of the mandibles. However, the Onychophora-Myriapoda-Hexapoda assemblage, also called Uniramia, shows like other arthropods, a reduction of the coelom, enlargement of the haemocoel, the synonymy of the "segmentation cavity" of the developing egg with the adult haemocoel, the haemocoelic perivisceral and pericardial spaces, the absence of fine vessels in the circulatory system and the dorsal tubular heart with paired ostia.

The structure and function of the blood cells are little understood in the Onychophora and Myriapoda, when compared with the extensive information available on the blood cells (haemocytes) of the Insecta. Jones (1962), proposed a classification of insect haemocyte types which appears less complex than those of earlier investigators. Recently, Jones' system of nomenclature and classification has been adopted for the haemocytes of several non-insect arthropods (Ravindranath, 1970, 1973, 1974a, 1974b, 1975; Sherman, 1973) and it was found that the Onychophora, Myriapoda, Crustacea and Arachnida have several haemocyte types which are similar to those of the Insecta (Ravindranath, 1977a, 1978; Gupta, 1979).

In onychophorans and myriapods, it is now fairly certain that one type of circulating blood cell is not a haemocyte, but may be the pericardial cell or nephrocyte which, in contrast to similar cells of insects, enters freely into the circulation (Campiglia and Lavallard, 1975; Seifert and Rosenberg, 1976; Rosenberg, 1978).

In the present chapter, an attempt is made: (1) to pool existing knowledge on the circulatory system and blood cell types of the Onychophora and Myriapoda (only the chilopods, diplopods and symphilids are dealt with in this chapter); (2) to correlate, wherever possible, fine structural with light microscopical descriptions of the cell types; (3) to describe the histochemical characteristics of the cytoplasmic inclusions; (4) to compare the blood cell nomenclature with the generally accepted haemocyte terminologies proposed for insects; and (5) to summarize the functional roles of the haemocytes of Onychophora and Myriapoda based on their structure and chemistry, as well as their behaviour, under different physiological conditions.

II. Structure of the circulatory system

A. Onychophora

The open circulatory system in onychophorans has been described by

Manton and Heatley (1937) in *Peripatopsis moseleyi* and *P. sedgwicki*. The heart is a dorsal tubular vessel devoid of an extension forming an anterior aorta, a feature unusual among arthropods. In every segment, the heart has a pair of cardiac ostia, each of which is in the form of a fissure. The heart narrows posteriorly and remains closed in the last segment of the body. No segmental arteries leave the heart.

The blood from the haemocoel reaches the pericardium partly through the ostia in the pericardial floor and partly through the intramuscular canal system. The pericardial floor is fused to the lateral musculature as in other arthropods. The supply of blood to the median and lateral haemocoelic cavities is from the anterior end of the heart, which extends above the anterior part of the pharynx and opens by a ventrally directed valve into the haemocoel. The pericardial floor here becomes non-existent, and so the heart directly supplies the haemocoel (Manton and Heatley, 1937).

B. Chilopoda

The circulatory systems of *Scolopendra* (Shukla, 1964; Varma, 1971), *Lithobius* (Biegel, 1922) and *Scutigera* (Demange, 1963) have been examined. In *Scolopendra*, there are both dorsal and ventral vessels. The dorsal tubular vessel or heart is supported by lateral muscles. There are 21 chambers in the heart, each with slit-like ostia. The first chamber lies in the second segment and has an anterior cephalic aorta extending to the brain where it branches and joins the ventral vessel forming an aortic arch. At each ostium, there is a pair of lateral vessels. The ventral vessel runs above the nerve cord and supplies blood to the legs. The pericardial septum in *Scolopendra* is a double layered membrane. In *Lithobius*, a pericardium is lacking. The heart of *Scutigera* has 13 pairs of ostia and from the anterior aortic arch, an artery arises and runs posteriorly and terminates in two swellings forming pulsatile organs, comparable to those of some insects.

The course of circulation in *Scolopendra* has been described by Shukla (1964). The blood is drawn in through the ostia by the dilation of the heart. When the heart is filled with blood, a steady wave of contraction passes forwards. The blood is carried to the cephalic arteries and then to the ventral vessel. From the arteries and ventral vessel the blood enters the spaces in the body cavity. The blood from the haemocoel is returned to the heart by way of the ostia.

C. Diplopoda

The details of the circulatory system in diplopods have been described in

Spirostreptus (Verhoeff, 1932), *Julus* (Rossi, 1902) and in *Thyropygus* (Krishnan, 1968), and reviewed by Verhoeff (1932) and Demange (1963). The heart is dorsal and tubular with segmentally arranged chambers. The first chamber lies in the second segment and has a short anterior aorta, which branches to form pairs of vessels. The first pair constitutes an aortic arch and the second pair extends posteriorly over the oesophagus where they fuse to form a median abdominal vessel. The anterior branches from this median vessel extend to the head and gnathochilarium. The entire system of arterial vessels arising from the median abdominal vessel has been described in *Spirostreptus* (Verhoeff, 1932). Each chamber of the heart bears a pair of ostia and a pair of ill-defined vessels. The pericardial septum lies immediately below the heart attached to the terga.

The course of circulation in *Thyropygus* has been described by Krishnan (1968). In the ventral vessel, the blood flows backwards and enters the body cavity. The blood from the haemocoel is returned to the heart by way of ostia. During systole, the blood flows anteriorly in the heart and passes into the cephalic artery supplying the head region.

D. Symphyla

In symphilids (Demange, 1963), the circulatory system is represented by a dorsal tubular heart. It has an anterior cephalic aorta. A vessel arises from it in the first segment and runs postero-ventrally.

III. Structure and classification of blood cells

Cells circulating in the haemolymph of the Onychophora and Myriapoda are grouped into two fundamental categories (Lavallard and Campiglia, 1975; Seifert and Rosenberg, 1976, 1977; Rosenberg, 1978).

(1) Cells without a basal lamina (or basement membrane), whose plasma membrane is directly in contact with the plasma, and which are called haemocytes.

(2) Cells separated from the plasma by a basal lamina, which covers the plasma membrane and encloses one to four cells, and which are called pericardial cells (Gaffron, 1885; Cuénot, 1949; Arvy, 1954; Lavallard and Campiglia, 1975). Schneider (1902), termed them "cellules lymphoides", although they are referred to as nephrocytes by a number of workers (Bruntz, 1903a,b; Zacher, 1933; Tuzet and Manier, 1959; Seifert and Rosenberg, 1976, 1977; Rosenberg, 1978).

These cells are often mistaken for haemocytes. Both the haemocytes and the pericardial cells are often found attached to the tissues.

A. Haemocytes

1. Onychophora

Information about the haemocytes of Onychophora is incomplete and is restricted to seven species. The number of cell types identified varies from two (Manton and Heatley, 1937), to four (Arvy, 1954; Grégoire, 1955; Tuzet and Manier, 1959) or five (Sundara-Rajulu *et al.*, 1970; Lavallard and Campiglia, 1975). These studies, however, do not provide any information about the physiological status of the animal under study.

In *Peripatus acacioi*, Lavallard and Campiglia (1975) have correlated the fine structure of the haemocytes with the morphology of cell types in the light microscope, and have also studied the histochemistry of the cytoplasmic inclusions. A summary of these results is presented in Table I. The blood cell nomenclature used by different authors and their equivalents in insects are indicated in Table II. Four cell types are commonly found in the Onychophora (Figs 1–10). These are prohaemocytes (Figs 5, 7), granular haemocytes (Figs 1, 2, 4, 7, 10), spherule cells (Figs 3, 7, 8, 9) and plasmatocytes (Figs 1, 6).

Histochemistry of the cytoplasmic inclusions of granular haemocytes and spherule cells showed that they differ in their chemical nature (Lavallard and Campiglia, 1975). The granules of granular haemocytes are acidophilic and contain a PAS positive neutral mucopolysaccharide. Lipid reactive sites are absent. The spherules of spherulocytes (spherule cells) contain basophilic protein and PAS positive lipoidal material. In addition to the aforementioned cell types, certain other cell types are also occasionally seen in the circulation, including macrophages (altered granular haemocytes according to Gupta, 1979), oenocytoids and cystocytes. Presence of oenocytoids in onychophorans, as has been claimed by Sundara-Rajulu *et al.* (1970), is doubtful, for the description and figure of oenocytoids fit precisely with those of pericardial cells (Lavallard and Campiglia, 1975). The cystocytes of onychophorans are comparable in their characteristics with those of chilopods, diplopods and insects (see Chapter 13).

2. Chilopoda

Previous information about the haemocytes of chilopods is meagre. The haemocytes of *Scolopendra* are classified into two (Duboscq, 1899; Kollmann, 1908) to seven (Ravindranath, 1970; Sundara-Rajulu, 1971a)

TABLE I. A summary of the general characteristics of the haemocyte types in *Peripatus acacioi* (Onychophora)[a].

Characteristics	Prohaemocytes	Macrophages	Granular haemocytes	Hyalocytes	Spherule cells
Size (μm)	8–12	10–12	10–12	10–16	8–30
Shape	round	polymorphic	polymorphic	round or oval	round or oval
Cell surface	smooth	irregular	irregular	smooth	smooth
Nature of cytoplasm	basophilic	basophilic	acidophilic	acidophilic	basophilic
Nucleus					
Position	central	central	central	eccentric	central
Shape	round/irregular	round/ovoid/ reniform/ pleurilobed	round/ovoid/ reniform/ pleurilobed	round/ovoid/ reniform	round/ovoid
Chromatin	aggregated in the periphery	aggregated in the periphery	aggregated in the periphery	distributed throughout	not observed
Perinuclear cisternae	not prominent	flattened	normal	prominent	normal
Nucleolus	not observed	well developed	not observed	not observed	not observed

Cytoplasmic inclusions					
Vacuoles-phagosomes	absent	present	absent	absent	—
Vacuoles-liposomes	absent	present	absent	absent	—
Granules-electron opaque	absent/rare	present	absent	rare/absent	—
Granules-electron dense	absent	rare	present	absent	—
Special inclusions	absent	absent	biclaved/reticulated electron-dense granules	absent	neutrophilic spherules present
Mitochondria	present	small	small	present	present
Rough E. R.	little	numerous	numerous	not prominent	not observed
Ribosomes	few	abundant	abundant	rare	abundant
Golgi complex	absent	well-developed	well-developed	absent	not observed
Microtubules	absent	present	—	absent	not observed
Mitosis	observed	no	observed	no	no
Endocytosis	nil	phagocytic	phagocytic	nil	pinocytic not phagocytic

[a] Based on the light microscopic and ultrastructural studies of Lavallard and Campiglia (1975).

TABLE II. A comparison of classification and nomenclature used by different authors for haemocytes of Onychophora and equivalent nomenclature followed for insect haemocytes.

Manton and Heatley (1937)	Arvy (1954)	Grégoire (1955)	Tuzet and Manier (1959)	Sundara-Rajulu Krishnan and Singh (1970)	Lavallard and Campiglia (1975)	Price and Ratcliffe (1974)
Peripatopsis moseleyi	*Peripatopsis capensis*	*Macroperipatus geayi* *Oroperipatus corradi* *Epiperipatus braziliensis* var. *Vagans*	*Peripatopsis moseleyi*	*Eoperipatus weldoni*	*Peripatus acacioi*	15 insect orders
Small round leucocyte	leucoblast	small round leucocyte	globule of Type I	prohaemocyte	prohaemocyte	prohaemocyte
—	leucocyte hyaline	hyaline leucocyte	globule of Type II	plasmatocyte	hyalocyte	plasmatocyte
Granular leucocyte	leucocyte granules eosinophiles	thinly granular haemocyte	globule of Type III	granular haemocyte	granular haemocyte	granular haemocyte
—	leucocyte granules cyanophilic	coarsely granular haemocyte	globule of Type IV	spherule cell	spherulocyte	spherule cell
—	—	fragile haemocyte	—	—	—	cystocyte
—	—	—	—	—	macrophage[a]	—
—	—	—	—	oenocytoid	circulating pericardial cell	oenocytoid

[a] Macrophage of Lavallard and Campiglia (1975) is not comparable to the cell type generally termed "plasmatocyte" as has been claimed by the authors. However it fits precisely with the plasmatocyte of *Calliphora erythrocephala* described by Zachary and Hoffman (1973) and the granulocyte of a decapod crustacean *Eriochier sinensis* (Bauchau and De Brouwer, 1974, see plates IIIa and IVa) vide text.

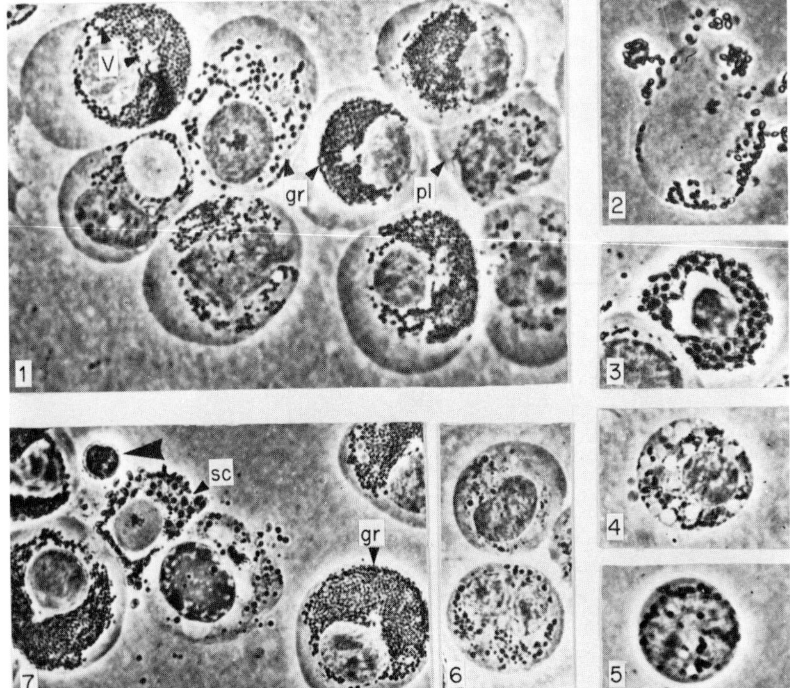

Figs 1–7. Haemocytes of *Peripatus* sp. (From Grégoire, 1955). ×800.

Fig. 1. Changes undergone by the granular haemocytes (gr) of *Peripatus* sp. in wet preparations. The cells degranulate and refractile vacuoles (V) appear in the cytoplasm. The degranulated cell may change in shape to appear like plasmatocytes (pl.).

Fig. 2. Granule discharge from a granular haemocyte.

Fig. 3. A spherule cell. Compare the size and appearance of the spherules with the granules of a granular haemocyte.

Fig. 4. A granular haemocyte discharging granules (or possibly an adipo-haemocyte?), showing variation in size of the phase-dark granules and numerous vacuoles or lipid droplets.

Fig. 5. Cell type comparable to prohaemocyte, showing large nucleus, thin rim of cytoplasm with phase dark granules and a few vacuoles.

Fig. 6. Two granular haemocytes after degranulation which appear like plasmatocytes.

Fig. 7. Arrow indicates cell type comparable to prohaemocyte. Grégoire considers it to be remnant of one of the cytolysed granular haemocytes. sc. spherule cell; gr. granular haemocyte.

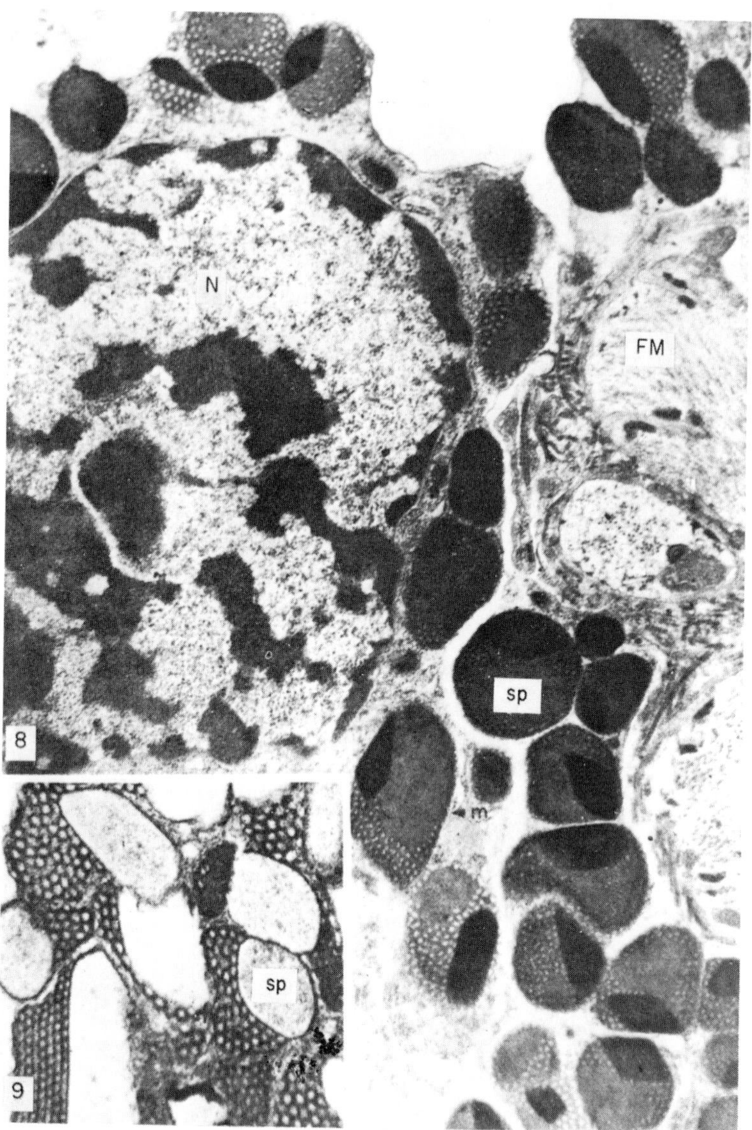

Fig. 8. Thin section of a spherule cell of *Peripatus acacioi* located adjacent to muscle fibre (FM). Note the complex structure of the spherules (sp). N, nucleus. (From Lavallard and Campiglia, 1975.) ×17 500.

Fig. 9. Spherule cell in which the lipid of the spherules (sp) has been extracted during embedding. (From Lavallard and Campiglia, 1975.) ×25 000.

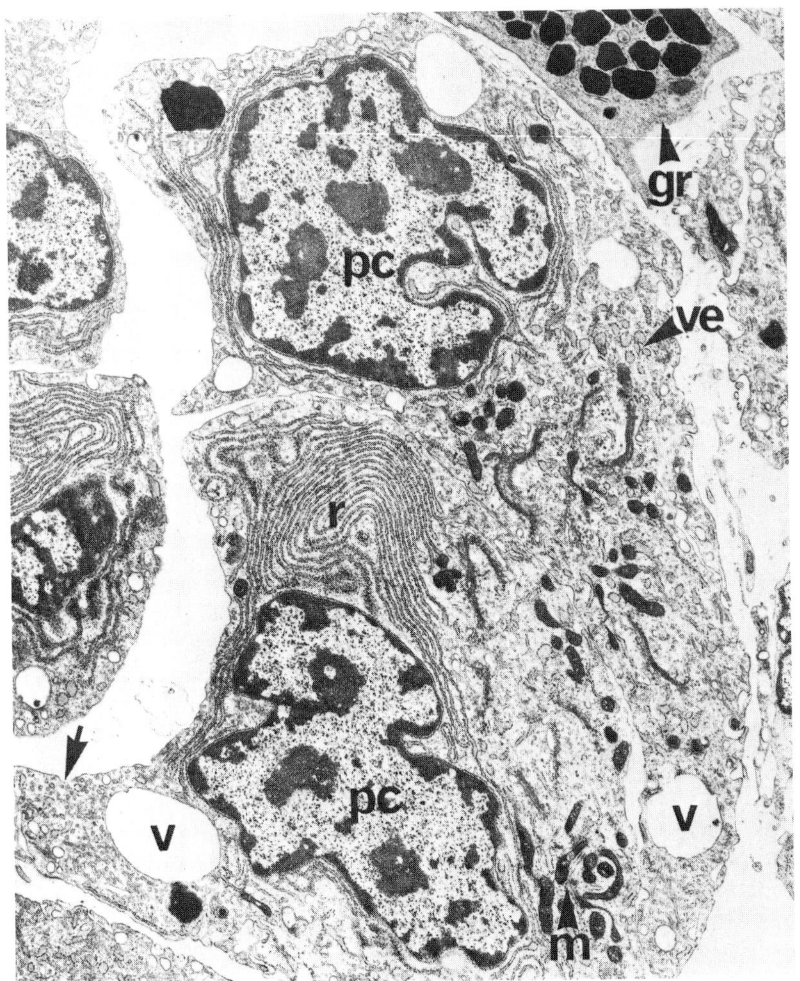

Fig. 10. Pericardial cells (=Nephrocytes) (pc) and a granular haemocyte (gr) of *Peripatoides leuckarti*. Pericardial cells have vacuoles (v), reticulate (r) and vesicular (ve) rough endoplasmic reticulum, mitochondria (m) and pinocytotic vesicles (arrow). (Original, courtesy Prof. G. Seifert and Dr J. Rosenberg.) ×8750.

morphologically different types, based on differences in size and shape of the cell and nucleus, on the general appearance and staining of the cytoplasm, and on the type, number, size and staining properties of the individual cytoplasmic inclusions. Recent investigators (Ravindranath, 1970; Sundara-Rajulu, 1971a) have used the insect haemocyte nomenclature of Jones (1962) to identify the cell types.

(*a*) *Prohaemocytes* (Fig. 13). These cells are the least common and are small and round, 7–10 μm in diameter, capable of putting out pseudopodia, and have a high nuclear/cytoplasmic ratio. The thin rim of cytoplasm is undifferentiated, encloses a few ribosomes, mitochondria, electron-dense granules and vacuoles. The nucleus usually contains large blocks of chromatin material. Prohaemocytes compare with the lymphocytes described by Duboscq (1899) and Kollmann (1908).

(*b*) *Granular haemocytes* (Figs 11, 12, 14, 15). These cells constitute 75% of the total cell population. They are highly refractile and in thin wet preparations are active and form hyaline cytoplasmic extensions, resembling the choanoleucocytes of annelids (Déhorne, 1925). The granular haemocytes are 11–14 μm in diameter with a central nucleus, which is masked by a large number of refractile granules (1·5 μm diameter). The granules are eosinophilic and stain yellow with iodine (Duboscq, 1899). In the electron microscope, the cell surface appears smooth and often shows pinocytosis. The cytoplasm contains a small amount of rough endoplasmic reticulum, numerous free ribosomes, mitochondria, variable numbers of electron-dense, and electron-lucent, round or filamentous granules and occasional vacuoles. The nucleus is often round or oval and sometimes indented. These cells resemble the granular leucocytes described by Duboscq (1899) and Kollmann (1908).

(*c*) *Plasmatocytes* (Fig. 11). These cells are seen only in light microscopy. They are not distinguishable from granular haemocytes in the electron microscope. In smears, their cytoplasm is basophilic containing small round eosinophilic inclusions. These cells are probably degranulated or degranulating granular haemocytes (see Ravindranath, 1978).

(*d*) *Cystocytes* (Figs 11, 12). These cells are round, characterized by a vacuolated cytoplasm, containing a few fine, round, phase-dark granules and a pycnotic shrunken nucleus. They are present in wet preparations but are rarely seen in smears or under the electron microscope. These cells are referred to as fragile hyaline haemocytes by Grégoire (1955, 1970). In wet preparation from *Scolopendra morsitans*, the granular haemocytes are seen to transform into cystocytes. The transformation involves swelling of the cells, vacuolization of the cytoplasm, loss of refractility of the granules, degranulation accompanied by reduction in the size of the nucleus, nuclear pycnosis, accompanied by increased uptake of basic and acidic dyes.

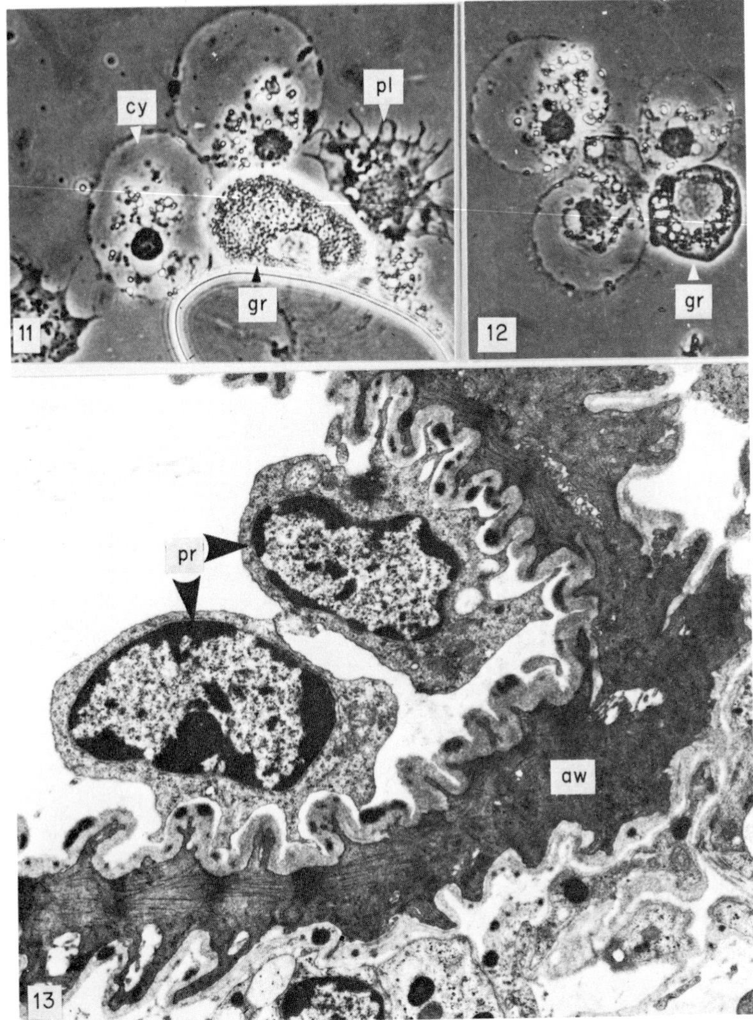

Fig. 11. Haemocytes of *Lithobius forficatus*. pl. plasmatocyte gr. granular haemocyte. cy. cystocyte with pycnotic nucleus. (From Grégoire, 1970.) ×600.

Fig. 12. Haemocytes in *Lithobius forficatus*. Note swelling, degranulation, formation of vacuoles, alteration in nuclear morphology and dispersion of granules in granular haemocyte (gr). (From Grégoire, 1955.) ×800.

Fig. 13. Prohaemocytes (pr) in close contact with the aortic wall (aw) in *Lithobius forficatus*. (Original, courtesy Prof. G. Seifert and Dr J. Rosenberg.) ×8700.

Occasionally, the whole cell shrinks giving it the appearance of a prohaemocyte.

(*e*) *Spherule cells*. These are round or ovoid, morula-like cells about 15–30 μm in diameter. The spherules are refractile under phase optics, stain with neutral red and measure 3–5 μm in diameter. These cells remain refractile for long periods in thin wet preparations and have not been examined under the electron microscope.

(*f*) *Adipohaemocytes*. These are oval cells about 7–10 μm in diameter and resemble fat body cells. The cytoplasm has fine phase-dark granules, refractile granules, phase-dark and phase-bright vacuoles similar in appear-

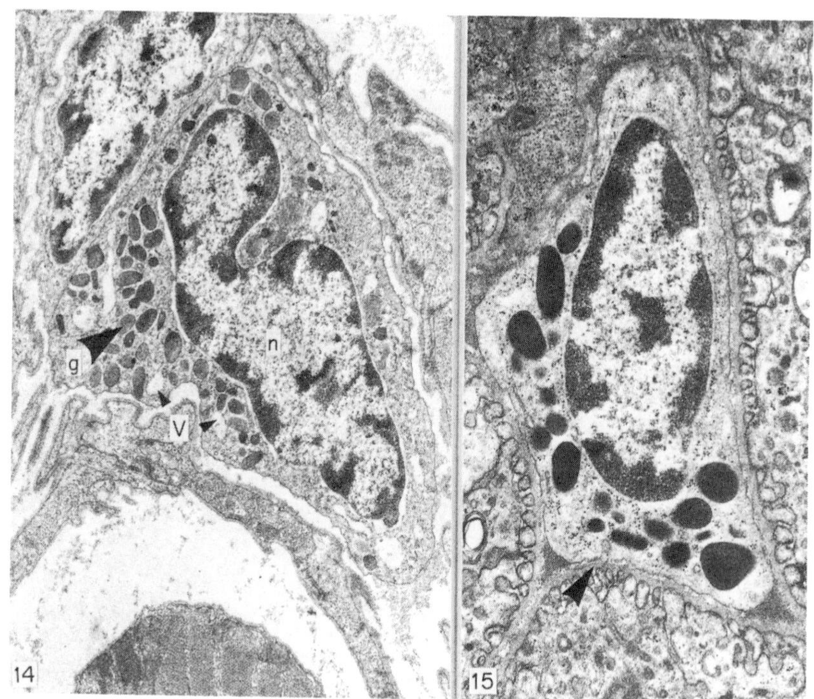

Figs 14, 15. Granular haemocytes of a chilopod, *Scutigera coleoptrata*.

Fig. 14. Granular haemocyte within a vessel, showing numerous granules (g), vacuoles (V), enlarged perinuclear cisterna and indented nucleus (n). (Original, courtesy Prof. G. Seifert and Dr J. Rosenberg.) × 13 800.

Fig. 15. Granular haemocyte within intercellular clefts of nephridia, showing electron-dense granules of different sizes. Arrow indicate formation of pinocytotic vesicles. (Original, courtesy Dr J. Rosenberg.) × 13 800.

ance to fat droplets. These cells have not yet been studied in the electron microscope.

(*g*) *Oenocytoids*. These are large oval, basophilic cells measuring 20–30 μm in diameter and are tapered at one end. The cytoplasm is homogeneous and the nucleus is eccentric. Often cytoplasmic inclusions form an irregular, finely granular net-work. These cells are often confused with oenocytes (Sundara-Rajulu, 1971a), the ectodermally derived acidophilic cells seen in some insects (see Chapter 13).

3. *Diplopoda*

The haemocytes of diplopods have been studied by a number of investigators (Bruntz, 1906a,b; Kollmann, 1908; Valeri, 1934; Palm, 1954; Tuzet and Manier, 1954; Grégoire, 1955; Grégoire and Jolivet, 1957; Krishnan, 1968; Gupta, 1968; Vostal, 1970; Sundara-Rajulu, 1971b; Ravindranath, 1970, 1973, 1977a; Krishnan and Ravindranath, 1973). The haemocytes are classified into 3–6 types by most of the workers. However, Ravindranath (1970, 1973), adopting the insect haemocyte nomenclature proposed by Jones (1962) for the haemocytes of millipedes, identified seven classes of haemocytes, namely, prohaemocytes, plasmatocytes, granular haemocytes, cystocytes, oenocytoids, spherule cells and adipohaemocytes. A cell type, however, comparable to the oenocytoid is rarely encountered in wet preparations. The characteristics of the different kinds of haemocytes are summarized in Table III. The histochemistry of the cytoplasmic inclusions of the haemocytes (Ravindranath, 1973) showed that the granules of granular haemocytes, cystocytes and adipohaemocytes are identical in their chemical nature and are basophilic, containing protein-acid mucopolysaccharide complexes. The spherules of spherule cells are strongly basophilic, metachromatic and are rich in acid mucopolysaccharides. The terminologies of blood cells used by different authors and their equivalents after adopting Jones (1962) nomenclature are given in Table IV. Haemocyte types seen in different species of millipedes are presented in Figs 16–25.

Information about the ultrastructure of diplopod haemocytes is mainly wanting. Only the granular haemocytes of *Craspedosoma rawlinsi* (Fig. 25) have been observed in the electron microscope (Seifert, unpublished). They contain numerous electron-dense granules, free ribosomes and rough endoplasmic reticulum. The ultrastructural features reveal a striking similarity with those of the granular haemocytes of other arthropods. In addition, liposomes may be present, recalling adipohaemocytes of insects (Jones, 1967; Neuwirth, 1973).

This lack of fine structural information does not allow comparisons to be made with the light microscope observations.

TABLE III. A summary of the general characteristics of the haemocyte types in the millipede, *Thyropygus poseidon* (Diplopoda: Myriapoda).[a]

Characteristics	Prohaemocytes	Plasmatocytes	Granular haemocytes	Cystocytes	Oenocytoids	Spherule cells	Adipohaemocytes
Size (μm)	3·5–8·0	10·0–16·5	15·0–19·0	12·0–17·0	8·0–12·0	10·0–35·0	25·0–40·0
Shape and appearance under phase optics	round, non-refractile	oval, polymorphic, non-refractile	oval, polymorphic, highly refractile	round, non-refractile	oval, non-refractile	round, refractile	irregular, refractile
Nature of cytoplasm	intensely basophilic, orthochromatic	basophilic, orthochromatic	basophilic orthochromatic	vacuolated, with poor affinity to basic dyes	highly meta-chromatic	weakly basophilic	weakly basophilic
Nucleus	central, chromatin granular and evenly distributed	central, occasionally eccentric	central occasionally eccentric	eccentric, occasionally lobulated chromatin dis-aggregated and marginated	eccentric	eccentric	eccentric
Cytoplasmic inclusions	present	granules scattered, non-refractile, bacciliform, acidophilic	granules, dense, highly refractile, bacciliform, acidophilic some granules become non-refractile.	granules round, both acidophilic and basophilic	not observed	spherules round, basophilic, metachromatic	granules and spherules are present
Behaviour in thin wet preparations	stable	ameoboid, degranulates, vacuolates and changes in shape, produces spike-like pseudopodia	amoeboid, degranulates, vacuolates and produces spike-like pseudopodia	undergoes alteration and bursts; causes no gelation of plasma	stable for long period	stable for long period	disintegrates

[a] Based on Ravindranath (1973).

TABLE IV. A comparison of classification and nomenclature used by different authors for the haemocytes of the Diplopoda.

Cattaneo, (1889)	Duboscq (1899)	Bruntz (1906b)	Kollman (1908)	Tuzet and Manier (1954)	Grégoire and Jolivet (1957)	Sundara-Rajulu (1971b)	Ravindranath (1973)
Glomeris sp.	*Glomeris* sp.	*Glomeris* sp.	*Schizophyllym mediterraneus*	*Schizophyllym rutilans* *Glomeris marginata*	*Scaphiostreptus acuticonus* *Spirostreptus virgator*	*Cingalobolus bugnioni*	*Thyropygus poseidon*
—	—	small cell (petits globules)	hyaline leucoyte stage I	petits leucocytes hyalines	—	prohaemocyte	prohaemocyte
—	—	gros globules	hyaline leucocyte stage II	leucocyte hyaline stages I and II	—	plasmatocyte	plasmatocyte
Leucocyte Granulations Refringentes	leucocyte granulations	leucocyte granulations	leucocyte granulations	granulocyte	granular haemocyte	plasmatocyte	granular haemocyte
—	—	leucocyte degenerescence	leucocyte degenerescence	globules se vacuolisant	explosive haemocyte (fragile haemocyte)	cystocyte	cystocyte
—	—	—	—	eleocyte	—	spherule cell	spherule cell
—	—	—	—	—	haemocyte cytoplasme sombre	oenocytoid	oenocytoid
—	—	—	—	—	—	adipohaemocyte	adipohaemocyte

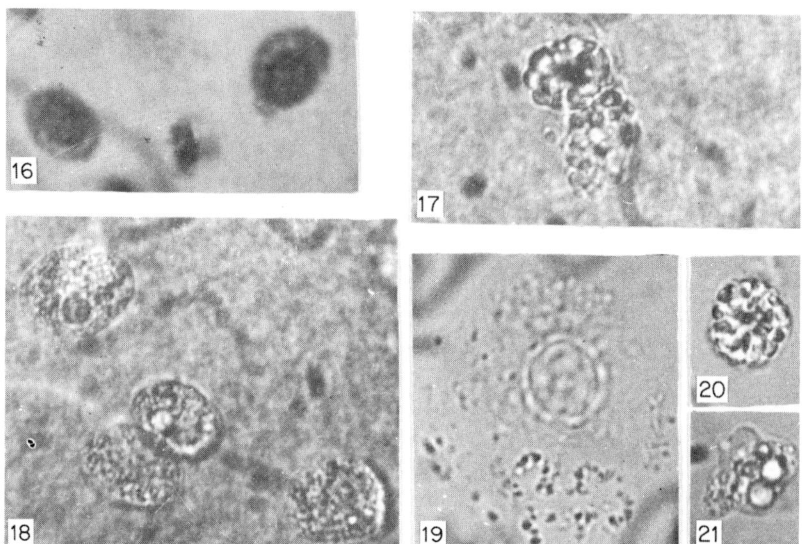

Figs 16–21. Haemocytes of the millipede *Thyropygus poseidon*.

Fig. 16. Prohaemocytes. ×600.

Fig. 17. Spherule cells. ×400.

Fig. 18. Granular haemocytes. ×400.

Fig. 19. Cystocyte liberating its granular content. ×400.

Fig. 20. Spherule cell. ×250.

Fig. 21. Adipohaemocyte. ×250.

Figs 22–24. Haemocytes of the millipede, *Spirostreptus virgator*. (From Grégoire and Jolivet, 1957.) ×800.

Fig. 22. Granular haemocytes at different stages of transformation (stages a, b and c). Note that highly refractile granules, surrounding the nucleus, lose their refractility (L–R) and are finally discharged.

Fig. 23. Oenocytoid (oe) and cystocyte (cy). Note the oval shape, dark cytoplasm and eccentric nucleus of the oenocytoid, the vacuolization of the cytoplasm and pycnotic nucleus of the cystocyte. Also note the formation of the meshwork (arrow) in the surrounding haemolymph suggestive of coagulation.

Fig. 24. Different stages in the transformation of granular haemocytes a few hours after bleeding. Note progressive nuclear shrinkage in cells a–e, loss of granules and bleb formation (arrows). Some cells continue to swell after degranulation.

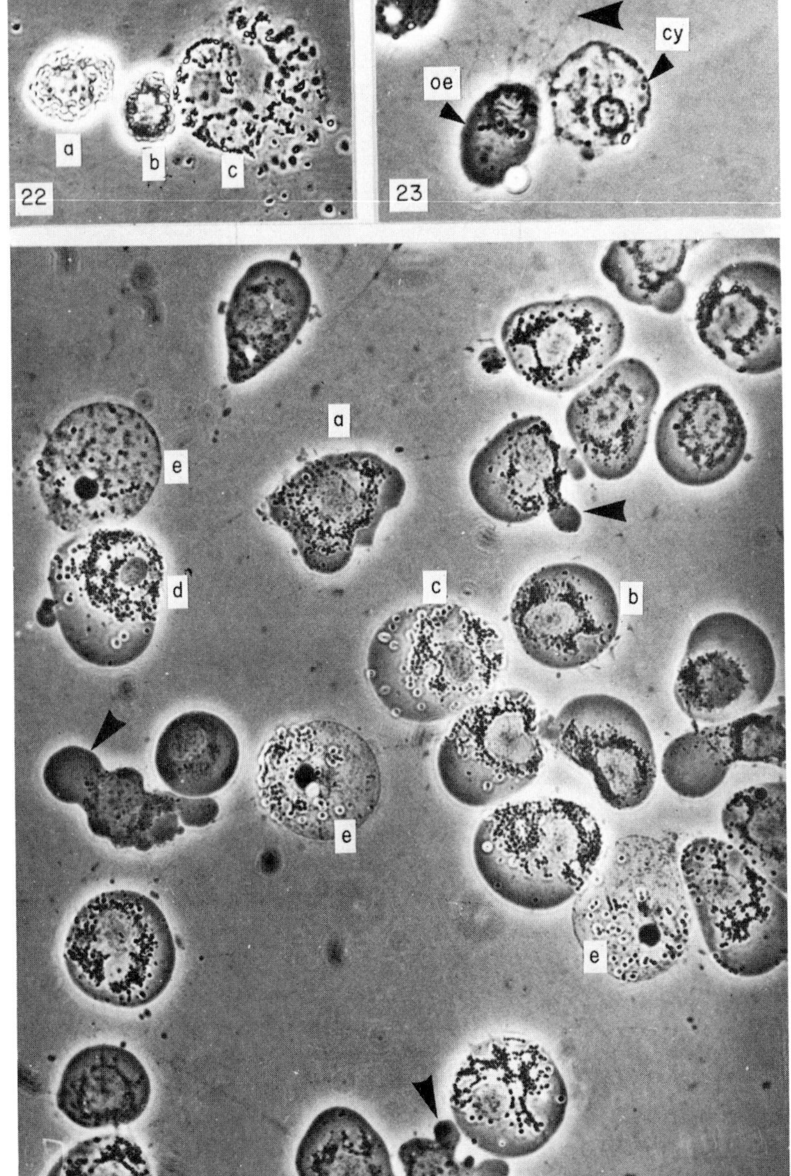

a
b
c
22
cy
oe
23
a
e
d
c
b
e
e
24

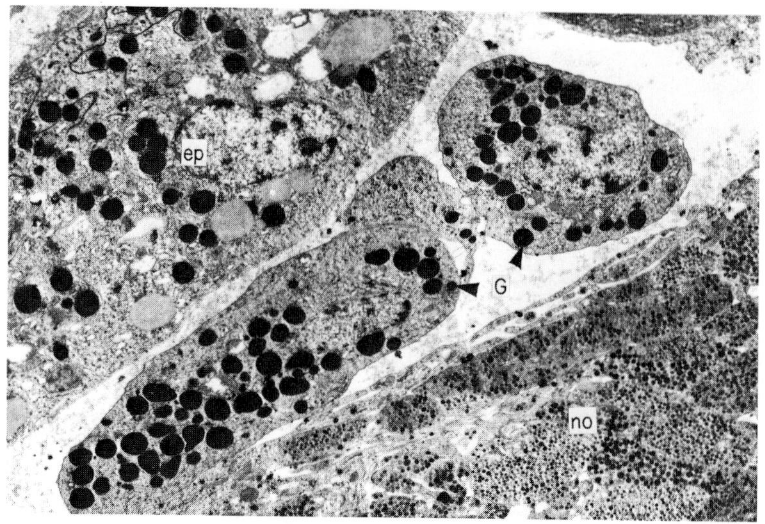

Fig. 25. Granular haemocytes of *Craspedosoma rawlinsi*, showing numerous electron-dense granules (G). ep, epidermal epithelium; no, neurohaemal organ. (Original, courtesy Prof. G. Seifert.) ×7600.

4. *Symphyla*

The haemocytes of a symphylan, *Scutigerella immaculata* have been studied by Gupta (1968, 1979). The blood of *S. immaculata* contains prohaemocytes, plasmatocytes, granular haemocytes, spherule cells, adipohaemocytes and cystocytes. No oenocytoids or pericardial cells were observed.

B. Pericardial cells

Pericardial cells or nephrocytes are commonly found in the circulating haemolymph. These cells are characterized by a basophilic cytoplasm, a large centrally located nucleus with one (Campiglia and Lavallard, 1975) or more (Arvy, 1954; Seifert and Rosenberg, 1977) nucleoli, extensive reticular or vesicular rough endoplasmic reticulum, a well-developed Golgi apparatus and numerous pinocytotic vesicles associated with cytoplasmic vacuoles (Fig. 10).

Detailed ultrastructural observations have been made in *Peripatus acacioi* (Campiglia and Lavallard, 1975) and in *Peripatoides leuckarti* (Fig. 10) (Seifert and Rosenberg, 1977). The most interesting aspect of cytology of pericardial cells is the formation of pinocytic and Golgi vesicles. These vesicles resemble coated vesicles described in insect pericardial cells by Bowers (1964). These are referred to as microvacuoles or pinosomes by Campiglia and Lavallard (1975), and as "Stachelsum-Vesickeln" by Seifert and Rosenberg (1977). In *P. acacioi*, two types of such vesicles are seen. One type has an electron-dense inner content and the other is electron-lucent.

In chilopods, the cytological characteristics of pericardial cells have been described in members of two families of Geophilomorpha, namely, *Haplophilus subterraneus* (=Himentariidae), *Clinopodes linearis* and *Necrophlaeophagus longicornis* (=Geophilidae) (Rosenberg, 1978). These cells are typical podocytes with enlarged intercellular spaces. Desmosome-like membrane specializations are prominent at the cell cortex. The cell surface has numerous tubular bodies. The fine structure of these cells resembles that of the pericardial cells of the Onychophora (described above). The presence of abundant coated vesicles, tubules and vacuoles are attributed to selective sequestration and transformation of haemolymph components.

In a millipede, *Orthomorpha gracilis*, Seifert and Rosenberg (1976) have described in detail the light microscopic and ultrastructural characteristics of pericardial cells. The basic cytological features are similar to the pericardial cells of Onychophora and Chilopoda. The endoplasmic reticulum, however, is smooth and weakly developed. The central region of the cells may contain one or more autolysosomes.

The pericardial cells appear to be analogous to the reticuloendothelial system of vertebrates (see Wigglesworth, 1970).

IV. Origin and formation of blood cells

A. Onychophora

Information concerning haemocytopoiesis is very scant in the Onychophora. Both prohaemocytes and granular haemocytes in circulation are observed to undergo mitotic division (Lavallard and Campiglia, 1975). The presence of haemocytopoietic tissues in *Peripatopsis moseleyi* has been reported by Arvy (1954). These tissues form three longitudinal bands, parallel to the body axis in the mid dorsal region; two bands lie on either side of the heart and a middle band surrounds the heart. Each band is made up of a layer of connective tissue, haemocytes and pericardial cells. The haemocytes primarily constitute prohaemocyte-like cells undergoing active mitotic division. The origin of other cell types and their inter-relationships are little understood.

B. Chilopoda

Embryologically, the blood cells proliferate from the ventrally-located median strand of mesoderm into the blood sinus (Heymons, 1901; Johannsen and Butt, 1941). The post-embryonic origin of blood cells is not thoroughly understood. Duboscq (1899) considered the small congregations of cells at the extremities of the laterodorsal or lateroventral vessels to be haemocytopoietic tissues. These formed a syncytial mass containing prohaemocytes and a few granular haemocytes. It is uncertain whether the prohaemocytes are precursors of the granular haemocytes, since the latter are often found to multiply by mitosis in the circulating haemolymph (Kollmann, 1908).

C. Diplopoda

Information about the haemocytopoietic tissues in diplopods is contradictory. For example, Bruntz (1906a) and Kollmann (1908) reported the absence of haemocytopoietic tissues, while Tuzet and Manier (1954) observed haemopoietic tissue in the dorsal vessel of *Glomeris marginata*. This projects into the cardiac cavity and gives rise to haemoblasts, which in turn differentiate into (hyaline) leucocytes, granulocytes and eleocytes. A study of the haemogram of *Thyropygus poseidon* during different stages in the moult cycle, also suggests the presence of haemocytopoietic tissue in diplopods (Ravindranath, 1974c). Dividing haemocytes have not been observed in the circulating haemolymph of diplopods, possibly haemocytes divide during specific times of the day (Ravindranath, 1977b). Ravindranath (1973), observed nuclear but no cytoplasmic division in the granular haemocytes of *T. poseidon*.

V. Functions of blood cells

The functions of haemocytes in onychophorans and myriapods are little understood. Detailed studies are required for a better understanding and appreciation of the functional roles of the different cell types. The three most commonly described functions are endocytosis, parasitic encapsulation and haemostasis.

A. Endocytosis

The term "endocytosis" is used to denote both phagocytosis and pinocytosis. In the literature, the expression phagocytosis is used freely, especially to imply endocytosis and to a limited extent vital staining. Both circulating and fixed haemocytes are found to accumulate colloidal substances such as trypan blue, neutral red, Congo red, Janus green, toluidine blue, bromphenol blue, iron and carbon (Kowalewsky, 1894, 1895; Duboscq, 1896; Bruntz, 1906a,b; Palm, 1954; Ravindranath, 1973). Kowalewsky (1894, 1895) investigated the phagocytic properties of *Scolopendra* sp. haemocytes by injecting bacteria, vertebrate blood, milk, iron saccharides and various dyes. Duboscq (1896), carried out similar experiments using erythrocytes, India ink and ammonium carminate. The amount of colloid concentrated by the haemocytes is known to vary with the substance injected. Thus in the diplopods *Glomeris*, *Julus* and *Polydesmus*, Bruntz (1906b) observed selective phagocytosis of Chinese ink by haemocytes from a mixture containing Chinese ink, ammonium carminate and indigo carmine. In the chilopods, *Lithobius*, *Pachymerium* and *Geophilus*, Palm (1954) observed haemocytes phagocytosing both ammonium and lithium carminate. Bruntz (1906b), has suggested that the accumulation of ammonium carminate in the haemocytes might be due to ingestion of disintegrating carminate-filled nephrocytes. Similarly, Palm (1954), attributed intense concentration of trypan blue in some of the circulating haemocytes to the uptake of dye-filled nephrocytes. In diplopods, Bruntz (1906a,b) recorded the phagocytosis of carbon particles in greater concentration by granular haemocytes than by plasmatocytes. Prohemocytes showed no signs of phagocytosis.

In a diplopod, *Strongylosoma* sp. Seifert (1932) observed that the granular haemocytes phagocytose Chinese ink and then enter the germinal follicles, ovary, testis and egg chambers. The above observations suggest that the haemocytes may selectively sequester colloidal substances and transport them to specific sites for utilization. Tanaka's (1961) ultrastructural observations on the mechanism of vital staining, revealed that the dyes may not only enter cells by penetrating the limiting membranes of phagocytic and pinocytic vacuoles but may also penetrate the outer plasma membrane directly.

B. Parasitic encapsulation

Encapsulation of internal metazoan parasites by the haemocytes is considered as one of the primary defence reactions in insects and other arthropods (Salt, 1963). In insects, capsules formed are usually made up of three layers (Nappi, 1975). Sheath encapsulation having the features of both cellular encapsulation and melanization is also common (Arnold, 1974). Sometimes, cellular encapsulation may not result in the melanization of the parasite (Ravindranath and Anantaraman, 1977).

The formation of sheath capsules has been recorded in two species of diplopods, *Floridobolus penneri* and *Narceus gordanus*, after infection with the acanthors of *Macracanthorhynchus ingens*, but no melanization has been reported (Bowen, 1967). No other information about the response of haemocytes to other kinds of parasites is available.

C. *Haemostasis*

In insects, haemocytes are known to play a major role in haemostasis in two ways; (1) by forming a cellular plug at the wound site and (2) by liberating clot promoting factors into the surrounding plasma which cause gelation. While Grégoire (1955), has shown that cystocytes bring about plasma gelation, a number of investigators believe that granular haemocytes also play a major role (see Grégoire, 1970). In spite of the occurrence of both cystocytes and granular haemocytes in the Onychophora, Chilopoda and Diplopoda, Grégoire (1955, 1970) reported that there is no plasma coagulation in these groups. It is not clear why the plasma of these groups fails to clot when exposed to air and probably, the only mechanism involved in haemostasis may be the formation of a cellular plug. In the symphylid, *Scutigerella immaculata*, however, Gupta (1968, 1979) reported plasma coagulation due to the release of cytoplasmic contents from cystocytes.

The haemocytes may also be involved in a number of activities in conjunction with other tissues, such as wound healing, phenol metabolism, basement membrane and cuticle formation. Information about wound healing is wanting in onychophorans and myriapods, although the role of haemocytes in phenol metabolism has been studied in diplopods.

D. *Phenol metabolism and cuticle formation*

The darkening of blood on exposure to air is due to oxidation of haemolymph diphenols by the action of a phenoloxidase in the haemocytes. The involvement of haemocytes in phenol metabolism, and thus in the process of melanization, during parasitic encapsulation and sclerotization of the cuticle, is indicated by the presence of phenoloxidase in the cytoplasm of these cells.

Dopa-oxidase has been reported in 10% of the haemocytes of spirobolid millipedes (Bowen, 1968). Furthermore, Krishnan and Ravindranath (1973) have located phenoloxidase in the granules of the granular haemocytes of three species of millipedes, *Thyropygus poseidon*, *Polydesmus* sp. and *Spirostreptus asthenes*. The results of the cytochemical characterization of the enzyme in the haemocytes reveal that the enzyme in the granules oxidizes diphenols, polyphenols and also tyrosine (Krishnan and Ravindranath, 1973).

It has also been suggested that the haemocytes are involved in cuticle formation during moulting in the millipede, *T. poseidon* (Ravindranath, 1974c). The degree of haemocytic response to moulting was assessed by combining differential counts with total haemocyte counts and estimates of blood volume (Ravindranath, 1974a). The results show that the total population of haemocytes during inter-moult, pre-moult and fresh moult was fairly constant. However, at post-moult there was a considerable increase in the total number of cells. The differential cell counts showed that the number of spherule cells decreased after ecdysis and histological sections revealed that large numbers had adhered underneath the epidermis secreting the new cuticle. Probably these cells are associated with the synthetic activities of the epidermal cell in producing the precursors of the new cuticle.

Finally, in female *Peripatopsis moseleyi*, Manton (1938) reported that the haemocytes accumulate underneath the cuticle which they may digest at the site of spermatophore deposition thus creating a passage for the entry of sperms from spermatophores into the haemocoel. They also probably repair the wound after sperm entry.

VI. Summary and concluding remarks

The haemocytes of the onychophorans and myriapods can be divided into several cell types based on their morphology and cytochemistry. It is, however, necessary to be aware of the changes a cell may undergo during various preparative techniques such as fixation which may alter their appearance and categorization. Therefore, the cell types should be named with caution. Jones' (1962, 1979) advice in this connection is highly pertinent; he recommends a nomenclature based on morphology, which is non-committal, rather than one on physiology since a variety of functions may be performed by the same cells, and also apparently different structural types may perform similar functions. There is also often a tendency to extend the terminologies used in vertebrate or mammalian haematology to arthropod haemocytes. To do so without a clear understanding of structure, chemistry and functions of the cell types leads to confusion.

The following salient findings emerge from an examination of the haemocytes of Onychophora and Myriapoda.

(1) The granular haemocyte is the most abundant cell type found in these arthropods.

(2) Cystocytes occur regardless of whether the haemolymph coagulates or not.
(3) The cystocytes probably represent the end cell stage of the granular haemocytes.
(4) Plasmatocytes are probably degranulated or degranulating granular haemocytes (Ravindranath, 1978).
(5) A cell type comparable with the prohaemocyte is seen in all the aforementioned arthropods. Sometimes a shrunken cystocyte appears as a prohaemocyte.
(6) Spherule cells are common. They are predominant during the pre-moult period.

The following information on onychophoran and myriapod blood cells is required: (1) ultrastructure; (2) cytochemistry of cytoplasmic inclusions; (3) qualitative and quantitative observations during different stages of the moult cycle, growth and physiological conditions; (4) functional capabilities of haemocytes in cellular immunity, coagulation and cuticle formation; (5) origin and formation of blood cells; and (6) the status of the pericardial cells.

Acknowledgements

I wish to thank Prof. Dr B. R. Seshachar, Centre for Theoretical Studies, Indian Institute of Science, Bangalore, and Prof. S. Somasundaram, Sir Theagaraya College, Madras, for critically reading the manuscript. I am most indebted to Prof. Dr G. Siefert, Dr J. Rosenberg and Dr Ch. Grégoire for providing me with prints and allowing me to reproduce their unpublished and published illustrations, and to Dr Lavallard for permission to reproduce his illustrations.

References

Arnold, J. W. (1974). *In* "The Physiology of Insecta" (M. Rockstein, Ed.), Vol. 5, pp. 201–254. Academic Press, New York.
Arvy, L. (1954). *Bull. Soc. Zool. Fr.* **79**, 13.
Bauchau, A. and De Brouwer, M. (1974). *J. Microsc.* **19**, 37–46.
Biegel, J. H. (1922). *Rev. Suisse. Zool.* **29**, 427–480.
Bowers, B. (1964). *Protoplasma* **59**, 351–367.
Bowen, R. C. (1967). *J. Parasitol.* **53**, 1092–1095.
Bowen, R. C. (1968). *Trans. Amer. Microsc. Soc.* 87, 390–392.
Bruntz, L. (1903a). *C.R. Acad. Sci. Ser. D.* **136**, 1148–1150.
Bruntz, L. (1903b). *Arch. Biol.* **20**, 217–422.

Bruntz, L. (1906a). *C.R. Soc. Biol.* **61**, 1–7.
Bruntz, L. (1906b). Archs Zool. exp. gén. **5**, 491–504.
Campiglia, S. and Lavallard, P. R. (1975). *Ann. Sci. Nat. Zool. Biol. Anim.* **17**, 93–120.
Cattaneo, G. (1889). *Boll. Scient.* **1**, 1–7.
Cuénot, L. (1949). *In* "Traite de Zoologie" (P. P. Grasse, Ed.), Vol. 6, pp. 3–37. Masson et Cie, Paris.
Déhorne, A. (1925). *C.R. Acad. Sci. Ser. D.* **180**, 333.
Demange, J. M. (1963). *In* "Les Arthropodes" Zoologie 2 Triage a part, pp. 411–486. Encyclopaedie de la pleiade.
Duboscq, D. (1896). *Zool. Anz.* **19**, 1–7.
Duboscq, D. (1899). Arch. Zool. exp. gén. **4**, 1–7.
Gaffron, E. (1885). *Zool. Beitr.* **1**, 33–60.
Grégoire, Ch. (1955). *Archs Biol.* **66**, 489–508.
Grégoire, Ch. (1970). *In* "The Haemostatic Mechanism in Man and Other Animals" (R. G. MacFarlane, Ed.), Vol. 27, pp. 45–75. Academic Press, London.
Grégoire, Ch. and Jolivet, P. (1957). *Smithson. Misc. Collect.* **134**, 1–35.
Gupta, A. P. (1968). *Ann. entomol. Soc. Am.* **61**, 1028–1029.
Gupta, A. P. (1979). *In* "Arthropod Phylogeny" (A. P. Gupta, Ed.), pp. 669–735. Van Nostrand Reinhold, New York.
Heymons, R. (1901). *Zoologica (N.Y.)* **13**, 1–244.
Johannsen, O. A. and Butt, F. H. (1941). *In* "Embryology of Insects and Myriapods", p. 462. McGraw-Hill, New York.
Jones, J. C. (1962). *Amer. Zool.* **2**, 209–249.
Jones, J. C. (1967). *Biol. Bull., Woods Hole* **132**, 211–221.
Jones, J. C. (1979). *In* "Insect Hemocytes: Development, Forms, Functions and Techniques" (A. P. Gupta, Ed.), pp. 1–15. Cambridge University Press, New York and London.
Kollmann, M. (1908). *Ann. Sci. Nat. Zool. Biol. Anim.* **9**, 1–238.
Kowalewsky, A. (1894). *Izv. Imp. Akad. Nauk* **4**, 1–7.
Kowalewsky, A. (1895). Archs Zool. exp. gén. **3**, 3–10.
Krishnan, G. (1968). "The Millipede *Thyropygus*". CSIR Zoological Memoirs—1. Publications and Information Directorate, New Delhi.
Krishnan, G. and Ravindranath, M. H. (1973). *J. Insect Physiol.* **19**, 647–653.
Lavallard, P. R. and Campiglia, S. (1975). *Ann. Sci. Nat. Zool. Biol. Anim.* **17**, 67–92.
Manton, S. M. (1938). *Philos. Trans. R. Soc. London, Ser. B.* **228**, 421–442.
Manton, S. M. and Heatley, N. G. (1937). *Philos. Trans. R. Soc. London, Ser. B.* **227**, 411–464.
Nappi, A. J. (1975). *In* "Invertebrate Immunity" (K. Maramorosch and R. E. Shope, Eds), pp. 293–326. Academic Press, New York.
Neuwirth, M. (1973). *J. Morphol.* **139**, 105–124.
Palm, N. B. (1954). *Ark. Zool.* **6**, 219–246.
Price, C. D. and Ratcliffe, N. A. (1974). *Z. Zellforsch. mikrosk. Anat.* **147**, 537–549.
Ravindranath, M. H. (1970). Comparative studies on the blood of chilopods and diplopods in relation to cuticle formation, pp. 1–140, Ph.D. Thesis, University of Madras.
Ravindranath, M. H. (1973). *J. Morphol.* **141**, 257–268.
Ravindranath, M. H. (1974a). *J. Morphol.* **144**, 1–10.
Ravindranath, M. H. (1974b). *J. Morphol.* **144**, 11–22.
Ravindranath, M. H. (1974c). *Physiol. Zool.* **47**, 252–260.

Ravindranath, M. H. (1975). *Biol. Bull., Woods Hole* **149**, 226–235.
Ravindranath, M. H. (1977a). *Cytologia* **42**, 743–751.
Ravindranath, M. H. (1977b). *Biol. Bull., Woods Hole* **152**, 415–423.
Ravindranath, M. H. (1978). *Dev. Comp. Immunol.* **2**, 581–595.
Ravindranath, M. H. and Anantharaman, S. (1977). *Z. Parasitenk.* **53**, 225–237.
Rosenberg, J. (1978). *Ent. Germ.* **4**, 24–32.
Rossi, G. (1902). "Organizzayione dei Myriapodi" Roma.
Salt, G. (1963). *Parasitology* **53**, 527–542.
Schneider, K. C. (1902). "Lehrbuch der vergleichenden Histologie der Tiere", pp. 988. G. Fischer Verlag, Jena.
Seifert, H. (1932). *Gegenbaurs morph. Jb* **25**, 1–7.
Seifert, G. and Rosenberg, J. (1976). *Zoomorphologie* **85**, 23–37.
Seifert, G. and Rosenberg, J. (1977). *Zoomorphologie* **86**, 169–181.
Sherman, R. G. (1973). *Can. J. Zool.* **51**, 1155–1159.
Shukla, G. S. (1964). *Agra Univ. J. Res. Sci.* **13**, 227–232.
Sundara-Rajulu, G. (1971a). *Cytologia* **36**, 515–521.
Sundara-Rajulu, G. (1971b). *Indian Zool.* **2**, 73–80.
Sundara-Rajulu, G., Krishnan, N. and Singh, M. (1970). *Zool. Anz.* **184**, 220–225.
Tanaka, M. (1961). *Proc. Japan Acad.* **1**, 44–60.
Tuzet, O. and Manier, J. F. (1954). *Bull. Biol. Fr. Belg.* **88**, 88–90.
Tuzet, O. and Manier, J. F. (1959). *Bull. Biol. Fr. Belg.* **92**, 7–23.
Valeri, O. M. (1934). *Memorie Soc. tosc. Sci. nat.* **43**, 1–7.
Varma, L. (1971). *J. Anim. Morphol. Physiol.* **18**, 111–120.
Vostal, Z. (1970). *Biol. Ceskoal.* **25**, 811–818.
Verhoeff, K. W. (1932). *In* "Dr. H. G. Bronns Klassen und ordnungan des Tierreichs", Vol. 5, pp. 1294–1305. Akademische Verlagsgesellschaft, Leipzig.
Wigglesworth, V. B. (1970). *J. Reticuloendothel. Soc.* **7**, 208–216.
Zachary, D. and Hoffmann, J. A. (1973). *Z. Zellforsch. mikrosk. Anat.* **141**, 55–73.
Zacher, F. (1933). *In* "Handbuch der Zoologie" (W. Kukenthal and T. Krunbach, Eds), Vol. 3, p. 864. de Gruyter Verlag, Berlin.

11. Chelicerates

R. G. SHERMAN

Department of Zoology, Miami University, Oxford, Ohio 45056, U.S.A.

CONTENTS

I. Introduction

The chelicerates represent a major subphylum of arthropods and include the major class of Arachnida (spiders, scorpions, etc.) and the smaller classes of Merostomata (horseshoe crabs) and Pycnogonida (sea spiders). The majority of the investigations of blood cells in these groups have been conducted on horseshoe crabs and spiders and to a lesser extent, the scorpions. For this reason, only these animals will be treated here.

II. Spiders

A. Structure of the circulatory system

The heart of spiders has a tubular shape and extends mid-dorsally along the anterior two-thirds of the abdomen, just beneath the exoskeleton (Petrunkevitch, 1933). It is held in position by suspensory ligaments which also serve to restore the heart to its diastolic volume after each heartbeat. There are from two to five pairs of ostia located along the lateral margins; the number is consistent for each species, but varies among the different families of spiders. The heartbeat is neurogenic; pacemaker impulses originate in the cardiac ganglion which is a thin, cord-like structure on the dorsal aspect of the heart (Bursey and Sherman, 1970).

The principal artery is the anterior aorta which supplies blood to all of the cephalothorax and the anterior portion of the abdomen. This vessel extends through the pedicel where it branches into two lateral aortas. These in turn divide into a cephalic artery which gives rise to vessels which supply the various components of the anterior region and into a descending branch which ultimately divides many times in a fan-like manner to give rise to arteries that supply the walking legs, etc. (Millot, 1949).

The abdomen receives blood via a posterior aorta and two or three pairs of lateral arteries that arise from the heart. Arterial blood accumulates in large sinuses; some of it passes through the book-lungs on its return course to the pericardial cavity, but some of the blood apparently by-passes the lungs and returns directly to the heart (Millot, 1949).

B. Structure and classification of haemocytes

Blood cells in the spiders have been described by several investigators in the past 90 years (Wagner, 1888; Deevey, 1941; Browning, 1942; Millot, 1949; Seitz, 1972a,b; Sherman, 1973). These cells were called leucocytes because their cytoplasm is colourless. The term haemocyte will be used instead, because as Seitz (1972a) pointed out, it is more neutral and conforms to terminology used generally for arthropods (see Chapter 1).

Table I summarizes the types of blood cells described by some of the early investigators who used a variety of light microscopic techniques. This table represents an updating of a similar one published by Browning (1942). The various blood cells can be grouped for the most part into three basic cell types for all of the species examined. Those shown in Category 1 in Table I all appear to be granular haemocytes which are typified by the presence of dense granules in the cytoplasm. Those in Category 2 all seem to be hyaline haemocytes which contain no particularly unique cytoplasmic granules. Category 3 are probably all leberidocytes of which there may be two different types. Deevey (1941) did not find a large vacuole in leberidocytes, but Kollmann (1908), Browning (1942) and Millot (1949) described one in cells that were present during moulting. Grégoire (1955) also reported a signet-shaped, large hyaline haemocyte with a vacuole in four species of spider. Deevey (1941) found that the cytoplasm of the leberidocytes contained tremendous quantities of glycogen. It seems possible that the glycogen may have been dissolved by the preparatory techniques employed by those investigators who reported the presence of vacuoles in this cell or that the cell may have released its contents prior to fixation. On the other hand, the vacuole may not be artefactual. This point must be reinvestigated, especially in light of the report of a vacuolated cell in scorpions (Ravindranath, 1974).

In addition to the three basic blood cell types, a variety of additional cells have been reported and these are listed in Category 4 of Table I. The so-called supplementary cells reported by Kollmann (1908) are probably not blood cells at all (Browning, 1942). The balloon cell type reported by Wagner (1888) may be one of the other basic cell types which has been distorted as a consequence of preparation for microscopy. Alternatively, it may by a cystocyte such as has been described for scorpions (Ravindranath, 1974). Deevey (1941) reported the presence of a "cyst-like" cell but she did not liken it to the balloon cell described by Wagner (1888) and Kollmann (1908). The "cells of Cuénot" contain needle-shaped protein crystals (Millot, 1949) which indicate that this cell actually may be a cyanocyte (Fahrenbach, 1970). The basophils and so-called cyst cells described by Deevey (1941) have not been found for certain in any other species of spider. It seems peculiar that one species of spider of the ten or so that have been studied should contain two completely different types of blood cell.

Descriptions of spider blood cells using electron microscopical techniques have been published by Seitz (1972a,b), Sherman (1973) and Midttun and Jensen (1978). Sherman (1973) recognized three basic types of haemocyte in

TABLE I. Types of spider blood cells described using light microscopic techniques.

Species studied	Category 1	Category 2	Category 3	Category 4	
	(granular haemocytes)	(hyaline haemocytes)	(leberidocytes)	(miscellaneous)	
Tarantula (species uncertain)	coloured cells	amoeboid cells	spherical cells	balloon cells	Wagner (1888)
Tegenaria atrica	granular haemocytes	hyaline haemocytes	vacuolar cells	supplementary cells	Kollmann (1908)
Tegenaria domestica *Amaurobius similis* *Tetragnatha extensa* *Aranea diadema* *Coelotes atropos*	granulous haemocytes	lymphocytes, hyaline haemocytes	vacuolar haemocytes	"cells of Cuénot"	Millott (1949)
Phormictopus canceriles	chromophobes, weak eosinophils, eosinophils	hyaline haemocytes	leberidocytes	basophils, "cyst cells"	Deevey (1941)
Tegenaria atrica	granulocytes	hyaline haemocytes	leberidocytes	—	Browning (1942)

the tarantula spider, *Eurypelma marxi*: granular haemocytes, oenocytoids and plasmatocytoids (plasmatocytes) (Figs 1–9). Granular haemocytes are the most abundant ones and measure approximately 10 × 25 μm (Fig. 1). They have numerous granules of varying electron-densities from 0·3–1·5 μm in diameter, which in some cases contain tubular structures (Fig. 2). The granules are bounded by a unit membrane and may undergo degradation (Fig. 3).

The oenocytoids described by Sherman (1973) actually appear to be cyanocytes (Figs 4, 5). These very large blood cells are about 20 × 50 μm, and contain a dense cytoplasm with many ribosomes and crystals of protein

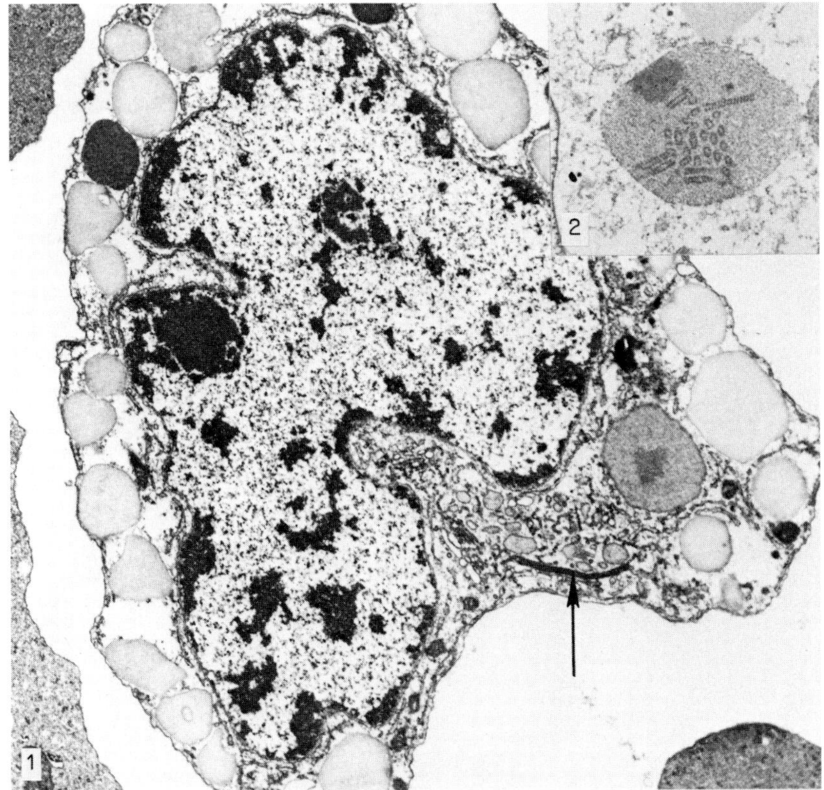

Fig. 1. Granular haemocyte in *Eurypelma marxi*. Numerous granules of varying density, Golgi complex (arrow) and many smaller granules and vesicles are present in the cytoplasm. ×9500.

Fig. 2. Granule in a granular haemocyte of *E. marxi* containing tubular structures. Note the periodicity of the tubular subunits. ×27 000.

which appear to be haemocyanin (Fahrenbach, 1970). The latter occur as rod-like structures which have been mis-identified as microtubules. Cyanocytes are not as prevalent in the blood near to the heart as are the granular haemocytes and plasmatocytes. Millot (1949) reported that they (cells of Cuénot) comprise only from 0 to 5% of the total blood cells. This may explain why they were not noted in the studies of Deevey (1941), Browning (1942) and Seitz (1972a,b).

The plasmatocytes (Figs 6, 7), so-named because of their similarity to such cells in insects, resemble the hyaline haemocytes described from light microscopic examination by previous investigators. They are 5–10 μm wide and 20–30 μm long and show numerous cytoplasmic extensions. Their main features are numerous small mitochondria, well-developed Golgi complexes, a stacked endoplasmic reticulum near the nucleus, a light staining cytoplasmic matrix, small granules and a general lack of large granular inclusions.

Leberidocytes are not noted by Seitz (1972a) or Sherman (1973). Subsequent examination of material obtained from *E. marxi* by the author

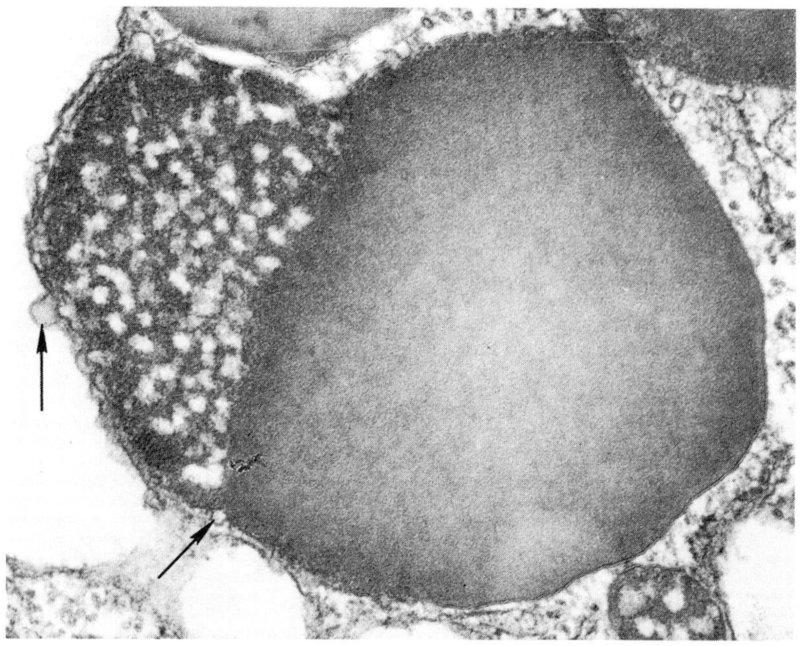

Fig. 3. A large dense granule in a granular haemocyte in *E. marxi*. The granule is bounded by a unit membrane and is in the process of degradation as evidenced by the exocytotic vesicles (arrows). ×76 000.

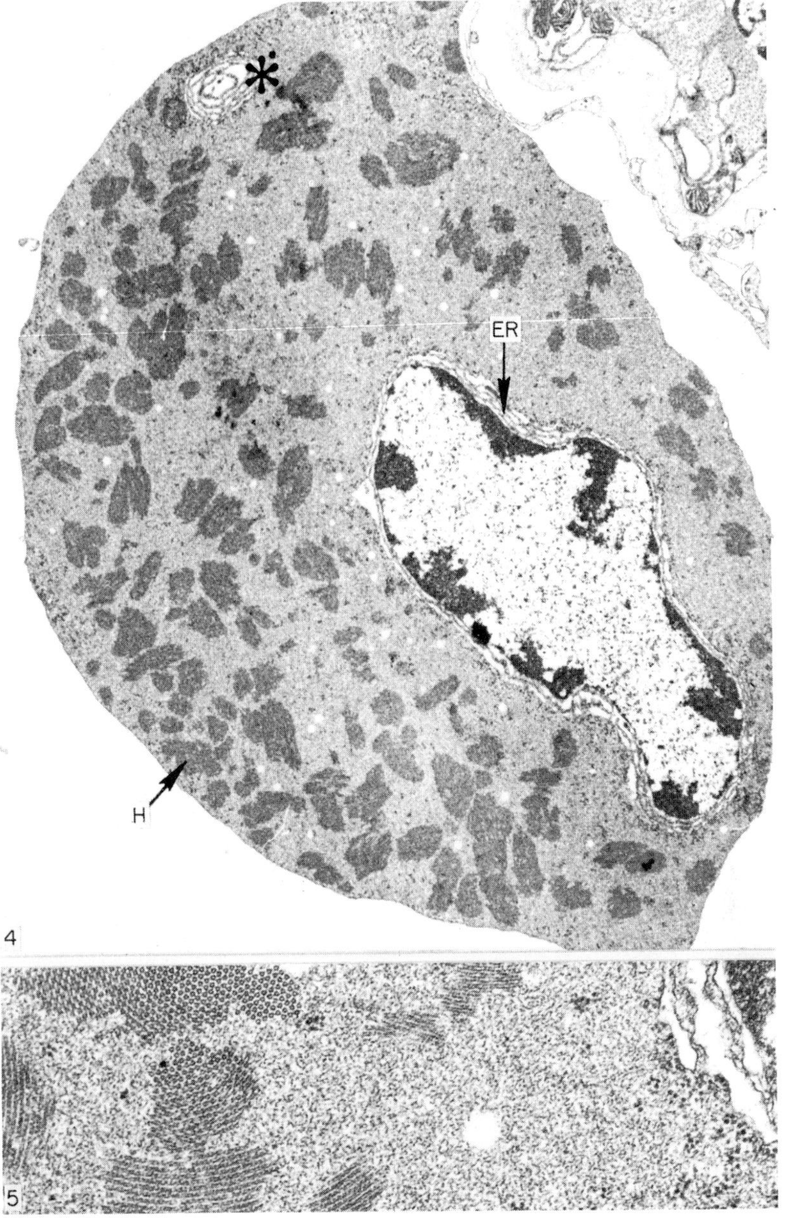

Fig. 4. Cyanocyte in *E. marxi*. The cytoplasm contains bundles of haemocyanin crystals (H). Numerous clear areas which may represent material that has been removed during tissue processing occur in the cytoplasm. Smooth endoplasmic reticulum (ER) surrounds the nucleus. Occasional whorls of ER (asterisk) occur distant to the nucleus. ×9400.

Fig. 5. Crystals of haemocyanin present in the cytoplasm of the cyanocyte in *E. marxi* are shown in higher magnification. ×36 000.

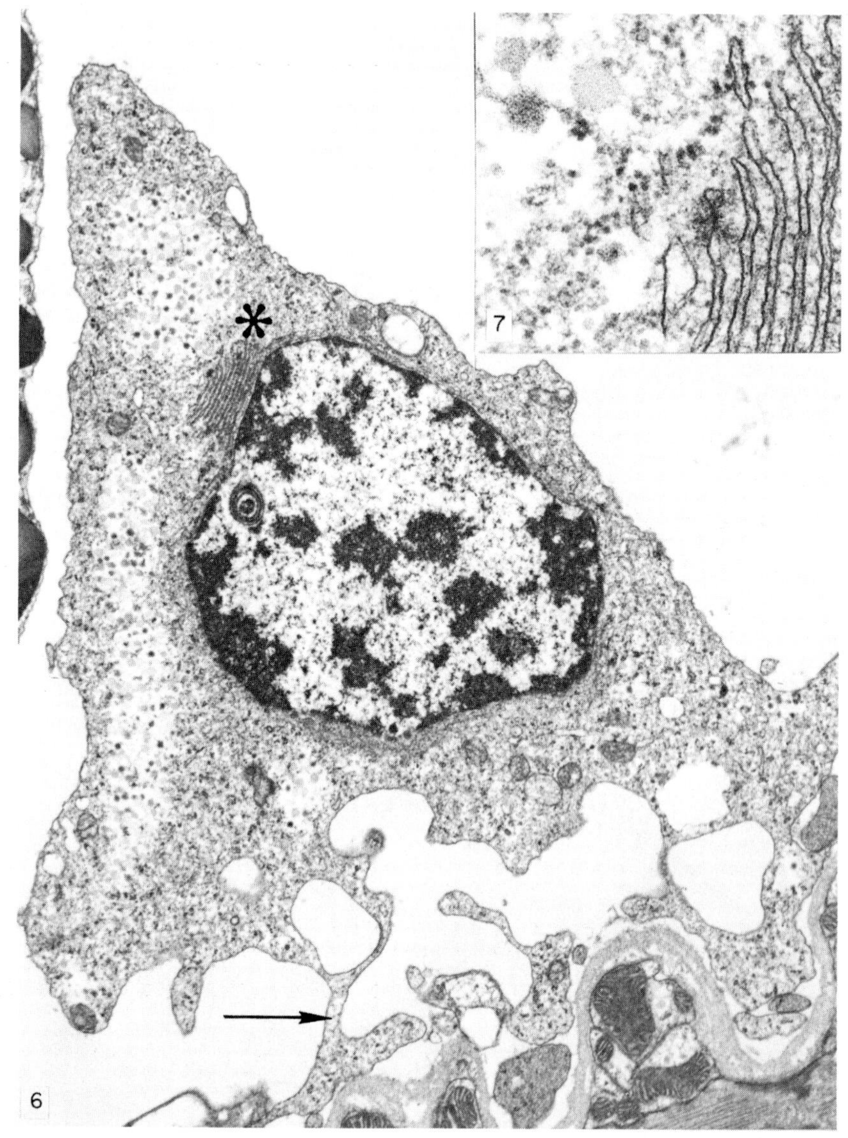

Fig. 6. Plasmatocyte in *E. marxi* containing a large number of small granules of varying density. Note the stacked endoplasmic reticulum (asterisk) and the narrow cytoplasmic extension (arrow). ×10 300.

Fig. 7. Enlarged view of the area near the asterisk in Fig. 6 which shows more clearly the stacked endoplasmic reticulum and the small granules. ×64 500.

has revealed the presence of another cell type which may indeed be a leberidocyte. It is a very large cell whose cytoplasm is devoid of the usual array of inclusions except for the presence of mitochondria and vast numbers of glycogen granules (Fig. 8). The cytoplasm is homogeneous and may contain polysaccharide material. This point needs to be investigated further using cytochemical techniques, but the appearance of this cell fits to some degree that described for leberidocytes by Deevey (1941).

Recently, Midttun and Jensen (1978) described a blood cell from 14 to 25 μm in diameter in *Pisaura mirabilis* and *Trochosa terricola* that resembles the oenocytoid haemocytes found in insects (Figs 9–11). Mature cells of this type contain large amounts of crystalloid material organized into numerous lamellae which have a crystal-like hexagonal lattice (Figs 10, 11). Apparently, these cells are capable of releasing the crystalloid material into the extracellular space.

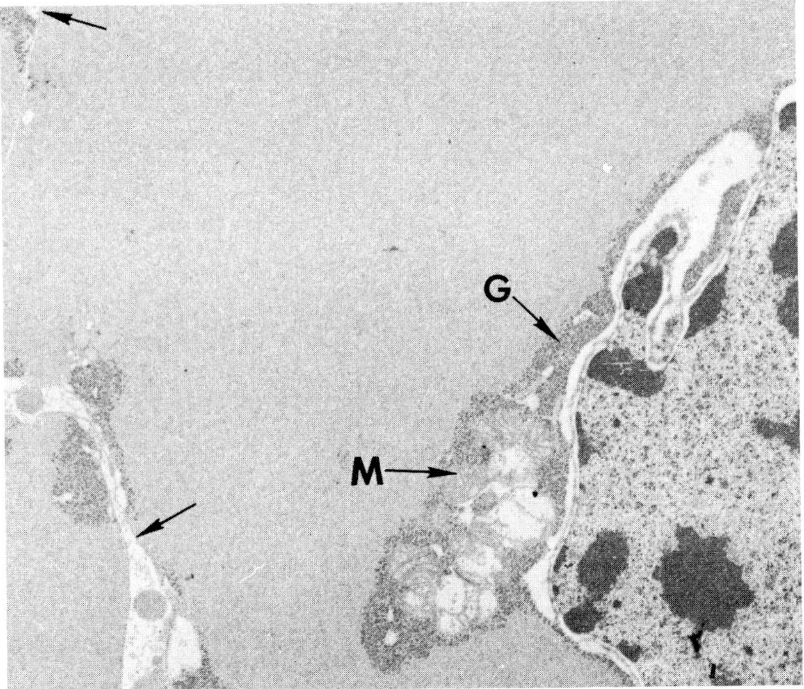

Fig. 8. A presumed leberidocyte in *E. marxi*. Mitochondria (M) and numerous glycogen granules (G) are present. Most of the cytoplasm is homogeneous. The cell membrane is denoted by the unlabelled arrows. ×8500.

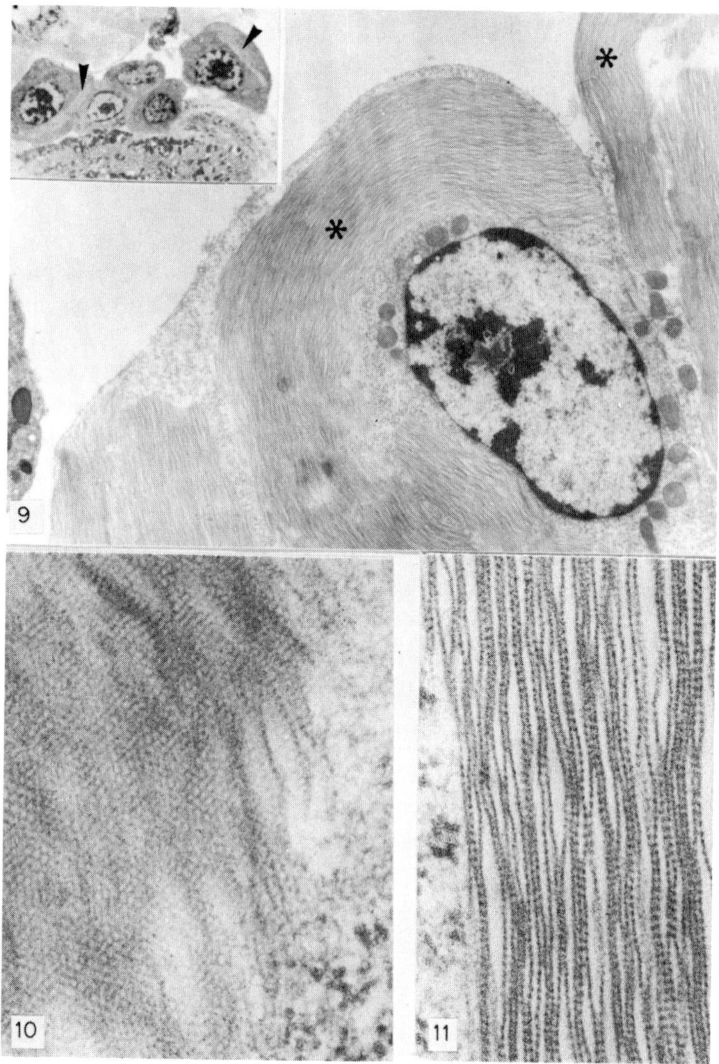

Figs 9–11. Oenocytoids in *Trochosa terricola* and *Pisaura mirabilis*.

Fig. 9. The most conspicuous feature is the crystalloid material (left asterisk) in the cytoplasm. This material is also found in the extracellular space nearby (right asterisk). ×4500. Insert: light micrograph of two oenocytoids (arrows) with crystalloid material. ×830. (Figs 9–11 courtesy of B. Midttun and H. Jensen.)

Fig. 10. Plane section view of the crystalloid material. ×93 000.

Fig. 11. Transverse section view of the crystalloid material. ×74 000.

Seitz (1972a) employed the transmission electron microscope to study the types of haemocyte present in embryonic specimens of *Cupiennius salei*. He recognized seven different types of haemocyte, based primarily on various stages in their differentiation (Figs 12–14).

(1) The prohaemocytes, which are found closely associated with the adventitia of the heart, are able to divide, and contain granular cytoplasm with a few mitochondria and small vacuoles.
(2) Haemocytes in the first stage of differentiation, with an increased number of mitochondria and initial development of the endoplasmic reticulum.
(3) Haemocytes in the second stage of differentiation, which have a larger

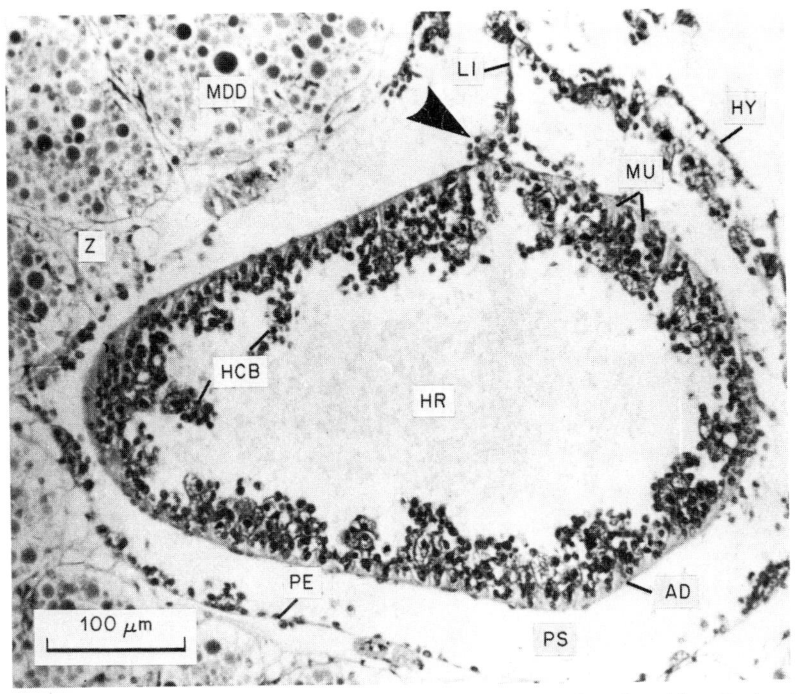

Figs 12–14. Sections through the heart of a five-month-old female spider *Cupiennius salei*. (From Seitz, 1972a.)

Fig. 12. Cuticle removed. Hypodermis (HY). Pericardium (PE) around the pericardial sinus (PS) which in turn is surrounded by the mid-intestine (MDD) and the intermediate tissue (Z). Adventitia (AD) forms a narrow band of tissue. Heart muscle (MU), ligament (LI). Haemocytes in genesis (HCB) in the wall of the heart (HR). Unlabelled arrow shows region of Fig. 13. Light micrograph.

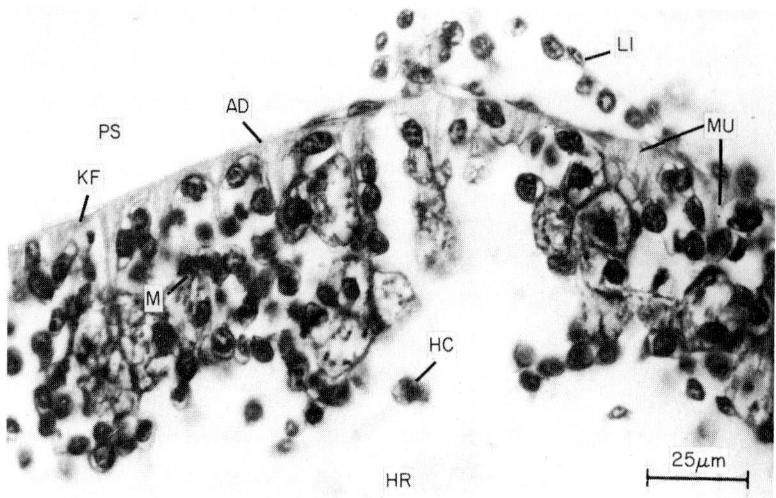

Fig. 13. Enlargement of Fig. 12 (region indicated by unlabelled arrow). Ligament (LI) passes through the pericardial sinus (PS) and ends in the stratum of collagen filaments (KF), lying between the adventitia (AD) and the heart muscle (MU). The heart muscle (MU) forms little septa projecting into the lumen of the heart (HR). Haemocytes in genesis (M) are situated near the septa. Light micrograph.

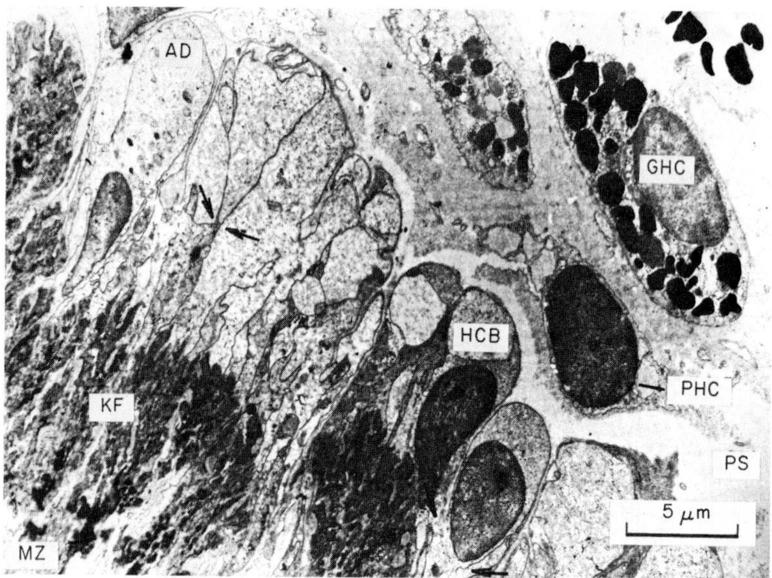

Fig. 14. Adventitia (AD) proliferating prohaemocytes (HCB). Extensions of these cells connect with the collagen filaments (KF) which are attached to the heart muscle (MZ). In the pericardial sinus (PS) there are free prohaemocytes (PHC) and granular haemocytes (GHC). Electron micrograph.

number of mitochondria and increased elaboration of the endoplasmic reticulum. A large Golgi apparatus is present with associated vesicles and occasional lysosomes.

(4) Granular haemocytes synthesizing protein, and characterized by a dense endoplasmic reticulum surrounding the nucleus. There are numerous polysomes and mitochondria in the cytoplasm. Numerous dense granules are present as are vacuoles presumably containing protein.

(5) Granular storing haemocytes, which are another form of the granular haemocyte. Mitochondria, many protein vacuoles and dense granules are also present.

(6) Phagocytes which are found primarily in organs undergoing decomposition and are rich in lysosomes, but have few other organelles.

(7) The dedifferentiated haemocytes which are cells like prohaemocytes, except larger.

Seitz (1972a) considers these cell types to be different stages in the progressive differentiation and subsequent dedifferentiation of the basic stem cell type, the prohaemocyte.

Table II shows an attempt to categorize the various types of spider blood cells that have been reported to date. It is possible to group most of the cells into six basic cell types. The additional cells mentioned earlier from light microscopic studies are not included. The table shows the relationship between each cell type reported from light microscopy to that reported using the transmission electron microscope. The cells Seitz (1972a) terms stage 1 differentiation haemocytes and dedifferentiated haemocytes have been categorized as plasmatocytes because they resemble the plasmatocytes described by Sherman (1973) and the hyaline haemocytes described by earlier investigators. The term plasmatocyte is used rather than hyaline haemocyte to bring spider blood cell terminology into conformity with that used for other arthropods (e.g. Jones, 1962).

TABLE II. Basic types of spider blood cell recognized by light and electron microscopy.

Light microscope	Transmission electron microscope
1. Lymphocyte	prohaemocyte
2. Hyaline haemocyte	plasmatocyte
3. Granular haemocyte	granular haemocyte
4. Leberidocyte	leberidocyte
5. "Cells of Cuénot"	cyanocyte
6. Oenocytoid	oenocytoid

The stage 2 differentiation haemocytes, the granular haemocytes synthesizing protein, the storing haemocytes and the phagocytes described by Seitz (1972a) are grouped into the granular haemocyte basic type. The prohaemocytes described by Seitz (1972a) appear to be identical to the lymphocytes described by Millot (1949). This basic cell type presumably is the stem cell for some of the other haemocytes. The scheme in Table II is a working one and will have to be modified as additional studies are conducted.

C. *Origin and formation of haemocytes*

1. Haemocytopoiesis

Haemocytopoiesis in spiders was described initially by Franz (1904). While analysing the structure of the heart wall in several spider species, including *Tegenaria derhami*, *Epeira quadrata* and *Attus rupicola*, he noted that the inner wall of the heart contained cells that had a different structure than the myocardial cells nearby. These cells formed an inner layer which some investigators considered to be an intima. Franz's observations, however, indicated that these cells did not constitute an intima, but instead are likely to be prohaemocytes. Other larger cells free in the lumen were similar in appearance to the prohaemocytes, and Franz (1904) suggested that these represented prohaemocytes that had detached from the heart wall and were capable of further differentiation.

Franz (1904) was unable to locate mitotic figures and suggested that blood cells once formed are not capable of replication. Therefore, it appears that mature cells differentiate from stem cells originating in the wall of the heart.

Seitz (1972a), using the transmission electron microscope, investigated the formation of haemocytes in the heart. He studied specimens of *Cupiennius salei* which were still in embryonic development. After three months of development, the heart had not completely differentiated. However, regions of the myocardial cell layer of the heart protruded into the lumen and were bound by cells that appeared to be prohaemocytes (Figs 12, 13). Unlike Franz (1904), Seitz (1972a) considers this layer to be an intima. Nonetheless, they are in agreement that this is a site of haemocytopoiesis. Cells in mitosis and amitosis were observed in this region.

Seitz (1972a) also found regions of the adventitia that showed club-like cytoplasmic branches which were embedded in the collagen fibril layer of the dorsal aspect of the heart (Fig. 14). These club-like branches also appear to be sites of prohaemocyte formation. Consequently, there are two sites of haemocyte formation in the heart; in the adventitia and along the inner wall of the heart. He envisaged that nuclei in the haemocytopoietic tissue multiply by amitosis and pass into the club-like cytoplasmic extensions which undergo constriction to form new free prohaemocytes. He also proposes that the prohaemocytes are themselves capable of division. There is no evidence for additional sites other than the heart itself for the formation of spider haemocytes.

2. *Differentiation of haemocytes*

All of the investigators of spider haemocytes are in agreement that the stem blood cell is the small hyaline haemocyte which Millot (1949) termed the lymphocyte and which Seitz (1972a,b) appropriately called the prohaemocyte. Millot (1949) and Kollmann (1908) reported intermediates between the basic cell types they described. Deevey (1941) described intermediates between hyaline haemocytes (=plasmatocytes) and basophils, between hyaline haemocytes and chromophobes, and between hyaline haemocytes and eosinophils. Deevey (1941) also states that leberidocytes differentiate from hyaline haemocytes and accumulate glycogen. A cell presumed to be an intermediate between a plasmatocyte and a granular haemocyte is shown in Fig. 15. These observations suggest that the prohaemocyte differentiates into the plasmatocyte which in turn may differentiate into one of the other basic cell types depending on the metabolic conditions in the spider.

The most extensive analysis of the differentiation of spider haemocytes was reported by Seitz (1972b) for *C. salei*. Seitz proposes a scheme to explain the differentiation and subsequent appearance of the haemocytes that he recognized (Table III). The prohaemocyte develops into the plasmatocyte which he terms "haemocyte in the first stage of differentiation". This cell soon differentiates into the next form which Seitz calls "haemocyte in the second stage of differentiation" which appears to be basically a more differentiated form of the plasmatocyte. At this point the haemocyte may follow one of two different lines of differentiation. It may develop into a "haemocyte undergoing synthesis" which appears to be an early form of the granular haemocyte. It then differentiates further into the "storing haemocyte" which again is a form of the granular haemocyte. Subsequently it differentiates into a "lysosome-rich haemocyte" which is a further stage of the granular haemocyte. Ultimately it undergoes dedifferentiation to what Seitz terms a dedifferentiated haemocyte. This cell appears to be a plasmatocyte. At this point the cell may be removed from the haemolymph through phagocytosis or undergo differentiation again to a haemocyte in the first stage of differentiation. If the haemocyte follows this line of differentiation, it re-enters the haemocyte differentiation cycle. Thus,

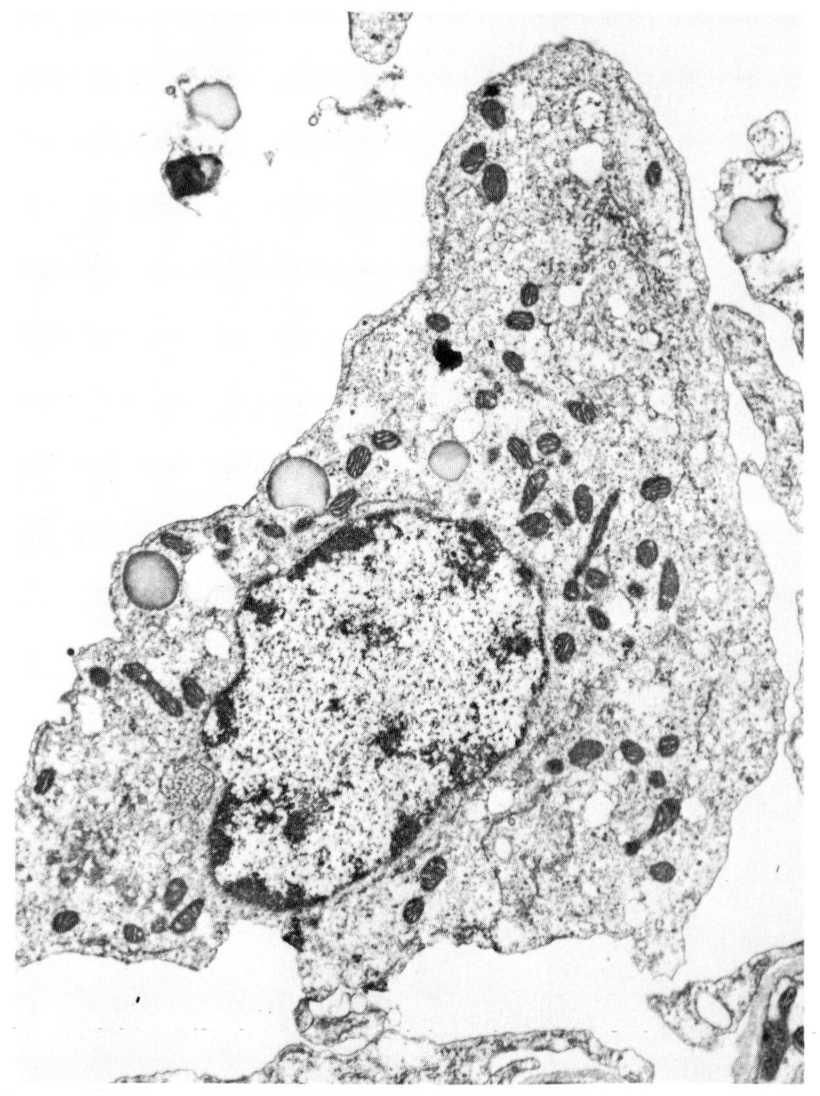

Fig. 15. A cell in *E. marxi* that shows characteristics of both a plasmatocyte and a granular haemocyte. It may be in transition from a plasmatocyte to a granular haemocyte. ×10 000.

according to Seitz, haemocytes that are well-differentiated may arise from the basic stem cell, the prohaemocyte, and from haemocytes that had undergone dedifferentiation and subsequently re-entered the differentiation cycle.

TABLE III. Scheme for haemocyte differentiation in spiders (Seitz, 1972b).

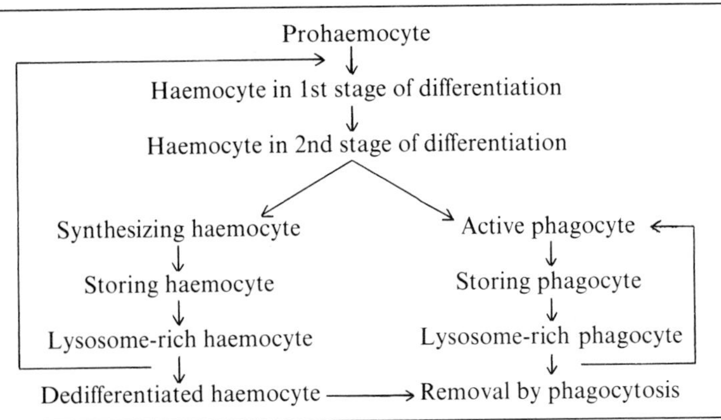

If the haemocyte in the second stage of differentiation follows the second line of differentiation, it develops into an active phagocyte which is another form of granular haemocyte (Table III). From this stage it develops into a storing phagocyte and ultimately into a lysosome-rich phagocyte. After this stage it may either be removed from the plasma through phagocytosis or re-enter this line of differentiation and become once again an active phagocyte.

Seitz (1972b) did not report the presence of oenocytoids, leberidocytes and cyanocytes in the species of spider that he studied. However, his scheme can be expanded to include these types of haemocyte by adding three additional lines of differentiation from the haemocyte in the second stage of differentiation. Which of the lines of differentiation were evoked would depend on the particular conditions in the spider. For example, during preparation for moulting the line of differentiation leading to the leberidocytes would be preferred, whereas in female spiders with exhausted ovaries the line of differentiation leading to lysosome-rich phagocytes would be stimulated (Seitz, 1972b). Needless to say, additional investigations should be conducted on this question.

3. *Blood cell percentages*

Millot (1949), Deevey (1941) and Browning (1942) studied the percentage of each cell type in the blood at different periods in the moult cycle. All three investigators agreed that during moulting, and in preparation for it, there is a dramatic decrease in the percentage of granular haemocytes and plasmatocytes in the blood while at the same time the percentage of leberidocytes is markedly increased.

There is little information on the total number of blood cells present in spider blood. Deevey (1941) found a mean of 11 025 blood cells per mm^3 of blood. This value might be low since right after death of the spider the value of 38 000 per mm^3 was obtained by her.

D. *Functions of haemocytes*

The granular haemocytes appear to have the most numerous functions. Seitz (1972b) provides evidence that the granular haemocytes are involved in the synthesis of protein, the storage and transport of reserve materials, and phagocytosis. By analogy with the function of granular haemocytes in the horseshoe crab, it is also possible that in spiders they contain the factors responsible for the clotting process. Grégoire (1952) briefly described blood clotting in spiders and noted the involvement of blood cells, but was unclear as to which types were involved. From his observations, it appears that these were either plasmatocytes or granular haemocytes.

Plasmatocytes are reported to be phagocytic by Deevey (1941). She also suggested that they play a primary role in the aggregation of other blood cells in clot formation. They may also differentiate into other blood cell types.

Leberidocytes are prominent during the moulting process. Browning (1942) suggested that they absorb water from the plasma which promotes an increase in total blood volume, thus facilitating the shedding of the old exoskeleton. Deevey (1941) proposes that the leberidocytes, because of their large quantities of glycogen, may function to transport glycogen to the newly forming cuticle during moulting.

The cyanocytes in the spider probably synthesize the respiratory pigment, haemocyanin (Boyd, 1937). Presumably, spider cyanocytes release haemocyanin into the haemolymph by cell rupture as has been suggested for cyanocytes in the horseshoe crab (Fahrenbach, 1970).

III. Scorpions

A. *Structure of the circulatory system*

The heart is tubular and extends the length of the pre-abdomen in a mid-dorsal position. There are seven pairs of ostia (Petrunkevitch, 1922; Randall, 1966), a pericardial sinus system, and suspensory ligaments. A cardiac ganglion is present and the heartbeat is probably neurogenic.

Blood leaves the heart through an anterior and a posterior aorta. The latter supplies blood to the post-abdomen. The anterior aorta extends into the cephalothorax and divides to form short aortic arches around the oesophagus. These in turn connect the aorta to the left and right thoracic sinuses near the brain (Millot, 1949). Two pairs of vessels arise from the aortic arches; one pair (cerebral) supplies blood to the suboesophageal ganglion and the other (cephalic) the chelicerae and nearby structures. Each thoracic sinus issues vessels to the appendages and they then unite to form the supraneural artery. This vessel is situated along the dorsal aspect of the ventral nervous system and it extends posteriorly the length of the animal. There is also a subneural artery situated beneath the nervous system which does not extend into the abdominal segments. It is connected with the supraneural artery by nine interneural arteries (Petrunkevitch, 1922).

Arterial blood flows into large ventral sinuses which are connected to the lungs. After oxygenation, the blood returns to the pericardial sinus via seven pairs of pulmonary veins (Millot, 1949).

B. Structure and classification of haemocytes

Kollmann (1908), described hyaline and granular haemocytes, as well as some other specialized cells in *Buthus occitans*, *Buthus australis*, *Scorpio maurus* and *Euscorpius flavicaudis*. Recently, an extensive light microcopic analysis describing the haemocytes in *Palamnaeus swammerdami* has been completed by Ravindranath (1974). He reported the presence of six basic types of blood cell:

(1) Prohaemocytes—these are small cells 7–12 μm in diameter with most of the cell volume occupied by the nucleus (Fig. 16). Few cell organelles are present.

(2) Plasmatocytes—these cells are usually 12–21 μm in size and show cytoplasmic extensions (Fig. 17). Many contain granules; some contain a large vacuole and are signet-ring-shaped. This point should be investigated further, since granular haemocytes in the horseshoe crab, *Limulus polyphemus*, form a large vacuole after granule release (Dumont *et al.*, 1966) and become signet-ring-shaped.

(3) Granular haemocytes—these cells are usually 18–25 μm in diameter, show cytoplasmic extensions, may have vacuoles and be completely filled with granules (Figs 18, 20).

(4) Cystocytes—these are 18–21 μm in diameter (Fig. 19). They contain a

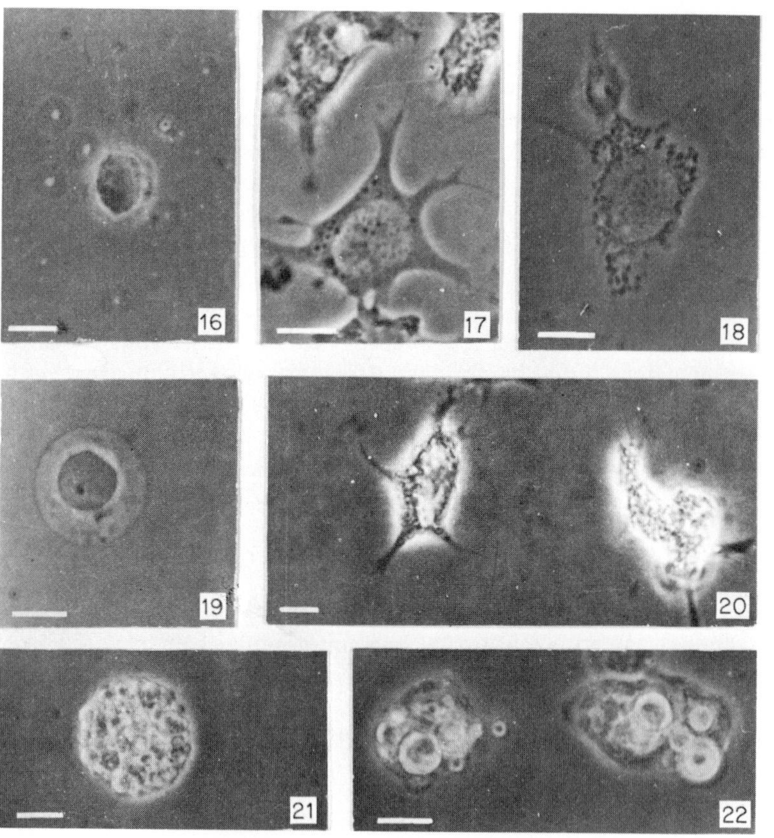

Figs 16–22. Haemocytes of the scorpion *Palamnaeus swammerdami*. Phase contrast. Scale bar = 10 μm. (From Ravindranath, 1974.)

Fig. 16. Prohaemocyte with large nucleus occupying most of cell.

Fig. 17. Plasmatocyte; note dark granules and pseudopodial extensions.

Fig. 18. Granular haemocyte; note numerous granules and cytoplasmic extensions.

Fig. 19. Cystocyte; note slightly eccentric nucleus and a few dark granules.

Fig. 20. Granular haemocytes with numerous granules and cytoplasmic extensions.

Fig. 21. Spherule cell; note refractile spherules masking nucleus.

Fig. 22. Adipohaemocytes containing different kinds of spherules, globules and granules.

few dark granules that stain with bromphenol blue, have an eccentric nucleus which is 5–8 μm in diameter and do not appear to be involved in coagulation. They may be similar to the cyst cells described in the spider, *P. canceriles*, by Deevey (1941) and to cystocytes in some insects (Ratcliffe and Price, 1974).

(5) Spherule cells—these are 15–21 μm in diameter with a nucleus of about 8 μm (Fig. 21). These cells characteristically contain refractile spherules about 1·5 μm in diameter. They are similar to spherule cells of some insects (Jones, 1962).

(6) Adipohaemocytes—these are large cells 40–45 μm long and about 20–22 μm wide (Fig. 22). They contain an eccentric nucleus about 6–8 μm in diameter. They also contain refractile globules of about 5 μm and spherules of about 2 μm. Some granules may also be present. Similar cells have been reported in insects (Jones, 1962).

The vacuolated plasmatocytes are regarded by Ravindranath (1974) to be possibly the same as the leberidocytes reported for spiders. Scorpion granular haemocytes are motile (Ravindranath, 1977). They are capable of forming vacuoles indicative of secretory activity and they undergo cytoplasmic fragmentation or clasmatosis (Ravindranath, 1977).

C. Origin and formation of haemocytes

Kollmann (1910) reported that the haemocytopoietic tissue in scorpions consists of a series of cell masses, presumably part of the lymphatic gland, that are attached to the nerve cord in the cephalothoracic and pre-abdomenal regions (Millot, 1949). The prohaemocytes may give rise to plasmatocytes, granular haemocytes, cystocytes and spherule cells (Ravindranath, 1977). Ravindranath (1974), did not note intermediate stages between the basic haemocyte types nor did he observe mitotic figures. These observations led him to suggest that differentiation of blood cells may not occur in the haemolymph of scorpions. He also suggested that each cell type may have a different cell lineage. Therefore, scorpions and spiders may differ in this respect.

D. Functions of haemocytes

Presumably, each type of scorpion haemocyte has functions similar to those described in spiders and in the horseshoe crab, but very little definitive information is available. Grégoire (1955) reported that he could detect no plasma transformations in blood samples obtained from scorpions. Nonetheless, the coagulation process is probably present in scorpions and presumably involves blood cells.

IV. Horseshoe crabs

A. Structure of the circulatory system

The heart is located mid-dorsally, just beneath the carapace and above the intestine (Patten, 1912). It begins near the eyes and extends posteriorly through the hinged region between the prosoma and opisthosoma; it ends near the middle of the abdomen. It is tubular in shape and held in position by suspensory ligaments. There are eight pairs of ostia located laterally, through which blood enters the heart from the pericardial sinus. The heartbeat is neurogenic and originates in the cardiac ganglion which is a thread-like cord that lies on the mid-dorsal surface of the heart.

Blood leaves the heart via eleven arteries. Three of these exit anteriorly, one from each lateral margin and one medially. Four pairs of arteries leave the heart laterally, one near each member of the anterior four pairs of functional ostia. The anterior medial artery (the frontal artery) carries blood to the anterior region of the cephalothorax. The other two anterior arteries (the aortic arches) curve ventrally and open into a vascular ring that forms a collar around the brain. From this vascular ring, blood may flow into the arteries that supply the appendages and nearby tissues or posteriorly through the ventral artery that forms a sheath around the ventral nerve cord. Of special note is the fact that the "ventral circulatory system" is perineural, in that it ensheaths the entire nervous system (Petrunkevitch, 1922).

The lateral arteries on each side of the heart empty into a collateral artery which gives off vessels to the lateral regions of the body as it courses longitudinally. The collateral arteries unite at a point mid-way in the abdomen to form the superior abdominal artery. This vessel supplies blood to the posterior region of the animal.

Arterial blood empties into large blood sinuses whereupon it is collected by a pair of large veins that extend longitudinally through the body. Branches of these veins carry the blood to the book-gills where it is oxygenated. It then flows into the pericardial sinus around the heart through five pairs of branchio-cardiac veins associated with the gill flaps (Shuster, 1978).

B. Structure and classification of haemocytes

Two basic types of haemocyte have been described in the blood of the horseshoe crab. These are the granular haemocytes, most often called the amoebocytes because of their motility, and the cyanocytes (Loeb, 1902;

Dumont *et al.*, 1966; Fahrenbach, 1970). Although the cyanocytes were found in horseshoe crab blood by Fahrenbach (1970), many recent workers still state mistakenly that the granular haemocyte is the only type of blood cell present.

Cyanocytes are observed only in small numbers in the general circulation of adult horseshoe crabs which may explain why they were not reported by earlier workers. They appear mostly in the blood sinuses associated with the compound eye, where they comprise 1–8 % of the circulating blood cells (Fahrenbach, 1970). They are more prevalent in the adult during moulting (Fahrenbach, 1970), and in the general circulation of embryonic horseshoe crabs (unpublished observation made independently by Daniel Gibson of Boston University and by the author).

Cyanocytes are characterized by the presence of vast numbers of ribosomes and aggregates of haemocyanin crystals (Figs 23, 24). They may extend up to 100 μm and be filled almost completely with haemocyanin crystals. These are liberated into the haemolymph by disruption of the cell (Fahrenbach, 1970).

Granular haemocytes are about 12 × 18 μm and are characterized by the presence of numerous dense granules (Fig. 25). These granules are ovoid and are about 0·5–1·5 μm in diameter. The cells display cytoplasmic extensions and are capable of undergoing extensive morphological changes (Dumont *et al.*, 1966). The cells should be termed granular haemocytes, rather than amoebocytes, to conform to terminology for other arthropods.

C. *Origin and formation of haemocytes*

Sites of haemocytopoiesis in the horseshoe crab are unknown. Fahrenbach (1970) suggests that cyanoblasts may arise in the hepatopancreas and then differentiate into mature cyanocytes. The site of formation of granular haemocytes is unknown. Loeb (1902) noted the presence of a small blood cell type with a thin film of protoplasm and pseudopodia. This cell might be a stem cell or perhaps a plasmatocyte, but this has not been confirmed.

Yeager and Tauber (1935) determined the total number of haemocytes present in *L. polyphemus* to be 30 000 per mm^3 for large adults and 14 600 mm^3 for small adults. These investigators found a mitotic index of less than 1 per 2000 haemocytes and, consequently, haemocyte production probably occurs in special haemocytopoietic tissue.

D. *Functions of haemocytes*

Cyanocytes synthesize haemocyanin (Fahrenbach, 1970) which is the blood respiratory pigment in horseshoe crabs (Redfield, 1934). The structure of haemocyanin has been studied extensively, but the details are beyond the scope of this chapter (see Levin, 1963; Fernandez-Morgan *et al.*, 1966).

The function of granular haemocytes has been fully investigated, beginning with the observations of Loeb (1902, 1903). These cells serve, in many ways, as the primary line of internal defence in the horseshoe crab (Cohen, 1979).

Granular haemocytes have the ability to detect bacterial endotoxin (Shirodkar *et al.*, 1960; Levin and Bang, 1964a; Stagner and Redmond, 1975), and to agglutinate several species of gram-negative bacteria (Bang, 1955; Pistole and Britko, 1978). They are capable of selectively killing certain

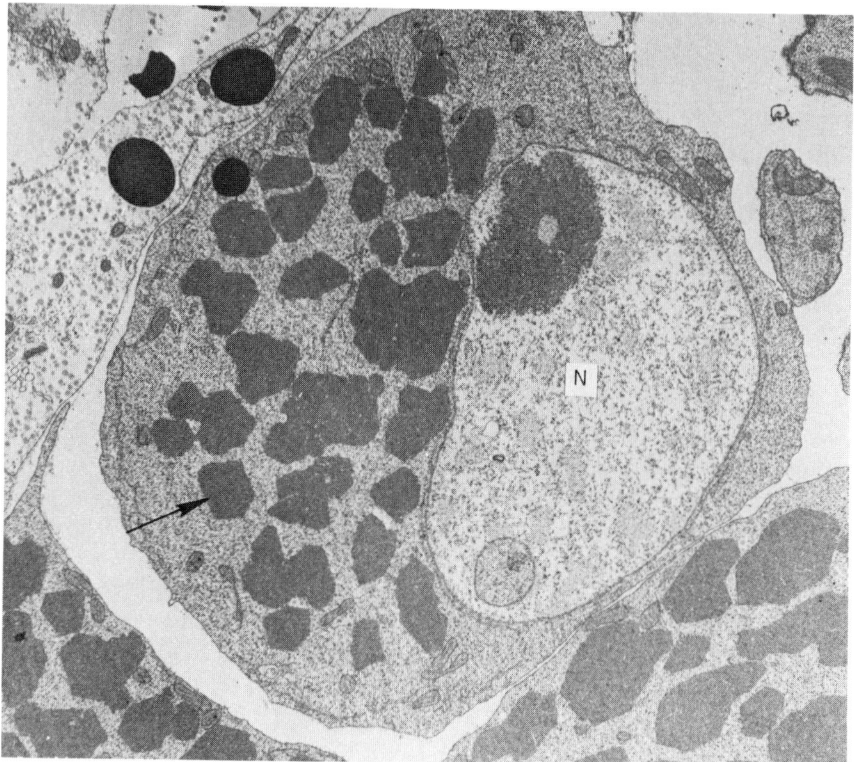

Fig. 23. Cyanocyte in the horseshoe crab *Limulus polyphemus*. This micrograph was obtained near the heart of an embryo about six-months-old. Note the aggregates of haemocyanin crystals (arrow). × 5250.

bacteria (Pistole and Britko, 1978; Nachum *et al.*, 1979) and are also involved in wound healing (Bursey, 1977).

The ability of granular haemocytes to form a clot in the presence of a very small amount of endotoxin, is the basis for a clinical test of endotoxin poisoning in humans (Levin and Bang, 1964a; Levin, 1967; Oberle *et al.*, 1974). However, some have questioned the usefulness of the *Limulus* lysate test in the diagnosis of endotoxaemia (Elin *et al.*, 1975). The potential of horseshoe crab blood extract as a biomedical resource has, however, received widespread recognition (Schofield, 1974; Pearson, 1978) and has simulated efforts to cultivate granular haemocytes *in vitro* (Pearson and Woodland, 1979). Furthermore, studies are underway on embryonic horseshoe crabs in an attempt to exploit them as a model biological system for the study of diseases (Bang, 1979).

There appears to be two main phases in the coagulation of horseshoe crab blood. The first is cellular clumping and the second is coagulation of the plasma (Levin and Bang, 1964b). The clumping of granular haemocytes presumably involves their ability to extend pseudopodia. Recent studies have utilized the motile abilities of the granular haemocytes for investigations of contact paralysis of pseudopodial activity (Armstrong, 1977).

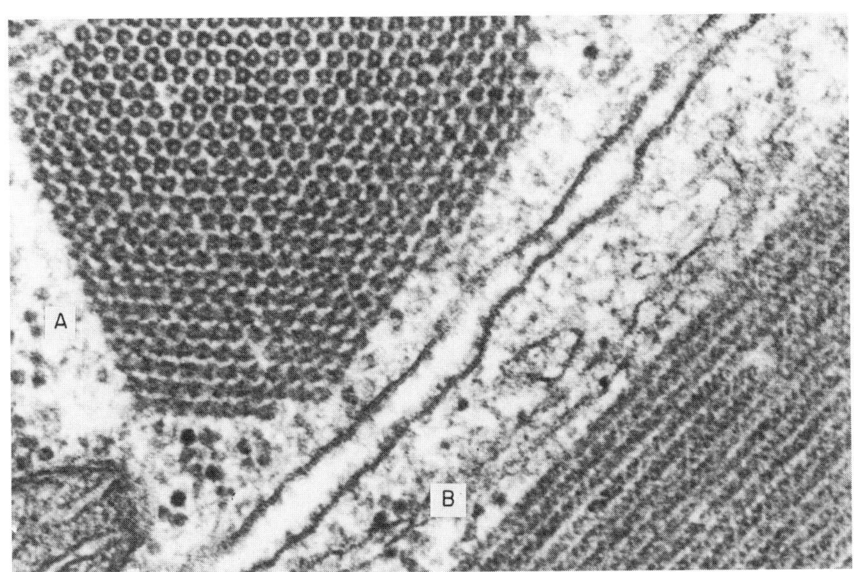

Fig. 24. A portion of two adjacent cyanocytes in *L. polyphemus* showing haemocyanin crystals in transverse view (cell A) and longitudinal view (cell B). ×86 400.

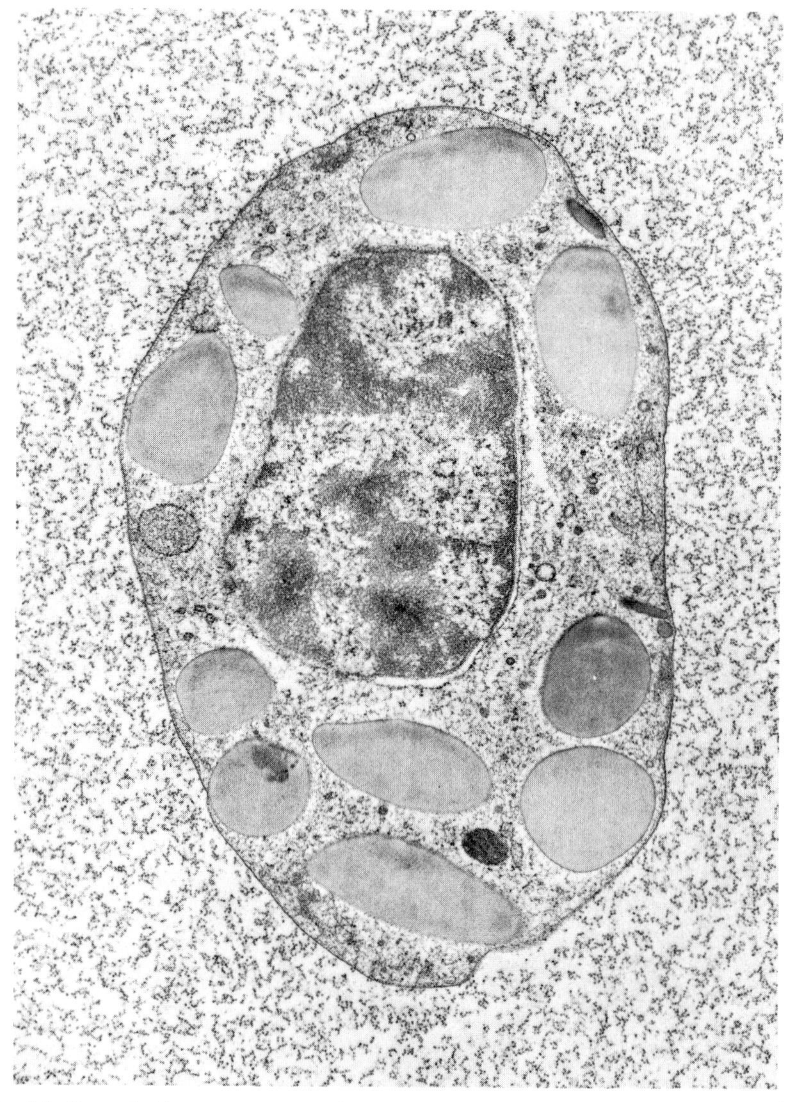

Fig. 25. Granular haemocyte (amoebocyte) in a *L. polyphemus* adult. Note the large granules in the cytoplasm. Haemocyanin free in the extracellular space is obvious around the cell. (Courtesy of R. L. Ornberg). $\times$ 19 000.

The ability of horseshoe crab blood to coagulate requires the presence of clottable proteins, the so-called coagulogens. Loeb's earlier studies (1902, 1903) indicated that these factors reside in the granular haemocytes. Subsequently, coagulogens present in granular haemocytes have been reported by several investigators (Levin and Bang, 1968; Solum, 1970a,b; Shishikura and Sekiguchi, 1978). Mürer *et al.* (1975) showed that the dense granules contain all of the factors required for the coagulation of blood, including the clottable proteins. This intracellularly located coagulation system is released when the cell undergoes degranulation (Dumont *et al.*, 1966; Solum, 1970b), whereupon it is enzymatically activated (Young *et al.*, 1972; Solum, 1973). The process of degranulation involves exocytosis which has been described recently by Ornberg and Reese (1978).

Clottable protein has also been localized in the cytoplasmic matrix of the granular haemocytes in the Japanese horseshoe crab, *Tachypleus tridentatus* (Shishikura *et al.*, 1977). Using a fluorescent antibody procedure, coagulogens were localized in the dense granules of only 15% of the granular haemocytes. In the remaining 85%, the coagulogens were localized free in the cytoplasm.

Finally, although much attention has been paid to the ability of horseshoe crab haemocytes to clot in response to endotoxin, the ability of these cells to ingest invading microorganisms is a subject of some dispute. Recently, however, Armstrong and Levin (1979) have shown conclusively that *Limulus polyphemus* blood cells are capable of phagocytosis and that this process occurs most efficiently in the absence of endotoxin. As a result, these authors postulate that the coagulation response deals with gram-negative bacteria while other foreign invaders are entrapped by phagocytosis.

V. Summary and concluding remarks

The present state of our knowledge of the basic types of blood cell that occur in three of the main chelicerate arthropod groups is shown in Table IV. The horseshoe crab contains the fewest number of basic cell types. However, the stem cell type or types have yet to be discovered for this animal. Furthermore, the fact that the plasmatocyte appears to be the first cell that differentiates from prohaemocytes in the spider and scorpion implies that a plasmatocyte-type cell may well be present in the horseshoe crab. On the other hand, it may be that the granular haemocyte differentiates directly from the basic stem cell in the horseshoe crab, by-passing the plasmatocyte stage in differentiation. Perhaps prohaemocytes will be found in the horseshoe crab once the location of haemocytopoiesis is discovered.

All three animal groups contain granular haemocytes. Cyanocytes have been found in spiders and horseshoe crabs and are presumably present in scorpions although this has yet to be reported. The finding that scorpions contain three basic cell types, not definitely shown to be present in spiders, is somewhat surprising. These cells, the cystocytes, spherule cells and adipohaemocytes, have been reported for some insects and eventually may be located in spiders. Furthermore, no electron microscopic studies have been conducted of scorpion blood cells and the studies that have been made have utilized blood removed from animals prior to fixation. Examination of scorpion blood cells should be undertaken in which the cells are fixed *in vivo*, as it is apparent from extensive studies on horseshoe crab granular haemocytes that unfixed blood cells may undergo tremendous morphological changes. Combined light and electron microscopical studies are also needed of both spider and scorpion blood cells in combination with cytochemical techniques. Furthermore, these studies should be conducted on animals in different physiological states such as during embryonic development and moulting.

TABLE IV. Basic types of haemocyte present in three chelicerate arthropods.

Cell type	Spiders	Scorpions	Horseshoe crabs
Prohaemocyte	x	x	—[a]
Plasmatocyte	x	x	—[a]
Granular haemocyte	x	x	x
Leberidocyte	x	—	—
Cyanocyte	x	—[b]	x
Cystocyte	?[c]	x	—
Spherule cell	—	x	—
Adipohaemocyte	—	x	—
Oenocytoid	x	—	—

[a] Likely to be present in horseshoe crabs, but not confirmed as yet.

[b] Likely to be present in scorpions, but not reported as yet.

[c] Deevey (1941) and Wagner (1888) reported a cell in spiders that may be a cystocyte.

Finally, it is unfortunate that most of the studies of blood cells conducted on chelicerate arthropods have involved only the spiders, scorpions and horseshoe crab. There are many other interesting chelicerates which must be examined if one is to ultimately gain the desired understanding of chelicerate blood cells.

Acknowledgements

The author expresses his appreciation to Prof. K. A. Seitz and Drs D. Gibson, W. H. Fahrenbach, H. Jensen, B. Midttun, R. L. Ornberg and M. H. Ravindranath for their assistance. Drs F. B. Bang and F. C. Pearson kindly provided copies of their unpublished manuscripts. Miss Krista McMullen provided expert assistance in the translation of articles into English. This article is dedicated to the late Frederick Lang.

References

Armstrong, P. B. (1977). *Exp. Cell Res.* **107**, 127–138.
Armstrong, P. B. and Levin, J. (1979). *J. Invertebr. Pathol.* **34**, 145–151.
Bang, F. B. (1955). *Bull. Johns Hopkins Hosp.* **98**, 325–337.
Bang, F. B. (1979). *In* "Biomedical Applications of the Horseshoe Crab (Limulidae)" (E. Cohen, Ed.). Alan R. Liss, Inc., New York.
Boyd, W. C. (1937). *Biol. Bull., Woods Hole* **73**, 181–183.
Browning, H. C. (1942). *Proc. Roy. Soc. Lond. B* **131**, 65–86.
Bursey, C. R. (1977). *Can. J. Zool.* **55**, 1158–1165.
Bursey, C. R. and Sherman, R. G. (1970). *Comp. Gen. Pharm.* **1**, 160–170.
Cohen, E. (1979). "Biomedical Applications of the Horseshoe Crab (Limulidae)". Alan R. Liss, Inc., New York.
Deevey, G. B. (1941). *J. Morph.* **68**, 457–491.
Dumont, J. N., Anderson, E. and Winner, G. (1966). *J. Morph.* **119**, 181–208.
Elin, R. J., Robinson, R. A., Levine, A. S. and Wolff, S. M. (1975). *New Eng. J. Med.* **293**, 521–524.
Fahrenbach, W. H. (1970). *J. Cell Biol.* **44**, 445–453.
Fernandez-Moran, H., VanBruggen, E. F. G. and Ohtsuki, M. (1966). *J. molec. Biol.* **16**, 191–207.
Franz, V. (1904). *Zool. Anz.* **27**, 192–204.
Grégoire, Ch. (1952). *Arch. Int. Physiol.* **60**, 100–102.
Grégoire, Ch. (1955). *Arch. Biol., Paris* **66**, 489–508.
Jones, J. C. (1962). *Amer. Zool.* **2**, 209–246.
Kollmann, M. (1908). *Am. Sci. Nat. Zool.* **8**, 1–238.
Kollmann, M. (1910). *Bull. Soc. Zool., France* **35**, 25–30.
Levin, J. (1967). *Fed. Proc.* **26**, 1707–1712.
Levin, J. and Bang, F. B. (1964a). *Bull. Johns Hopkins Hosp.* **115**, 265–274.
Levin, J. and Bang, F. B. (1964b). *Bull. Johns Hopkins Hosp.* **115**, 337–345.
Levin, J. and Bang, F. B. (1968). *Thrombos. Diathes. Haemorrh.* **19**, 186–197.
Levin, O. (1963). *Arkiv Kemi* **21**, 29–35.
Loeb, L. (1902). *J. Med. Res.* **7**, 145–158.
Loeb, L. (1903). *Biol. Bull., Woods Hole* **4**, 301–318.
Midttun, B. and Jensen, H. (1978). *Acta Zool. (Stockh.)* **59**, 157–167.
Millot, J. (1949). *In* "Traite de Zoologie" (P. Grasse, Ed.), Vol. VI, pp. 639–646. Masson et Cie, Paris.
Mürer, E. H., Levin, J. and Holme, R. (1975). *J. Cell Physiol.* **86**, 533–542.
Nachum, R., Watson, S. N., Sullivan, J. D. Jr. and Siegel, S. E. (1979). *J. Invertebr. Pathol.* **33**, 290–299.

Oberle, M. W., Graham, G. G. and Levin, J. (1974). *J. Pediatr.* **85**, 570–573.
Ornberg, R. L. and Reese, T. S. (1978). *Biol. Bull., Woods Hole* **155**, 460.
Patten, W. (1912). "The Evolution of the Vertebrates and Their Kin." P. Blakiston's Sons and Co., Philadelphia.
Pearson, F. C. (1978). *The Maritimes* **22**, 4–6.
Pearson, F. C. and Woodland, E. (1979). *In* "Biomedical Applications of the Horseshoe Crab (Limulidae)" (E. Cohen, Ed.). Alan R. Liss, Inc., New York.
Petrunkevitch, A. (1922). *J. Morph.* **36**, 157–189.
Petrunkevitch, A. (1933). *Trans. Connect. Acad. Arts Sci.* **31**, 299–389.
Pistole, T. G. and Britko, J. L. (1978). *J. Invertebr. Pathol.* **31**, 376–382.
Randall, W. C. (1966). *J. Morph.* **119**, 161–180.
Ratcliffe, N. A. and Price, C. D. (1974). *J. Morph.* **144**, 485–498.
Ravindranath, M. H. (1974). *J. Morph.* **144**, 1–10.
Ravindranath, M. H. (1977). *Cytologia* **42**, 743–751.
Redfield, A. C. (1934). *Biol. Rev.* (*Cambridge*) **9**, 175–212.
Schofield, M. (1974). *Woods Hole Notes* **6**, 1–4.
Seitz, K.-A. (1972a). *Zool. Jb. Anat.* **89**, 351–384.
Seitz, K.-A. (1972b). *Zool. Jb. Anat.* **89**, 385–397.
Sherman, R. G. (1973). *Can. J. Zool.* **51**, 1155–1159.
Shirodkar, M. U., Warwick, A. and Bang, F. B. (1960). *Biol. Bull., Woods Hole* **118**, 324–337.
Shishikura, F. and Sekiguchi, K. (1978). *J. exp. Zool.* **206**, 241–246.
Shishikura, F., Chiba, J. and Sekiguchi, K. (1977). *J. exp. Zool.* **201**, 303–308.
Shuster, C. N., Jr. (1978). "The Circulatory System and Blood of the Horseshoe Crab." Report #14, U.S. Dept. Energy, Fed. Energy Reg. Comm., Washington, D.C.
Solum, N. O. (1970a). *Thrombos. Diathes. Haemorrh.* **23**, 170–181.
Solum, N. O. (1970b). *Symp. Zool. Soc. Lond.* **27**, 207–216.
Solum, N. O. (1973). *Thrombos. Res.* **2**, 55–70.
Stagner, J. I. and Redmond, J. R. (1975). *Mar. Fish. Rev.* **37**, 11–19.
Wagner, W. (1888). *Ann. Sci. Nat. Zool.* **6**, 280–389.
Yeager, J. F. and Tauber, O. E. (1935). *Biol. Bull., Woods Hole* **69**, 66–70.
Young, N. S., Levin, F. and Prendergast, R. A. (1972). *J. Clin. Invest.* **51**, 1790–1797.

12. Crustaceans

A. G. BAUCHAU

Département de Biologie Animale, Facultés Universitaires de Namur, Belgium

---

I. Introduction

Crustacea, like other arthropods, have an open vascular system. For this reason, the blood has properly been called haemolymph. Accordingly, the numerous blood cells carried by the circulatory fluid should be termed haemocytes instead of leucocytes or lymphocytes so as to prevent any confusion with particular blood cells of vertebrates.

As early as 1824, crustacean haemocytes were described by Carus and ever since have been studied along two main lines of investigation: the first has been directed toward the characterization of different morphological types of cells while the other has sought to determine their particular role in blood clotting. Considerable progress is now also being made in crustacean pathology and immunology. Since an open circulatory system is more susceptible to repeated intrusions from the surrounding environment, interest in haemocytes has been revived and enlarged because of their implication in wound-repair and defence mechanisms against parasites like fungi, viruses, rickettsiae, bacteria, protozoa, helminths and even other crustaceans. (Vago, 1966; Sawyer, 1969; Rabin, 1970; Bonami *et al.*, 1971; Vivares, 1972–73; Kellog *et al.*, 1974; Nyhlen and Unestam, 1975; Johnson, 1977a,b).

The aim of the present chapter is to offer an overview of the rapidly expanding field of research on crustacean haemocyte structure and functions.

II. Structure of the circulatory system

The crustacean heart develops from a dorsal blood vessel. In most entomostracans and lower malacostracans, it is still a long and slender tube with a single muscle layer and paired lateral ostia. However, in more advanced malacostracans, the heart differentiates as a short but large pentagonal chamber, dorsally located in the thorax above the respiratory organs which supply the oxygenated haemolymph. The walls are thickened by several layers of crossing muscle strands. It is suspended in a pericardial space by means of fibrous ligaments with a short band of muscle fibres attached to their outer extremities so as to secure diastolic relaxation (Fig. 1).

Elastic but non-muscular arteries leave the heart. They have valves which prevent the blood from flowing back into the cardiac cavity. They penetrate the pericardial membrane and after a variable number of branching processes deliver the haemolymph to irregular spaces or *sinuses*, scattered throughout the body. An exchange of substances then takes place between the circulatory fluid and the surrounding tissues and organs. The network of venous sinuses, typically bounded by a membrane, drains all the blood to a median ventral sinus from which it flows into the gills. Efferent branchio-cardiac veins bring it back to the pericardium by means of three wide non-valved openings. The blood enters the heart through three pairs of valved ostia and is expelled again into the arteries.

Current evidence indicates that most crustacean hearts have a pacemaker ganglion although in primitive forms they seem to be myogenic.

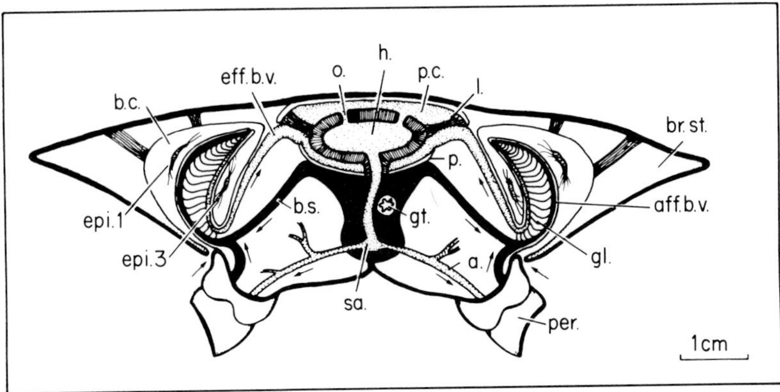

Fig. 1. Diagrammatic transverse section through the thorax of the crab *Carcinus maenas* to show the blood circulation system. Arrows indicate direction of blood flow. a, artery; aff.b.v, afferent branchial vessel; b.c, branchial chamber; br.st, branchiostegite; b.s, branchial sinus; eff.b.v, efferent branchial vessel; epi. 1, epipodite of 1st maxilliped; epi. 3, epipodite of 3rd maxilliped; gl, gill; gt, gut; h, heart; l, suspensory ligament; o, ostium; p, pericardium; p.c, pericardial cavity; per, pereiopod; s.a, sternal artery.

III. Structure and classification of haemocytes

Several attempts made in the past to establish a convenient classification of haemocytes have resulted in a state of confusion in the literature. These attempts were unsuccessful for two principal reasons. The first stems from a lack of logical guidelines in classification schemes. When some categories are defined on pure morphological criteria while others are derived from functional properties, resulting nomenclatures are not founded on sound rational. A lack of sufficient caution in sampling procedures has been a second reason contributing to the discrepancies in haemocyte classification. Haemocytes are very reactive cells which undergo considerable transformations when removed from the haemocoel. Cell shape, in particular, is so labile that it cannot be accepted as a valid distinctive feature.

More recent classifications have tried to overcome these shortcomings. A large number of anticoagulants have been used to preserve the cells in their native state. The best ones available seem to be EDTA (although effective for a few hours only) and *N*-ethyl-maleimide. When histological studies are carried out, rapid and effective fixation has been shown to be imperative. The next logical and practical steps are to define morphological types at both the light and electron microscope levels, to further characterize them biochemically and, subsequently, to investigate their physiological properties.

TABLE I. Haemocyte types

Type	Shape	Nucleus	Endoplasmic reticulum	Free ribosomes	Golgi	Granules
Hyaline cell	round to oval	central, round and large	smooth, rough and scarce	present	0 or 1	0 or few
Semi-granular cell	oval to spindle-shaped	central or eccentric, oval and lobed	smooth, rough and abundant	abundant	1 or more	moderate
Granulocyte	oval	eccentric and kidney-shaped	smooth, rough and moderate	moderate	0 or 1	abundant

Although under different names, at least three broad classes of haemocytes have been recognized (described below) by a variety of authors from examinations of wet mounts and/or histological and thin sections. Whenever sufficient details are provided, some synonymous haemocyte terms are suggested as in Table I. Cell sizes vary with species as shown in Table II; granule sizes change too according to cell types and species (Table III).

Hyaline cells (Figs 2, 3, 4) are the smallest of the cell types, with a large, central nucleus, surrounded by a generally basophilic cytoplasmic fringe. The cytoplasm contains scarce endoplasmic reticulum, free ribosomes, one or no Golgi and none or few small, round, membrane-bound granules. In

Lysosomes	Mitochondria	Synonyms—authors
	moderate	pale amoeboïd cell (Halliburton, 1885) amibocyte hyaline (Cuénot, 1891) explosive corpuscle (Hardy, 1892) hyaline thigmocyte (Tait and Gunn, 1918) hyaline lymphoid cell (George and Nichols, 1948) leucocyte hyalin (Arvy, 1952) lymphoïd cell (Toney, 1958) hyaline cell (Wood and Visentin, 1967; Bauchau and De Brouwer, 1972; Bodammer, 1978) gerinnungszellen (Stang-Voss, 1971) prohaemocyte (Ravindranath, 1974) prohyalocyte (Cornick and Stewart, 1978) phagocytic cell (Smith and Ratcliffe, 1978)
present	abundant	thigmotactic amebocyte (George and Nichols, 1948) monocyte (Toney, 1958) phagocytierende amöbocyten (Stang-Voss, 1971) small granulocyte (Wood and Visentin, 1967) semi-granular (Bauchau and De Brouwer, 1972) hyalocyte (Cornick and Stewart, 1978) intermediate cell (Bodammer, 1978)
present	abundant	eosinophilic corpuscle (Hardy, 1892) acidophilic granule cell (George and Nichols, 1948) explosive refractile granulocyte (Toney, 1958) eosinophil, ovoid and spindular basophil (Hearing and Vernick, 1967) large granulocyte (Wood and Visentin, 1967) granulären amöbocyte (Stang-Voss, 1971) granulocyte (Bauchau and De Brouwer, 1972) granulocyte, plasmatocyte, cystocyte (Ravindranath, 1974) eosinophilic granulocyte (Cornick and Stewart, 1978) refractile cell (Smith and Ratcliffe, 1978)

TABLE II. Haemocyte size (in μm).

Species	Hyaline	Semi-granular	Granulocyte	Lipo-protein	Authors
			Cell types		
Helleria brevicornis	5–6	11–12	11–13		Hoarau (1976)
Orconectes virilis	7–10	9–18	18–35		Wood and Visentin (1967)
Astacus astacus	max. 30	max. 30	max. 50		Stang-Voss (1971)
Cambarus bartoni	8–11	7–9	15–18		Toney (1958)
Homarus americanus	11–13	7–10·8	16·8–25·2		Toney (1958)
			7·3–13·9 (eosinophil) 8·4–11·5 (ovoid basophil) 9·3–14·4 (spindular basophil)		Hearing and Vernick (1967)
	8·4–8·5	8·6–20·9	9·1–24·8		Cornick and Stewart (1978)
Callinectes sapidus	6–7	6–7	14–14		Toney (1958)
	7–13	13·5–19·5	13·4–15·7		Bodammer (1978)
Carcinus maenas	5–6		10–12		Johnston *et al.* (1973)
	7	7	8–10	30–45	Sewell (1955)
			10–15		Chassard-Bouchaud and Hubert (1975)
Carcinus mediterraneus	6–7		10–13		Durand (1973)
Eriocheir sinensis	6–8		13–18	45	Bauchau and De Brouwer (1972)
Pachygrapsus marmoratus	6·5–10	8–13	15		Arvy (1952)
	6–7		8–12		Charmantier (1971)
Macropipus depurator	4·5–6	6–7	7–10		Durand (1973)

TABLE III. Granule size (in μm).

Species	Hyaline	Semi-granular	Granulocyte	Authors
Helleria brevicornis		0·2–1·2	max. 1·5	Hoarau (1976)
Astacus astacus	0·1–0·5		max. 3	Stang-Voss (1971)
Cambarus bartoni			2	Toney (1958)
Homarus americanus			1	Toney (1958)
			0·53–0·74	Hearing and Vernick (1967)
Callinectes sapidus			0·7	Toney (1958)
	0·13–0·55	0·15–0·63	0·33–1·4	Bodammer (1978)
Carcinus maenas			0·1–1	Chassard-Bouchard and Hubert (1975)
Carcinus mediterraneus			0·8–1	Durand (1973)
Eriocheir sinensis	0·2–0·5	0·2–1·5	0·3–2·6 max. 4	Bauchau and De Brouwer (1972)
Pachygrapsus marmoratus			max. 1·5	Arvy (1952)
Macropipus depurator			0·8	Durand (1973)

wet, unfixed preparations, these cells readily exhibit pseudopodial extensions.

Granulocytes (Figs 2, 5, 6) are the largest cells with small, eccentric, kidney-shaped nuclei. A Golgi is present most of the time. A dominant rough as well as a smooth endoplasmic reticulum are restricted to around the nucleus and along the cell border. Free ribosomes are scattered in a cytoplasm literally filled with large, membrane-bound granules. These are electron-dense and usually strongly acidophilic while the cytoplasm is basophilic. Granulocytes of *Homarus americanus* have been divided into eosinophils and ovoid or spindular basophils by Hearing and Vernick (1967). Cornick and Stewart (1978), working on the same species, found mostly eosinophils (Table I); they mentioned a chromophobic granulocyte whose granules did not stain or were only faintly basophilic, even though these two categories looked exactly the same in wet mounts. Comparable variations have often been recorded and related to age or functional alterations, with little evidence upon which to base such an assumption (Wood and Visentin, 1967).

Semi-granular cells (Figs 2, 7, 8) as described by Bauchau and De Brouwer (1972), are an intermediate cell type between the two cell types described above. They are intermediate in size between hyaline cells and granulocytes and have a central or eccentric, spherical or lobed, nucleus which is smaller than that of the hyaline cell but larger than the nucleus from a granulocyte. They also contain free ribosomes, smooth and rough endoplasmic reticulum, more developed than in the two other types, and two or more Golgi producing a fairly large number of eosinophilic granules which are sparsely dispersed in the cytoplasm. In general, the granules have an opaque homogeneous texture but some are heterogeneous and may even contain many tubular or microfibrillar aligned formations, myelin bodies and phagosomes also occur and represent secondary lysosomes.

These three main types apparently form a continuous differentiation series with many intermediate forms. A regularly decreasing nucleo-cytoplasmic ratio as well as an increasing number of granules argue in favour of this hypothesis. This concept was first proposed by Cuénot (1891) and has been generally supported by subsequent work (Bruntz, 1907; Arvy, 1952; Wood and Visentin, 1967; Charmantier, 1971; Stang-Voss, 1971; Bauchau and De Brouwer, 1972; Gibert, 1972; Hoarau, 1976; Bodammer, 1978).

An ingenious reverse evolution series, however, has been recently advanced by Vranckx and Durliat (1977). Granulocytes would be the only native circulating cell type and, because of their extreme lability, any particular stress (as in removal from the haemocoel) would readily initiate a degranulation process, giving rise to a population of semi-granular and finally hyaline cells. This interpretation is in agreement with the work of

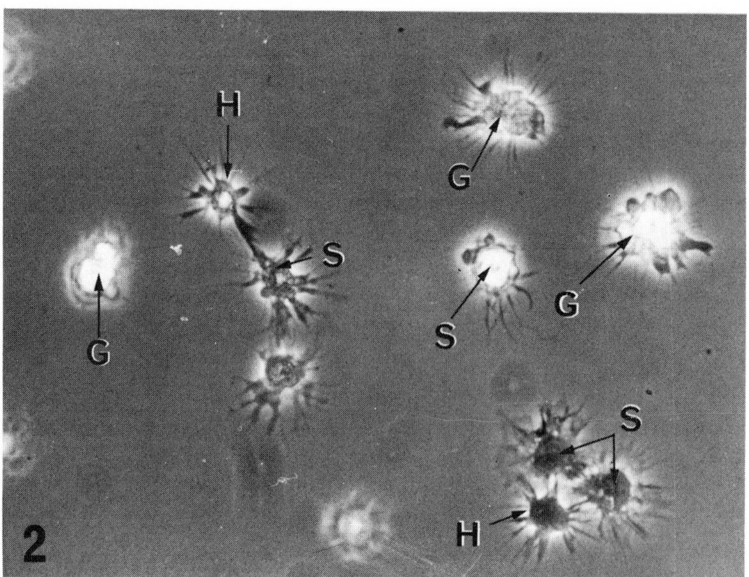

Fig. 2. The three haemocyte types of *Eriocheir sinensis* sending out pseudopods and forming clusters of cells, 5 min after their deposition on a glass plate. H, hyaline cell; G, granulocyte; S, semi-granular cell. Phase contrast ×400.

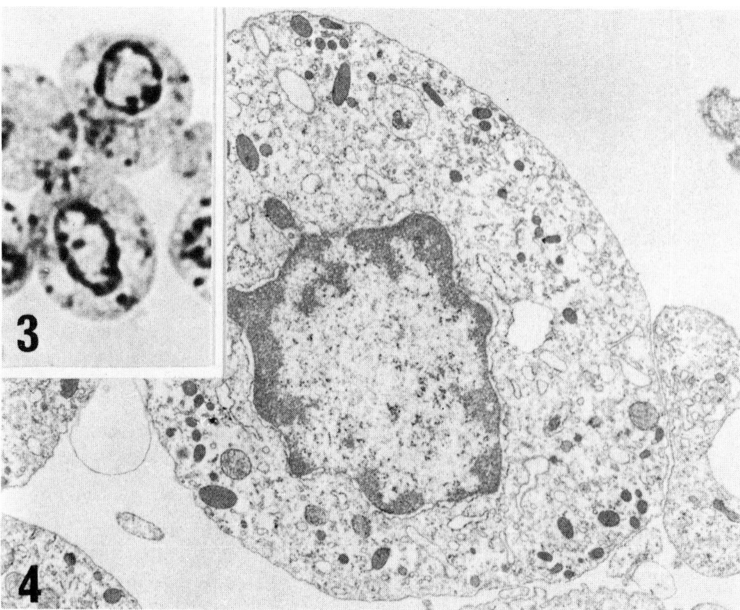

Fig. 3. Hyaline cells of *E. sinensis* typically with some small granules scattered in the cytoplasm. ×2000.
Fig. 4. Hyaline cell of *E. sinensis*. ×9400.

Lochhead and Lochhead (1941) who found only granulocytes in the haemolymph of *Artemia salina*. Moreover, all cell types of *Homarus americanus* and *Astacus astacus* as described, respectively, by Hearing and Vernick (1967) and Stang-Voss (1971) have a definite number of granules. This hypothesis, however, needs further substantiation. A few specific points may, however, briefly be stated: would an advanced stage of degranulation be followed by cell decay? Hyaline cells could hardly be considered as decaying, as their high nucleo-cytoplasmic ratio is normally associated with young cellular stages and their nuclear ultrastructure has a perfectly regular outline, in sharp contrast to degenerating nuclei of known degranulated granulocytes (compare Figs 3, 4 with Fig. 22). Furthermore, semi-granular cells are characterized by their Golgi bodies, responsible for granule production; this seems rather strange in a degranulation hypothesis unless degranulated granulocytes are assumed to recover and readily resume the production of new granules. Such an assumption, however, has yet to be proven. Finally, hyaline cells have shown to be discharged from

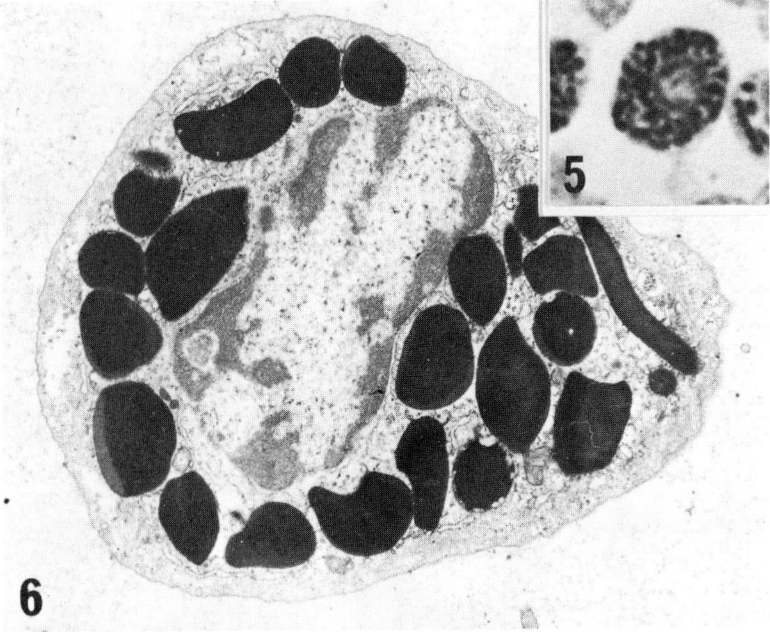

Fig. 5. Granulocyte of *E. sinensis* packed with large granules. ×1000.
Fig. 6. Granulocyte of *E. sinensis*. Note large granules of different shapes which are electron-dense. ×10 500.

haemopoietic nodules (Ghiretti-Magaldi *et al.*, 1977) suggesting that they are the basic cells from which the other types develop.

Other proposed nomenclatures are briefly discussed. Johnston *et al.* (1973) divided *Carcinus maenas* haemocytes into two morphological series called α- and β-cells. The growth series of α-cells may easily be considered as equal to the three basic types mentioned above. The poorly described β-cells, however, are somewhat obscure. They were seldom observed intact and could not be identified under the electron microscope. They could possibly be related to a final mature stage of granulocytes which are known to be very labile.

Ravindranath (1974) tried to extend to Crustacea the classification scheme proposed by Jones (1962) for insects. Seven haemocyte types were recorded in *Ligia exotica*. The first one, prohaemocytes of hyaline cells, was further subdivided into five subclasses, depending on a central or eccentric nucleus and on particular staining affinities. A few selected criteria (location of nucleus, staining of cytoplasm and granules, kinds of granules)

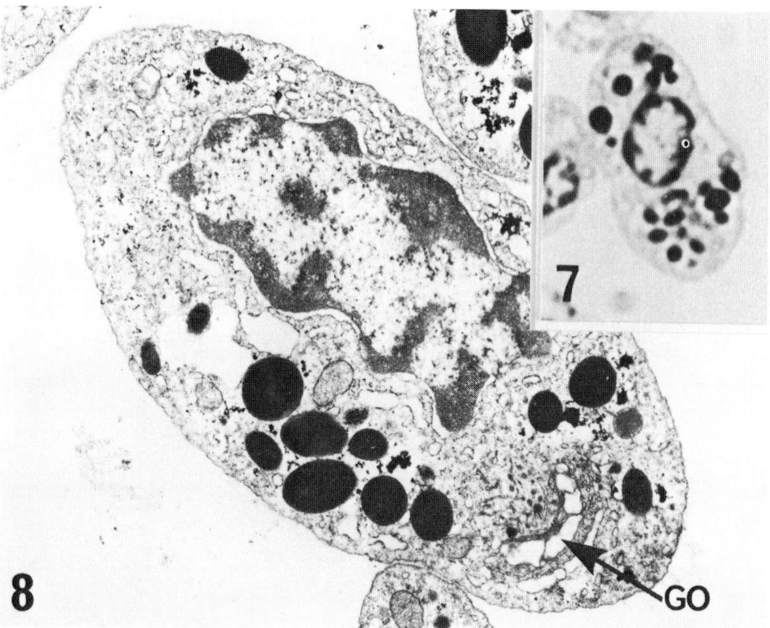

Fig. 7. Semi-granular cell of *E. sinensis* with granules dispersed in the cytoplasm. × 2000.

Fig. 8. Semi-granular cell of *E. sinensis* with granules of different sizes produced by a Golgi complex (GO) × 11 900.

served to distinguish the six other types: plasmatocytes, granulocytes, cystocytes, oenocytoids, spherule cells and adipohaemocytes. Whether or not these classes are sufficiently characteristic to be valid in other groups of Crustacea remains an open question. Ravindranath (1977a) himself finds it difficult to separate plasmatocytes from granulocytes in *L. oceanica* and *Emerita asiatica* and considers that plasmatocytes and cystocytes are "modified versions of granulocytes", which could readily be produced by alterations in the hydrogen ion concentration (Ravindranath, 1975, 1977b). In that case, one wonders why they should not belong to a basic class of granulocytes.

Besides the three main types of haemocytes mentioned earlier, one or more of the following have been identified in some Crustacea by a few carcinologists:

Lipo-protein cells were found by Sewell (1955) in *C. maenas*. They are larger but originate from hyaline or semi-granular cells. One vacuole gradually increases in size, confining the cytoplasm to the periphery and displacing a flattened nucleus to one corner. A fine granular lipo-proteinaceous material aggregates into dense refractile bodies (2–12 µm). This kind of cell appears in large numbers towards the end of the C_4 stage, as defined by Drach (1939) and Drach and Tchernigovtseff (1967). They are attached below the epidermis during the D stages and disappear completely after ecdysis (B stages). They seem to be responsible for the secretion of the non-chitinous epicuticle, prior to moulting. A comparable cell has been found in females of *Eriocheir sinensis* (Fig. 9), prior to egg-laying (Bauchau and De Brouwer, 1972) and could possibly be the same as the adiop-haemocytes of *L. oceanica* (Ravindranath, 1974).

According to Vranckx and Durliat (1977), it is not a true haemocyte but rather a fat body cell entering the circulation in its final maturation stage.

Cyanocyte is the name given by Fahrenbach (1970) to blood-cells of *Limulus polyphemus*, which synthesize and store haemocyanin as crystalline cytoplasmic bodies. Ghiretti-Magaldi *et al.* (1973) noticed a positive immunoreaction for haemocyanin in some granulocytes of *C. maenas*. The proteinaceous material is confined in granules, which in many instances contain a crystalline substructure. As with all other blood cells, the cyanocytes stem from haemoblasts and leave the haemopoietic organ (see section on origin and formation of haemocytes, below). However, they do not really enter into the circulation but become attached to connective tissue strands surrounding the ophthalmic artery, the fore-gut and the caecae of the hepatopancreas. Typical cyanocytes thus complete their differentiation in close connection with mesodermal structures. One or more compact granules of haemocyanin increase in size and progressively invade the whole cytoplasm (Figs 10, 11). Ultimately the nucleus becomes pycnotic while

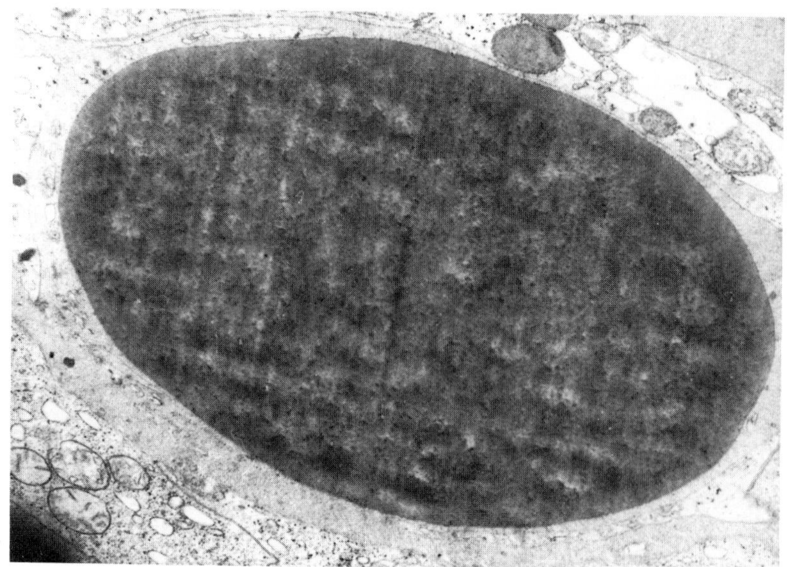

Fig. 9. Lipo-protein cell of *E. sinensis* with one large lipo-proteinaceous body. ×11 500.

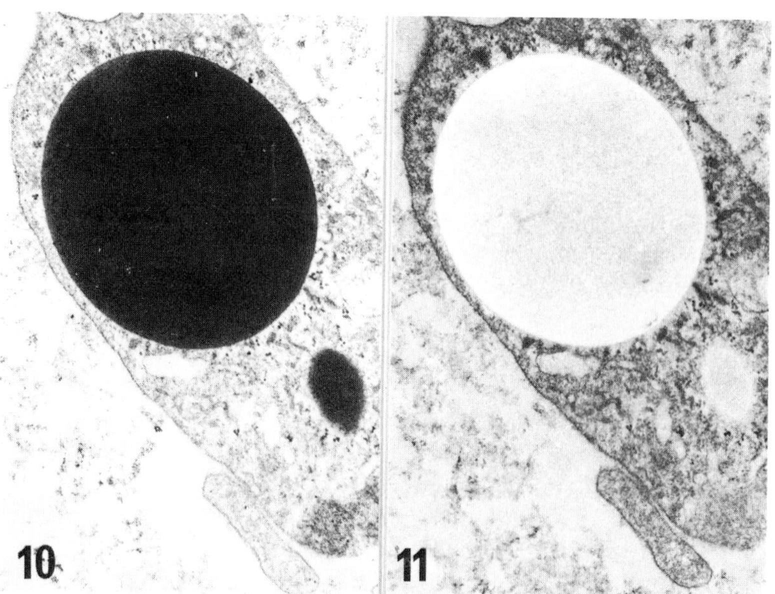

Fig. 10. Circulating cyanocyte of *E. sinensis* with one large granule of haemocyanin. ×19 500.

Fig. 11. The same cyanocyte as in Fig. 10 after treatment with pepsin. The proteinaceous content of the granule has been entirely digested. ×19 500.

mitochondria and other organelles are removed through autophagy. Once the plasma membrane is broken, haemocyanin is released into the blood by a kind of holocrine secretion (Ghiretti-Magaldi *et al.*, 1977).

Other data may be mentioned here because they indicate that at least some circulating granulocytes are still capable of haemocyanin synthesis. Stang-Voss (1971) detected the presence of copper in the granulocytes from *A. astacus* and Durliat and Vranckx (1976a) identified by electrophoresis and immunoelectrophoresis haemocyanin as one of the three soluble proteins in haemocyte homogenates. Likewise, Mengeot *et al.* (1977) recognized by electrophoresis different bands of cupro-proteins in isolated granule homogenates from the lobster, *Homarus vulgaris*. These cupro-proteins are probably some form of haemocyanin (Martin *et al.*, 1977). Furthermore, paracrystalline bodies were found in some granulocytes of *E. sinensis* (Fig. 12). (Bauchau and De Brouwer, 1972) and of *C. maenas* (Chassard-Bouchaud and Hubert, 1975). These observations make circulating granulocytes plausible candidates for the synthesis of haemocyanin. Whether all or only some of them are capable of this particular metabolism awaits further research.

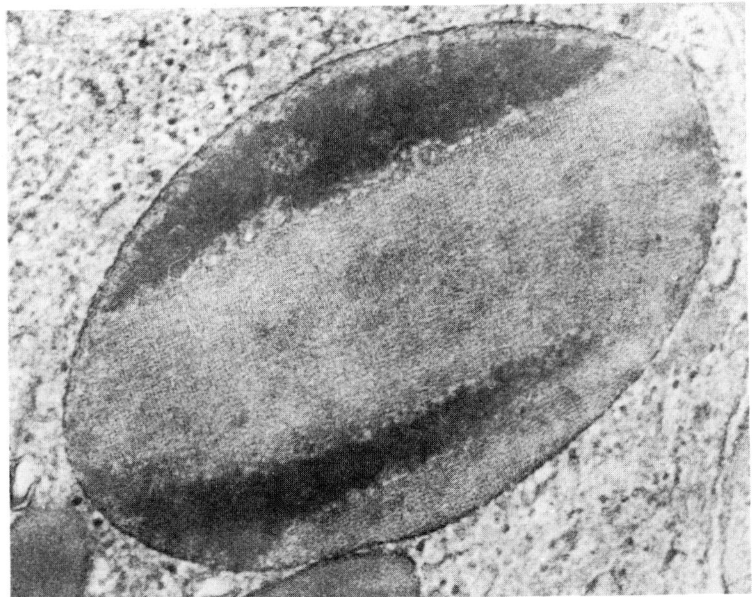

Fig. 12. Granule of *E. sinensis* granulocyte with a paracrystalline formation in its centre and on one side, flanked with electron-dense amorphous material. × 32 700.

IV. Cytochemical analysis of haemocytes

The structural analysis of cell types may be substantially complemented by cytochemical examination. Unfortunately, much of the available data comes from weakly specific staining tests which do not provide a solid basis for classification. By means of specific histochemical techniques, however, significant information has been collected about the chemical content of granules.

Williams and Lutz (1975b), divided the haemocytes of *C. maenas* into two types, one with glycogen-containing granules and another with non-glycogen polysaccharide containing-granules. This has not been confirmed by other investigators although Johnson *et al.* (1973), also working on *C. maenas*, noticed glycogen deposits in haemocytes, however, all electron micrographs located the glycogen stores in the cytoplasm of hyaline cells or between the granules of granulocytes. Glycogen was also shown to be present in the cytoplasm of haemocytes in *Orconectes virilis* (Wood and Visentin, 1967) *E. sinensis* (Bauchau *et al.*, 1975) *Pachygrapsus marmoratus* Arvy, 1952) and *A. salina* (Lochhead and Lochhead, 1941) but it was never found in the granules themselves (Fig. 13).

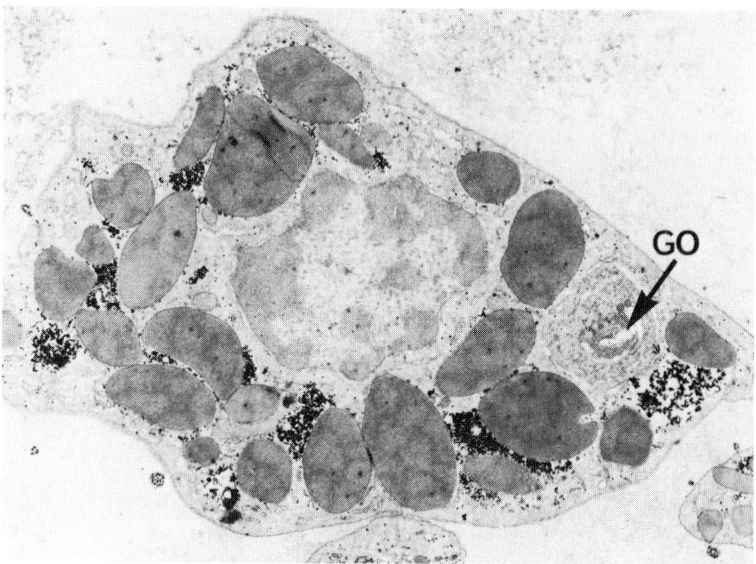

Fig. 13. Granulocyte of *E. sinensis* with numerous dense glycogen deposits between the granules. Golgi complex (GO). ×9200.

Using specific staining techniques and enzymatic digestion methods (pepsin, trypsin, pronase and amylase), the granules of *E. sinensis* granulocytes have been shown to contain large amounts of basic proteins as well as non-glycogen carbohydrates (Bauchau *et al.*, 1975) (Figs 14, 15). The latter has been tentatively identified as chitin by Johnston and Davies (1972) but this is doubtful. Neutral mucopolysaccharides comprise the bulk of the granule content although in some species acid mucopolysaccharides may also be found (Dall, 1965). In addition, some variation in the response to staining and digestion indicates that the granule population is not perfectly homogeneous and this conclusion is in agreement with electrophoretic patterns of isolated granules (Mengeot *et al.*, 1976, 1977). Although lipids are present in all cell types, they do not accumulate in granules, with the exception of lipo-protein cells.

A systematic examination of the enzyme content of haemocytes has hardly been attempted. The available data may be summarized as follows: mitochondrial enzymes are ubiquitous; non-specific esterases are found only in semi-granular cells and granulocytes; leucine acyl naphthylamidase

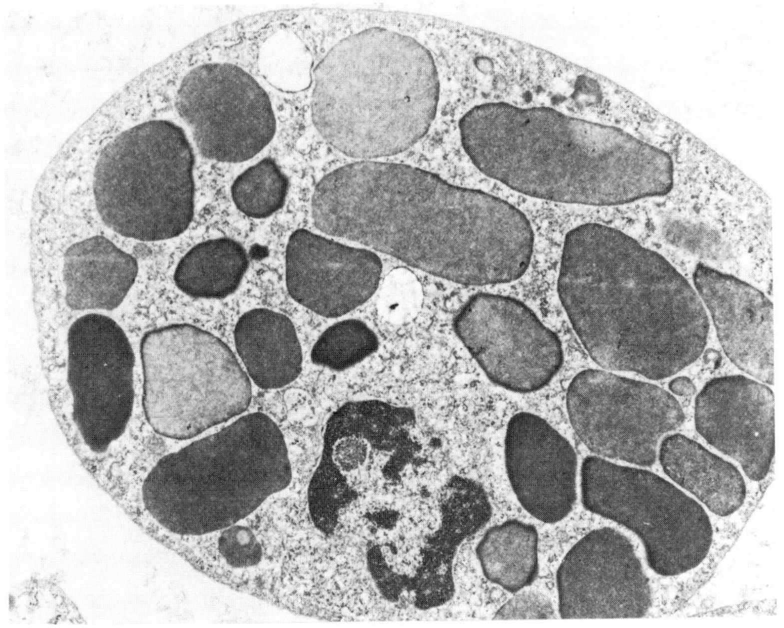

Fig. 14. Granulocyte of *E. sinensis* after digestion by pepsin. The granular density has been considerably reduced. ×9200.

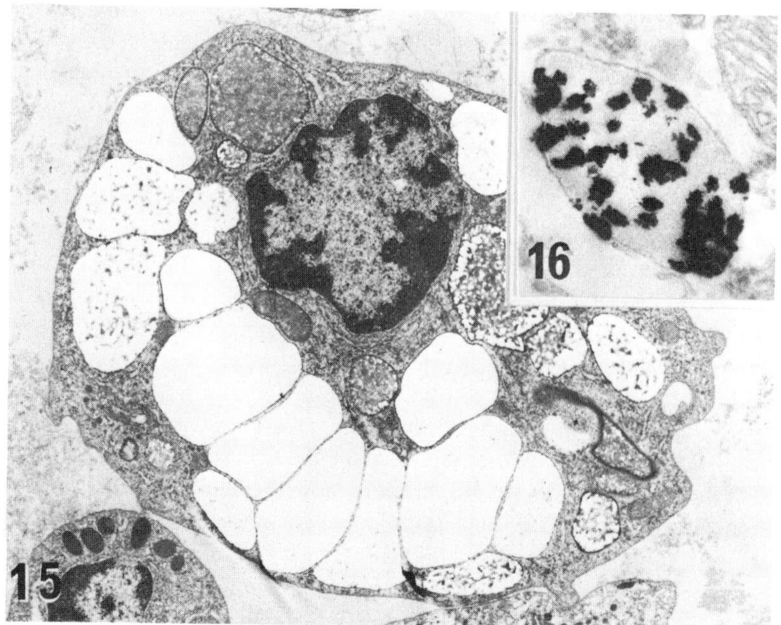

Fig. 15. Granulocyte of *E. sinensis* after digestion by amylase. The granular content has been partially or completely dissolved. × 7000.
Fig. 16. Granule of *E. sinensis* showing acid phosphatase activity. × 18 150.

is found in hyaline cells and granules; acid phosphatase titre is higher in haemocytes than in plasma (it has been localized in electron micrographs within some granules (Fig. 16); acid β-*N*-glucosaminidase, amylase and protease have also been recorded (Wood and Visentin, 1967; Horn and Kerr, 1969; Chassard-Bouchard and Hubert, 1975; Bauchau *et al.*, unpublished). Phenoloxidase activity is found in granulocytes but not in hyaline cells of *Cancer pagurus*, a maximum occurring from C_2 to C_4 and from A_1 to B_1, while no activity is detected during the D stages (Decleir and Vercauteren, 1965).

V. Origin and formation of haemocytes

Most Crustacea have a distinct haemopoietic organ, made up of a series of nodules surrounded by a thin sheath of connective tissue. It is found in close vicinity to the ophthalmic artery, and in the Natantia lies at the base of the rostrum (Demal, 1956), but in the Reptantia spreads extensively over the dorsal and lateral walls of the fore-gut (Cuénot, 1897; Kollmann, 1908; Fischer-Piette, 1931; Charmantier, 1972).

In each nodule, stem-cells or haemoblasts with large nuclei and hyaline cytoplasm are easily recognized, and undergo regular mitoses producing small hyaline daughter-cells (Fig. 17) which leave the nodule and migrate into the general body cavity.

Variations in the mitotic index during the inter-moult cycle in normal and eyestalkless *Pachygrapsus marmoratus* are summarized in Table IV (Marrec, 1944; Charmantier, 1972). A hormonal control of haemopoietic activity has rightly been advocated, since removal of the sinus gland in the eyestalk induces a marked increase in mitoses, probably under the influence of the Y-organ once it has been freed from the sinus gland inhibition (Matsumoto and Tongu, 1966; Charmantier-Daures, 1973b).

In some primitive species (e.g. *Chirocephalus* sp. and *Argulus* sp.), circulating haemocytes may still divide (Debaisieux, 1952, 1953), but in more advanced forms this occurs exceptionally, if at all, and the number of circulating blood cells depends on the mitotic rate in the haemopoietic

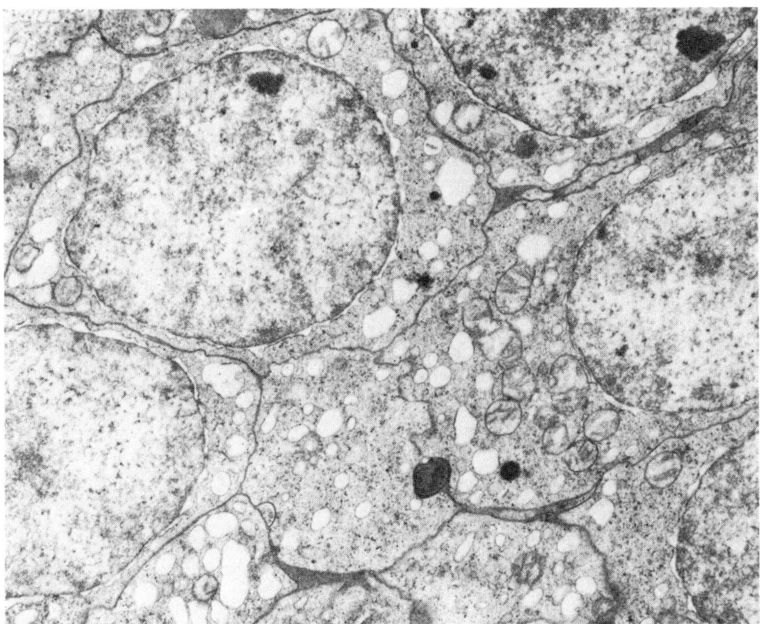

Fig. 17. Haemoblasts in the centre of a haemopoetic nodule of *E. sinensis*. ×9400.

TABLE IV. Mitotic index variations of the haemopoietic organ of normal and eyestalkless *Pachygrapsus marmoratus*, during the inter-moult cycle (according to Charmantier-Daures, 1973b).

Inter-moult stages	Mitotic index (%) Normal crab	Eyestalkless crab
A	0·84	1·91
B–C_1	1·26	2·65
C_2–C_3	2·08	3·78
C_4	0·56	2·07
D_0	1·44	2·58
D_1	1·24	2·07
D_2	1·54	2·67
D_3	1·42	3·43

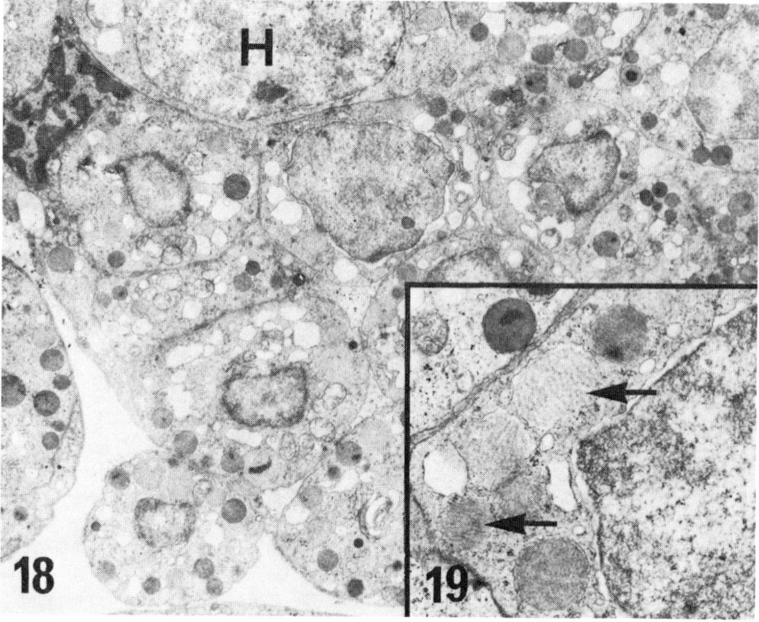

Fig. 18. Border of a haemopoietic nodule of *E. sinensis*, showing one haemoblast (H) surrounded by more or less differentiated haemocytes containing some small granules. ×4500.

Fig. 19. Part of a differentiating haemocyte in a haemopoetic nodule of *E. sinensis*, with many granules filled with a microtubular material (arrows). ×13 400.

organ. However at ecdysis, the water influx triggers a huge liberation of the haemocytes stored in nodules during D stages.

When different species are compared, the number of circulating haemocytes shows wide variations (Yeager and Tauber, 1935; Drach, 1939; Bauchau and Plaquet, 1973). Moreover, particular physiological states (e.g. stage of ova or sperm maturation) as well as various stresses (fasting, temperature, intensive regeneration, parasitism, etc.) also temporarily affect the number of circulating cells (Bauchau and Plaquet, 1973; Charmantier-Daures, 1973a; Hamann, 1975).

Circulating hyaline cells are thought to progressively differentiate into granulocytes (George and Nichols, 1948; Charmantier, 1972), but this problem does not seem to be definitely settled. In *A. salina* (Lochhead and Lochhead, 1941), *Palaemon* sp., (Demal, 1956) and *P. marmoratus* (Arvy, 1952), some haemocytes at the periphery of nodules already have a few, rather small, partially eosinophilic, granules. In a preliminary ultrastructural investigation of *E. sinensis* haemopoietic tissue, intermediate stages between hyaline cells and fully-developed granulocytes were apparent (Fig. 18). A few granules were electron-opaque, but most of them were filled with a microtubular material arranged in regular parallel rows (Fig. 19) (Bauchau, unpublished). In *C. maenas*, haemopoietic nodules contain haemocytes at various stages of differentiation so that mature granulocytes, as well as hyaline cells, are released into the blood (Ghiretti-Magaldi *et al.*, 1977). These observations leave no doubt about the occurrence of a more or less advanced differentiation process in the haemopoietic organ itself but do not exclude the possibility of further differentiation in circulating cells.

VI. Functions of haemocytes

A. Haemolymph coagulation and wound repair

Halliburton (1885) and Hardy (1892) discovered that a category of fragile haemocytes, termed "explosive corpuscles" were involved in blood coagulation in Crustacea. They were supposed to secrete a "fibrin-ferment" which initiated, or at least participated in, the formation of a clot. After much comparative work, different patterns of coagulation became apparent, depending on the role played by two simultaneous and coordinated processes, cell agglutination and gelation of the plasma. Tait (1911) suggested a classification into three basic types of coagulation:

A type: haemocytes simply agglutinate without any subsequent gelation of the plasma (*C. pagurus*, *Maia squinado*).

B type: cell agglutination is followed by a general gelation of the plasma (*Palaemon serratus*, *H. vulgaris*, *Macropipus puber*, *C. maenas*).

C type: the gelation process is at first limited to the periphery of a few insignificant cell clots but subsequently affects the whole of the remaining plasma (*Isopoda*, *Astacus fluviatilis*, *Palinurus vulgaris*).

Many descriptions of coagulation in different species have been reviewed by Grégoire (1970). The crab, *E. sinensis*, which belongs to the intermediate B type, has been chosen here as an example because it has been studied by light and electron microscopy (Bauchau and De Brouwer, 1974). A two-step reaction is clearly indicated. The agglutination of adjacent haemocytes produces an extensive cellular network by means of numerous elongated pseudopods adhering to whatever cell they come in contact with (Fig. 2). Hyaline and semi-granular cells are the first to react and are the most active in the process (Fig. 20), although granulocytes too are implicated. A more or less complete gelation of plasma occurs simultaneously with the release of material contained in large vacuoles within hyaline and semi-granular cells (Fig. 21). In granulocytes, the reaction is somewhat slower but more sustained. The granules dissolve gradually, either within vacuoles or *in situ*,

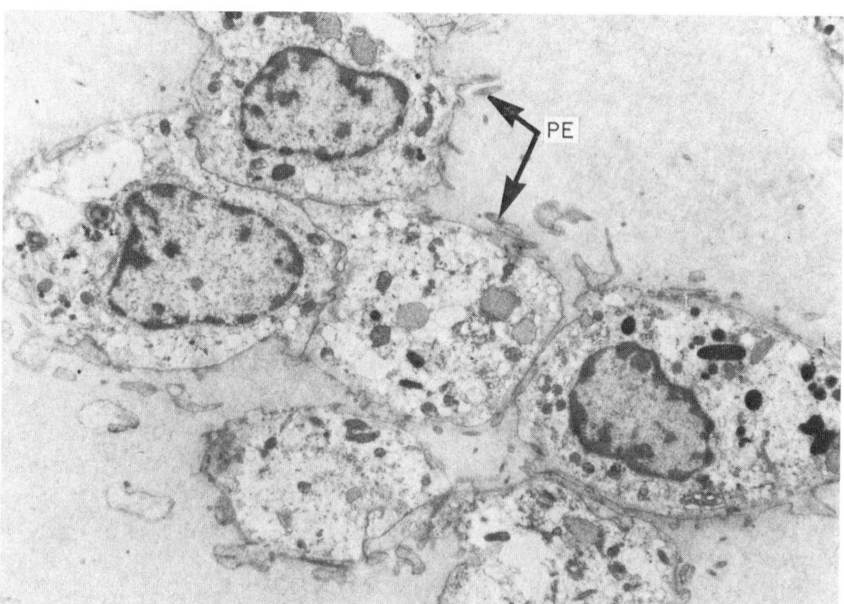

Fig. 20. Agglutinated hyaline and semi-granular cells of *E. sinensis* with many pseudopods (PE); the surrounding plasma is gelated. ×4200.

and their contents are expelled into the plasma. This could bring about a more extensive coagulation. The cytoplasm is finally reduced to a thin rim around an enlarged and degenerating nucleus (Fig. 22).

Comparable experiments by Wood *et al.* (1971) with *O. virilis*, identified the factor or one of the factors released from the blebs of hyaline cells, as well as from granulocytes, as a glyco- or muco-protein. The nature of this or these factors remains a controversial question. The "fibrin-ferment" of Hardy (1892), better named "coagulin" by Nolf (1909), is the most obvious candidate. This unstable and thermolabile protein has been identified in the lobster as an intracellular transglutaminase which, once secreted into the plasma, catalyses the formation of peptide bonds between so-called "fibrinogen" molecules and is thus responsible for the clotting process (Laki, 1972; Lorand, 1972).

Whether or not "fibrinogen" is present in the blood before any haemocytic intervention occurs is a matter of dispute. Available data are conflicting.

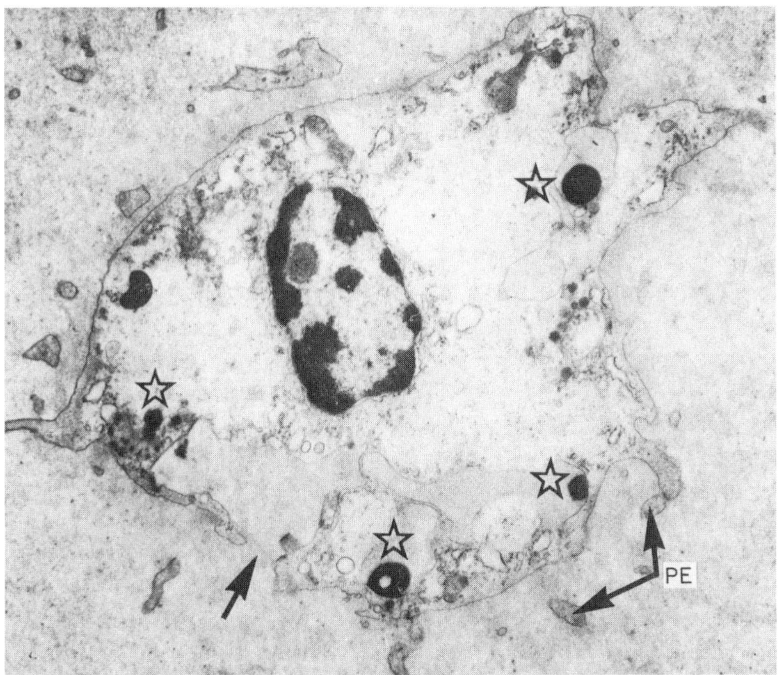

Fig. 21. Semi-granular cell of *E. sinensis*, 15 min after haemolymph coagulation. Several granules (stars) are being dissolved in large vacuoles which are emptying into the medium (arrow). Pseudopodial extensions (PE) are conspicuous. ×4900.

For example, in some cases, the existence of a clottable plasma protein has been demonstrated (*Homarus* sp., Duchateau and Florkin, 1954; *H. americanus*, Stewart *et al.*, 1966; *Panulirus interruptus*, Fuller and Doolittle, 1971a, 1971b; Doolittle and Fuller, 1972; *Gammarus* sp., *Asellus* sp., *Oniscus* sp., Jazdzewski *et al.*, 1975; *Astacus leptodactylus*, Durliat and Vranckx, 1976b; *M. puber*, Vendrely *et al.*, 1977), while in other cases it could not be found by electrophoresis (*Gecarcinus lateralis*, Stutman and Dolliver, 1968; *Cancer irrotatus*, *Cancer borealis*, *Hyas coarctatus*, Stewart and Dingle, 1968; *O. virilis*, Wood and Karpawich, 1972).

These conflicting data, however, could be reconciled if fibrinogen titres, too low to be detected, are responsible for the negative responses in electrophoregrams. Such an assumption is not unlikely because large variations in concentrations between species are well documented and significant fluctuations have even been recorded during the inter-moult cycle (Morrison and Morrison, 1952; Vendrely *et al.*, 1977). This would provide a convenient explanation for the different coagulation types proposed by Tait (1911). In the A type reaction, the plasma fibrinogen titre would be low, while in B and C types it would be high enough to allow the formation of an extensive clot.

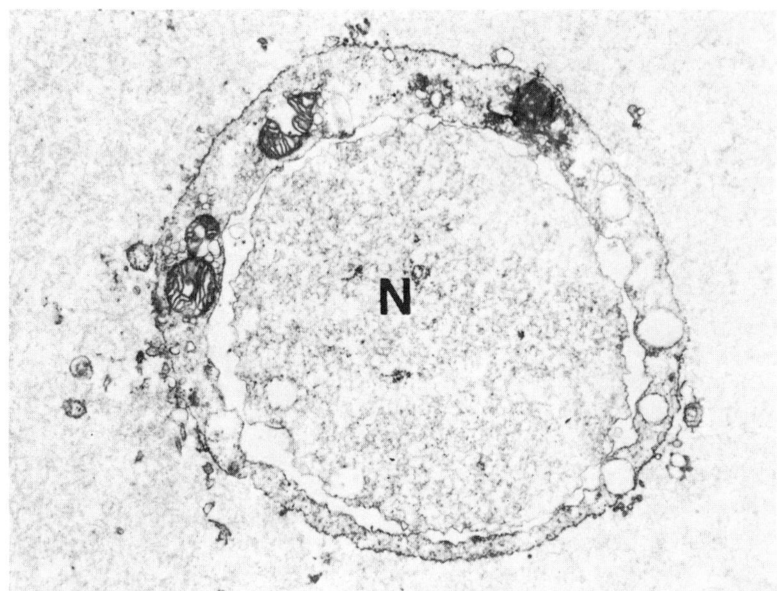

Fig. 22. Granulocyte of *E. sinensis* reduced to a thin rim of cytoplasm around a degenerating nucleus (N). ×9400.

Recently, substantiating information has been provided by the work of Durliat and Vranckx (1976b). They identified a clottable protein in the plasma of *A. leptodactylus* and, in addition, found it in a monomeric form in the haemocytes. Monomers are converted into dimers or polymers when secreted. Whether they may be stored in some particular site within the blood cells is unknown. If future work localizes at least some monomers on the cell membrane, a ready-made mechanism of agglutination would be at hand. Indeed, coagulin, when released, could catalyse the formation of peptide bonds not only between clottable proteins of the plasma (gelification) but also between membrane-localized monomers of adjacent cells (agglutination). The two-step coagulation system of Crustacea would then receive a satisfactory biochemical explanation (Bauchau and Mengeot, 1978).

Haemolymph coagulation is an adaptive mechanism of great value for the survival of organisms with an open vascular system. A rapid occlusion of any open wound inflicted to the exoskeleton is imperative to stop bleeding and prevent further intrusion of microorganisms. This is evidenced even after autonomy, when the distal side of the preformed diaphragm is coated by a thick clot of blood.

An injury to the carapace elicits a haemocyte reaction. The damaged tissues are temporarily replaced by a network of haemocytes and fibrinogen strands which, in order to secure a tighter seal, soon melanize due to granulocyte phenoloxidase. Under this protective blackish cap, epidermal cells regenerate and secrete a new cuticle, restoring the integument integrity (Bazin and Demeusy, 1972; Fontaine and Lightner, 1973).

B. Phagocytosis

Phagocytosis is one of the more common cellular defence reactions. Microorganisms or particulate matter introduced into the body cavity can soon be found in the cytoplasm of haemocytes. Damaged or decaying cell debris may also be engulfed (Metchnikoff, 1884; Pixell-Goodrich, 1928; Chassard-Bouchaud and Hubert, 1975; Shivers, 1977). This blood clearing procedure is very effective although in *H. americanus* the bacterium, *Aerococcus viridens*, var. homari (formerly *Pediococcus homari*, formerly *Gaffkya homari*), represents a notable exception because it is not destroyed following phagocytosis and continues to multiply to induce a fatal septicaemia (Cornick and Stewart, 1968). Furthermore, some species of viruses, rickettsiae, bacteria and protozoa can live in the haemocoel without being phagocytosed. The ciliate *Anophrys* sp., for example, invades the bloodstream of *C. maenas*, digests the circulating haemocytes and causes the death of the crab. *Maia squinado*, however, is resistant to the same infection, except prior to moulting (Bang, 1967).

Each type of haemocyte has the capability to phagocytose, although hyaline and semi-granular cells appear more active than granulocytes (Figs 23, 24). Some functional specialization though may be present as in the blue crab *Callinectes sapidus*, in which *Paramoeba perniciosa* is exclusively engulfed by hyaline cells while Gram-negative bacteria are taken up by both hyaline cells and granulocytes (Johnson, 1976, 1977b).

Phagocytosis is apparently a simple phenomenon, but, in fact, a large number of external and internal parameters make a sequential analysis rather complicated. Some factors are clearly inhibitory, such as acidic pH or low temperatures (below 10°C). Discrimination between self and non-self is another crucial step. In several invertebrates, the mediation of serum proteins has been advocated. At least some Crustacea are known to have hetero-agglutinins in their blood, which might well be essential in recognition of non-self (Ghidalia *et al.*, 1975; Schapiro, 1975).

In the crayfish *Parachaeraps bicarinatus*, for example, bacteria as well as human and sheep erythrocytes are scarcely or not phagocytosed at all unless

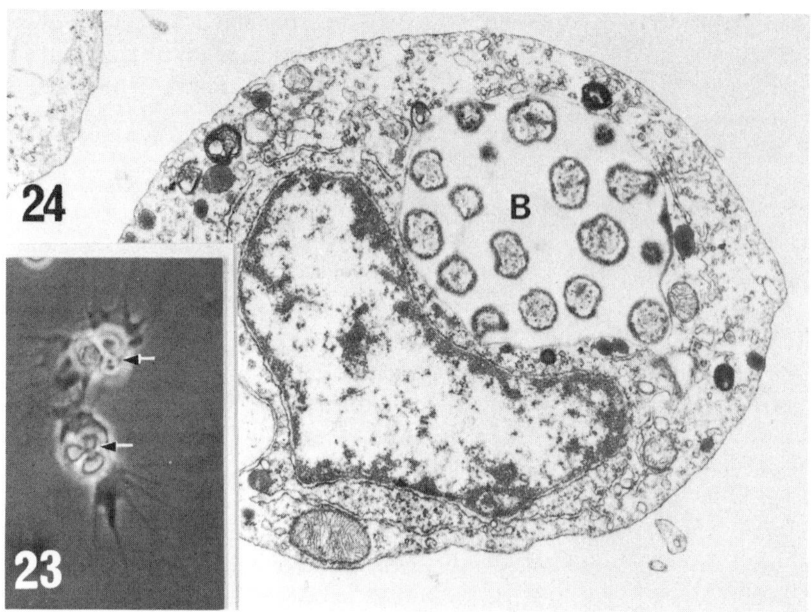

Fig. 23. Hyaline cells of *Carcinus maenas* with two or three phagocytosed yeast cells (arrows). Phase contrast ×600.

Fig. 24. Hyaline cell of *E. sinensis* with many bacteria (B) in a phagosome. ×11 700.

they are pre-treated with crayfish serum. The purified agglutinin also shows opsonic activity, suggesting that the naturally occurring haemagglutinins are responsible for the opsonic activity of crayfish haemolymph (McKay and Jenkin, 1970a,b; Tyson and Jenkin, 1973, 1974). Comparable results have been obtained in the lobster, *H. americanus* (Paterson and Stewart, 1974; Paterson *et al*., 1976). Moreover, natural agglutinins are synthesized by the lobster haemocytes and afterwards released into the blood (Cornick and Stewart, 1973, 1978).

Levels of phagocytosis have been measured *in vitro*. After 1 h, 10% of *P. bicarinatus* haemocytes had phagocytosed one or more erythrocytes (McKay and Jenkin, 1970b) while only 2% was reported in *H. americanus* after 2 h (Paterson and Stewart, 1974) and a similar level was also found in *C. maenas* (Bauchau and Mars, unpublished). After 3 h, Smith and Ratcliffe (1978) recorded in *C. maenas* higher rates with different bacteria (*ca*. 5% and 3% for *Bacillus cereus* and *Aerococcus viridens* var. homari, respectively; *ca*. 15% for *Moraxella* sp.) but sheep erythrocytes were not phagocytosed at all. These levels are low in comparison with other invertebrates, such as molluscs, but they probably represent only a conservative estimate of *in vivo* rates. Moreover, one phagocyte frequently ingests more than one foreign body, and when the total number of haemocytes is taken into account even a 2% level represents a substantial phagocytic capability (Paterson *et al.*, 1976). Inadequate opsonization procedure may be responsible for low levels of phagocytosis obtained *in vitro* since twice as many phagocytic cells were found by Schapiro *et al.* (1977) when bacteria were opsonized with lobster plasma instead of serum. In *C. maenas*, pre-incubation of Gram-positive bacteria in serum did not enhance phagocytosis whereas the rate of uptake of *Moraxella* sp., a Gram-negative bacterium, was even depressed, although the recognition phase of phagocytosis was enhanced (Smith and Ratcliffe, 1978).

Whether contact with non-self is made by chance or whether some chemical stimulus attracts blood cells from a distance is not known. Definite membrane receptors have neither been isolated nor well characterized in crustacean haemocytes although a theoretical model has been presented (Parish, 1977). Once contact has been established, the haemocyte membrane may invaginate, elongated pseudopodia or large cytoplasmic veils are produced to surround particles or droplets of haemolymph and give rise to phagosomes. The mechanism of the membrane reaction is not clear although Ca^{2+} seems necessary and microfilaments which normally form a network beneath the cell membrane are probably involved because their disruption by cytochalasin B (10 μg/ml) inhibits phagocytosis (Bauchau and Mars, unpublished). Further work is needed to elucidate the ultrastructure of the reaction.

Subsequent events such as fusion with lysosomes, enzymatic activities in the phagosomes, exocytosis or storage of degraded material, as well as the fate of phagocytes, are still poorly documented in Crustacea.

C. Capsules and nodules

A clear distinction has been drawn by Maupas (1899) between encapsulation and encystment. A capsule is made up of cells laid down by the host around any foreign body introduced into its tissues, while a cyst is a protective covering made by a parasite about itself. All Crustacea so far investigated are capable of encapsulation.

The following account is based on an ultrastructural study of capsules formed in the crab, *C. maenas*, by implanting nylon threads or pieces of human hair into the haemocoel (Bauchau and De Brouwer, unpublished).

At a very early stage, the capsule looks like a homogeneous mass of spherical blood cells. After a period of about 5 h, three concentric layers may be recognized (Fig. 25) (see also Chapter 13). The inner layer, about ten cells thick, adheres closely to the implant surface. The innermost flattened cells become necrotic and small beads of melanin are deposited principally along the cell membranes and around the nuclei (Fig. 26). When

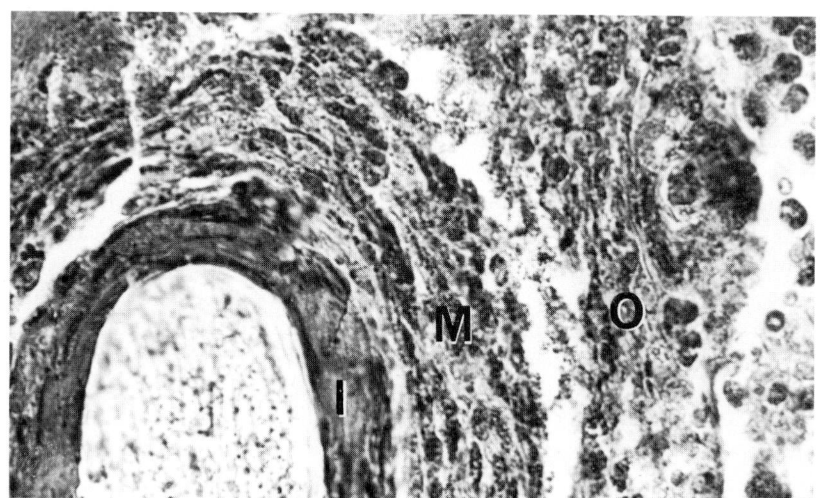

Fig. 25. Capsule formed around a piece of hair introduced into the haemocoel of the crab, *C. maenas*. Note the three layers of the capsule. I, inner; M, middle; O, outer layer. ×200.

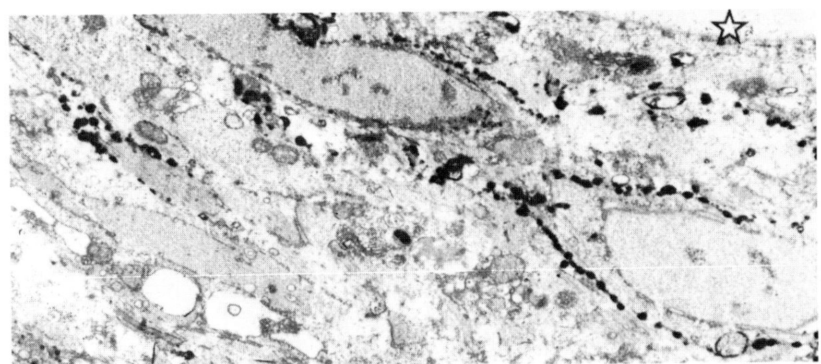

Fig. 26. Inner layer of a capsule in *C. maenas* with necrotic flattened cells and small beads of melanin along the cell membranes and nuclei. Star indicates the location of the implanted nylon thread. ×9000.

the capsule is subjected to mechanical stresses by nearby muscles or organs, it breaks leaving clumps of cellular debris.

The middle layer accounts for about half of the capsule thickness (Fig. 27). The three basic cell types are present as flattened, interdigitating haemocytes, which are sometimes held together by a dense intercellular collagen-like substance. They do not show any sign of necrosis and cytoplasmic granules may be replaced by bundles of microtubules. Intercellular spaces are filled with a microfilamentous material which frequently masks the membrane profiles.

Five or six layers of spherical haemocytes form a loosely connected outer region. These cells have the same fine structure as free blood cells and

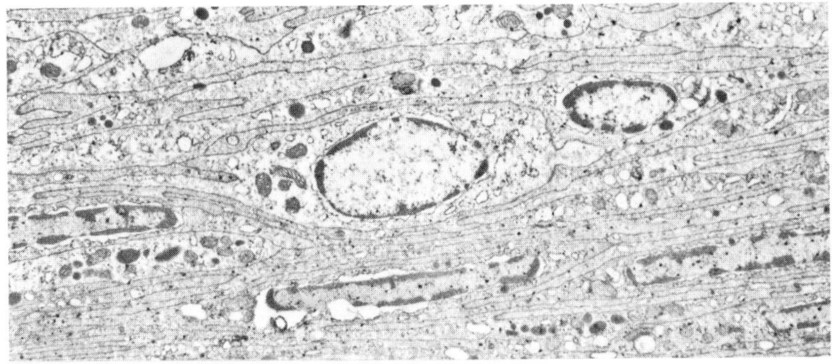

Fig. 27. Middle layer of the same capsule as in Fig. 26. Flattened but healthy haemocytes are tightly interdigitated. ×5400.

may return to the blood stream (Fig. 28). In the neighbourhood of muscles, though, they may be flattened too.

Phagocytosis of injected bacteria or yeast cells has been observed in *C. maenas*, but the most common reaction is encapsulation and nodule formation (Smith and Ratcliffe, 1980a,b; Bauchau and Mars, unpublished). Clumps of bacteria readily initiate the formation of small capsules or of nodules. The latter combines capsule segregation with the phagocytic activity of some haemocytes. Nodules are always heavily melanized (Fig. 29). These observations are in agreement with previous reports made in studies on *Astacus* sp. by Cuénot (1895) and in *Carcinus* sp. by Poisson (1930).

Hyphae of *Aphanomyces astaci* are always encapsulated by blood cells of healthy *A. astacus* and *Pacifastacus leniusculus* (Unestam and Weiss, 1970). As soon as haemocytes make contact with a parasite hypha, they attach to it and additional blood cells are likewise trapped by chance contact with small pseudopodial extensions protruding from the aggregated cells. Within the capsule, granulocytes release their contents of granules which seem to be responsible for covering the nearby hypha with a thin refractile layer. Within a few hours, this layer becomes melanized. The melanin-forming enzyme, a polyphenoloxidase, as well as its substrate originate from the granules (Unestam and Nylund, 1972).

Substances in the cell walls of various organisms are capable of activating

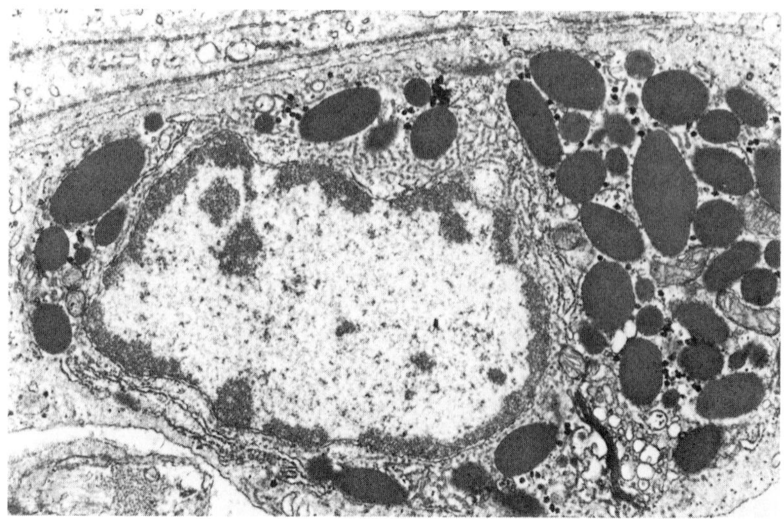

Fig. 28. A granulocyte from the outer layer of the same capsule as in Figs 26, 27 with an unaltered ultrastructure. ×8700.

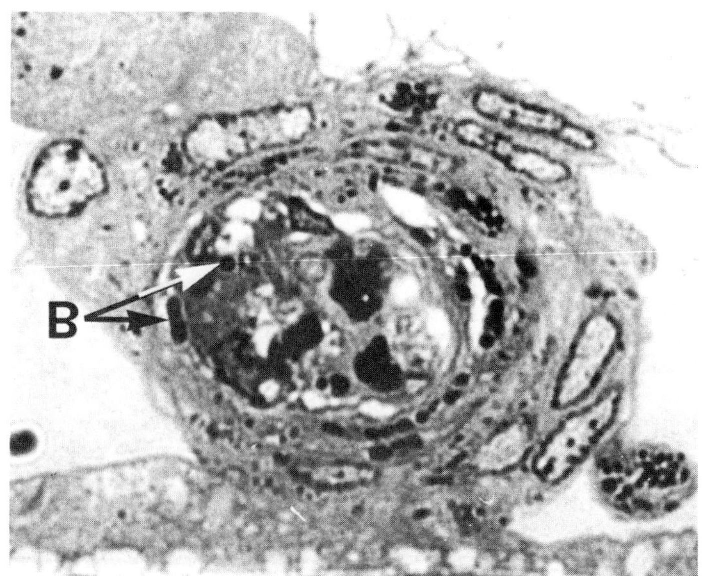

Fig. 29. Melanized nodule in *C. maenas* formed around bacteria (B). Note necrotic melanized core (From Smith and Ratcliffe, 1980a.) ×2000.

phenoloxidase but cellulose, chitin and nylon are ineffective (Unestam, 1976; Unestam and Beskow, 1976; Unestam and Ajaxon, 1976; Unestam and Söderhäll, 1977).

The same type of immunological reaction has been recorded in different species of shrimps (De Backer, 1961–62; Fontaine *et al.*, 1975; Solangi and Lightner, 1976; Poinar and Hess, 1977). Even the most successful parasite of *C. maenas*, *Sacculina carcini*, elicits a haemocytic reaction. Granulocytes stick to the sacculine roots and cover them by a collagen-like film originating from the granules. However, the parasite does not seem to be affected and remains healthy (Hubert *et al.*, 1976).

D. Transport and synthesis of carbohydrates

Crustacean haemolymph contains large amounts of various kinds of polysaccharides. The neutral or acidic mucopolysaccharides are packed in membrane-bound granules, while glycogen stores although scattered in the cytoplasm of the three basic cell types, are found more abundantly in semi-granular cells and granulocytes (Johnston *et al.*, 1973; Bauchau *et al.*, 1975; Bodammer, 1978).

^{14}C-labelled glucose is actively incorporated as polysaccharide in *C. maenas* haemocytes (Johnston and Davies, 1972). In *H. americanus*, an injection of cAMP produces a marked rise of the glucose level in the blood and at the same time depletes the haemocyte glycogen stores, however, after 24 h glycaemia and the glycogen deposits return to normal (Trausch, Isenborghs and Bauchau, unpublished). Blood cells may thus regulate the blood sugar level according to particular needs. On starvation, glycogen is depleted and increases after feeding (Williams and Lutz, 1975a).

Chitin or a chitin precursor has been proposed as one of the other polysaccharides stored in haemocytes (Dall, 1965; Johnston *et al.*, 1973) which could be used at moult in the production of the new exoskeleton. This could be one of the reasons for an increase in the number of circulating haemocytes at that time (Bauchau and Plaquet, 1973).

E. Moulting and vitellogenesis

A significant increase in the number of circulating haemocytes occurs in *E. sinensis* during definite physiological conditions such as moulting or gonadal activity. It is tempting to interpret these variations as being indicative of an as yet undetermined role played by the blood cells in these processes (Bauchau and Plaquet, 1973). This hypothesis has not been proved correct at the present time although some data support it. Busselen (1971), for example, discovered that during vitellogenesis haemocyanin and another serum protein were incorporated into the eggs of three species of crabs (*C. maenas*, *E. sinensis* and *Portunus holsatus*). Haemocyanin may be produced by haemocytes as indicated under section III and although the origin of the other protein has not been traced the blood cells could possibly be involved.

New information also points to some impressive similarities between blood and integument proteins. Ghidalia *et al.* (1976) compared, by electrophoresis and immuno-reaction, proteins extracted from calcified cuticle, epidermis and the sera of male *Macropipus puber*. One antigenically identical protein was shown to be shared by the epidermis and serum during a brief period preceding and following ecdysis (from the end of C_4 or beginning of D_0 to the end of A). By means of more elaborate immunological techniques, Durliat and Vranckx (1978) and Vranckx (1978) also established that many plasma proteins were present in the soft integument of *Astacus leptodactylus* as well as in the calcified cuticle. The plasma "fibrinogen", synthesized, as the monomer in haemocytes, was specifically identified in the soft integument. If the other proteins could unambiguously be related to blood cells, a leading role in the physiology of crustacean moulting could clearly be assigned to the haemocytes. Further results leading to similar conclusions have recently been provided by Herberts *et al.* (1978) working with *Carcinus mediterraneus*.

F. *Free amino acid pool*

The haemocytes of *C. maenas* contain a pool of free amino acids, which is large in comparison to their concentrations in the plasma (Evans, 1972). It could play a significant role in osmotic regulation in these cells, when the euryhaline crab moves into a medium of differing salinity (Schoffeniels and Gilles, 1970).

Taurine, alanine and glutamine are strikingly more concentrated in blood cells than in muscle or nerve tissues; more specifically, the taurine molecule alone accounts for 50% of the pool in the haemocytes. Since an inhibitory effect of taurine on crustacean nerve impulses is well documented (Kravitz *et al.*, 1963a,b), Evans suggests that one possible function of haemocytes could be to maintain a low level of free taurine in the plasma and thus prevent any interference with the transmission of nerve impulses. In addition, this strongly anionic molecule would help to balance the high internal concentration of potassium ions in the haemocytes.

VII. Summary and concluding remarks

A critical evaluation of available data concerning the morphology of haemocytes favours the concept of a developmental series leading from poorly differentiated hyaline cells to mature granulocytes with intermediate semi-granular cells. The structural characteristics reflect more a functional flexibility than a rigid classification into separate cell types. Whether each morphological pattern can be shifted to another in response to physiological demands or whether a one-way sequence is part of the life-cycle of individual cells is still unknown. A similar interpretation has been advocated by Scharrer (1972) for insect blood cells. In Crustacea, further investigations of haemopoiesis would be of great value. Fragments of haemopoietic tissues have been successfully cultured previously (Fischer-Piette, 1931); if repeated, such experimental cultures would help in tracing the relationship between stem-cells and basic circulating blood cell types. A more extensive knowledge of their enzyme content would also shed greater light on the nature of the differentiation processes.

Haemocytes are committed to an unexpected wide range of physiological activities. This consideration, though, should not conceal an underlying functional harmony. Indeed haemocytes act as security officers in charge of preserving the individual autonomy of crustaceans in a changing and often hostile environment.

Phagocytosis serves to dispose of small foreign particles. Larger bodies and parasites are sequestered in capsules and nodules. Any breakage of the exoskeleton initiates the formation of a blood clot securing a temporary protective cover. Damaged cells are then engulfed while surrounding epidermal cells regenerate and secrete a new cuticle, thus restoring the integument.

Immunochemical investigations point to an even more significant relationship between haemocyte and epidermal cell functions. At least some of the proteins identified in the epidermis, cuticle and haemocytes are antigenically identical. Whether the antigenic similarity results from a resorption of old cuticle material prior to moult or from a secretion of proteins delivered by haemocytes to epidermal cells and subsequently incorporated into the new exoskeleton is not definitely settled but the latter possibility seems likely. Fibrinogen is of particular interest in this respect because it has not only been found in haemocytes as the monomer and in plasma as the dimer but has also been identified in the soft and calcified integument of *Astacus leptodactylus* (Durliat and Vranckx, 1978). Ghidalia *et al.* (1976), however, could not extract it from the calcified cuticle of *Macropipus puber*. A possible passive diffusion of blood material soaking into the new cuticle should also be taken into consideration. The problem is thus still open and offers an exciting field for further inquiries.

It has been suggested that chitin or a chitin precursor is produced by haemocytes (Johnston *et al.*, 1973) but a more convincing demonstration by means of labelled carbohydrates would be useful. On the other hand, the amount of glycogen deposits in haemocytes exceeds their own needs and may be used to modify glucose levels in the blood in response to physiological demand. Haemocyanin, too, seems to be synthesized in some blood cells. These considerations could well validate the concept of haemocytes acting as "free circulating hepatocytes" put forward by Johnston *et al.* (1971).

Finally some observations may indicate an involvement of haemocytes in endocrine activity. Chassard-Bouchaud and Hubert (1975) noticed their large number in close vicinity to and inside the Y-organ, and in fact they have even been mistaken for a second kind of Y-organ cell (Madyastha and Rangneker, 1972). In *C. maenas* parasitized by *Sacculina*, they are actively engaged in phagocytosis of decaying Y-organ cells (Hubert *et al.*, 1976). The question of their role in ecdysone production or transfer to target-organs remains unanswered at the present time.

In summary, because of their functional flexibility, haemocytes perform a large number of specific tasks. Their analysis is still far from complete but there remains no doubt that future investigations will underline their significant role in crustacean physiology.

Acknowledgements

I am most indebted to Drs V. Smith and N. A. Ratcliffe for providing me with Fig. 29. The credit for preparing the illustrations of this review goes to M. B. de Brouwer, E. Passelecq-Gérin and J. Collet. I sincerely appreciate the secretarial assistance of Mrs M. C. Simoens-Lefevere.

References

Arvy, L. (1952). *Am. Sc. Nat. Zool.* (Serie 11) **14**, 1–12.
Bang, F. B. (1967). *Feder. Proc.* **26**, 1680–1684.
Bauchau, A. G. and De Brouwer, M. B. (1972). *J. Microsc.* (*Paris*) **15**, 171–180.
Bauchau, A. G. and De Brouwer, M. B. (1974). *J. Microsc.* (*Paris*) **19**, 37–46.
Bauchau, A. G. and Mengeot, J. C. (1978). *Archs Zool. exp. gén.* **119**, 227–248.
Bauchau, A. G. and Plaquet, J. C. (1973). *Crustaceana* **24**, 215–223.
Bauchau, A. G., De Brouwer, M. B., Passelecq-Gérin, E. and Mengeot, J. C. (1975). *Histochemistry* **45**, 101–113.
Bazin, F. and Demeusy, N. (1972). *C.R. Acad. Sci. Paris* **274D**, 2603–2605.
Bodammer, J. E. (1978). *Cell Tiss. Res.* **187**, 79–96.
Bonami, J. R., Vago, C. and Duthoit, J. L. (1971). *C.R. Acad. Sci. Paris* **272D**, 3087–3088.
Bruntz, L. (1907). *Archs Zool. exp. gén.* (Serie 4) **7**, 1–67.
Busselen, P. (1971). *Comp. Biochem. Physiol.* **38A**, 317–328.
Carus, D. C. G. (1824). "Von den äuszeren Lebensbedingungen der heisz- und kaltblütigen Thiere". Leipzig.
Carmantier, M. (1971). Influences neuroendocrines sur l'organe leucopoiétique et l'hemolymphe en fonction du cyole d'intermue chez *Pachygrapsus marmoratus* (Fabricius 1787), Décapade Brachyoure. *Thèse Univ. Montpellier.* 76 pp.
Charmantier, M. (1972). *C.R. Acad. Sci. Paris* **275D**, 683–686.
Charmantier-Daures, M. (1973a). *C.R. Acad. Sci. Paris* **276D**, 2553–2556.
Charmantier-Daures, M. (1973b). *Bull. Soc. Zool. France* **98**, 221–231.
Chassard-Bouchaud, C. and Hubert, M. (1975). *C.R. Acad. Sci. Paris* **281D**, 807–810.
Cornick, J. W. and Stewart, J. E. (1968). *J. Fish. Res. Board. Can.* **25**, 695–709.
Cornick, J. W. and Stewart, J. E. (1973). *J. Invertebr. Pathol.* **21**, 255–262.
Cornick, J. W. and Stewart, J. E. (1978). *J. Invertebr. Pathol.* **31**, 194–203.
Cuénot, L. (1891). *Archs Zool. exp. gén.* (Série 2) **9**, 13–90.
Cuénot, L. (1895). *Archs Biol.* **13**, 243–303.
Cuénot, L. (1897). *Archs Anat. microsc.* **1**, 153–192.
Dall, W. (1965). *Austr. J. Mar. Freshw. Res.* **16**, 163–180.
De Backer, J. (1961–62). *Ann. Soc. R. Zool. Belgique* **92**, 141–151.

Debaisieux, P. (1952). *La Cellule* **54**, 253–294.
Debaisieux, P. (1953). *La Cellule* **55**, 245–290.
Decleir, W. and Vercauteren, R. (1965). *Cah. Biol. Mar.* **6**, 163–172.
Demal, J. (1956). *La Cellule* **56**, 87–101.
Doolittle, R. F. and Fuller, G. M. (1972). *Biochem. Biophys. Acta.* **263**, 805–809.
Drach, P. (1939). *Ann. Inst. Oceanog.* **19**, 103–391.
Drach, P. and Tchernigovtseff, C. (1967). *Vie et Milieu* **18**, 597–607.
Duchateau, G. and Florkin, M. (1954). *Bull. Soc. Chim. Biol.* **36**, 295–305.
Durand, J. (1973). Recherches sur la culture des cellules et d'organes de crustacés décapodes marins. Applications à quelque problèmes biologuiques et cytopathologiques. *Thèse Univ. Montpellier.* 183 pp.
Durliat, M. and Vranckx, R. (1976a). *Biol. Bull., Woods Hole* **151**, 467–477.
Durliat, M. and Vranckx, R. (1976b). *C.R. Acad. Sci. Paris* **282D**, 2215–2218.
Durliat, M. and Vranckx, R. (1978). *Comp. Biochem. Physiol.* **59B**, 123–128.
Evans, P. D. (1972). *J. exp. Biol.* **56**, 501–507.
Fahrenbach, W. H. (1970). *J. Cell Biol.* **44**, 445–453.
Fischer-Piette, E. (1931). *Archs Zool. exp. gén.* **74**, 33–52.
Fontaine, C. T. and Lightner, D. V. (1973). *J. Invertebr. Pathol.* **22**, 23–33.
Fontaine, C. T., Bruss, R. G., Sanderson, I. A. and Lightner, D. V. (1975). *J. Invertebr. Pathol.* **25**, 321–330.
Fuller, G. M. and Doolittle, R. F. (1971a). *Biochemistry* **10**, 1305–1310.
Fuller, G. M. and Doolittle, R. F. (1971b). *Biochemistry* **10**, 1311–1315.
George, W. C. and Nichols, J. (1948). *J. Morphol.* **83**, 425–443.
Ghidalia, W., Lambin, P. and Fine, J. M. (1975). *J. Invertebr. Pathol.* **25**, 151–157.
Ghidalia, W., Montmory, C., Vicomte, M., Lambin, P. and Fine, J. M. (1976). *Cah. Biol. Mar.* **17**, 157–164.
Ghiretti-Magaldi, A., Milanesi, C. and Salvato, B. (1973). *Experientia* **29**, 1265–1267.
Ghiretti-Magaldi, A., Milanesi, C. and Tognon, G. (1977). *Cell diff.* **6**, 167–186.
Gibert, J. (1972). *Crustaceana* Suppl. 3, 342–350.
Grégoire, Ch. (1970). *In* "The Haemostatic Mechanism in Man and Other Animals". *Sympos. Zool. Soc. London* No. 27, 45–74. Academic Press, New York and London.
Halliburton, W. E. (1885). *J. Physiol.* **6**, 300–335.
Hamann, A. (1975). *Z. Naturforsch.* **30c**, 850.
Hardy, W. V. (1892). *J. Physiol.* **13**, 165–190.
Hearing, V. and Vernick, S. H. (1967). *Chesapeake Sc.* **8**, 170–186.
Herberts, C., Andrieux, N. and De Frescheville, J. (1978). *Can. J. Zool.* **56**, 1735–1743.
Hoarau, F. (1976). *J. Microsc. biol. Cell.* **27**, 47–52.
Horn, E. C. and Kerr, M. S. (1969). *Comp. Biochem. Physiol.* **29**, 493–508.
Hubert, M., Chassard-Bouchaud, C. and Bocquet-Vedrine, J. (1976). *C.R. Acad. Sci. Paris* **283D**, 789–792.
Jazdzewski, K., Gondko, R. and Alikhan, M. A. (1975). *Zool. Polon.* **25**, 73–80.
Johnson, P. T. (1976). *J. Invertebr. Pathol.* **28**, 25–36.
Johnson, P. T. (1977a). *J. Invertebr. Pathol.* **29**, 201–209.
Johnson, P. T. (1977b). *J. Invertebr. Pathol.* **29**, 308–320.
Johnston, M. A., Davies, P. S. and Elder, H. Y. (1971). *Nature* **230**, 471–472.
Johnston, M. A. and Davies, P. S. (1972). *Comp. Biochem. Physiol.* **41B**, 433–443.

Johnston, M. A., Elder, H. Y. and Davies, P. S. (1973). *Comp. Biochem. Physiol.* **46A**, 569–581.

Jones, J. C. (1962). *Amer. Zool.* **2**, 209–249.

Kellog, S., Steenbergen, J. F. and Schapiro, H. C. (1974). *Aquaculture* **3**, 409–413.

Kollmann, M. (1908). *Ann. Sci. Nat. Zool.* (Série 9). **8**, 1–240.

Kravitz, E. A., Kuffler, S. W., Potter, D. D. and Van Gelder, N. M. (1963a). *J. Neurophysiol.* **26**, 729–738.

Kravitz, E. A., Kuffler, S. W. and Potter, D. D. (1963b). *J. Neurophysiol.* **26**, 739–751.

Laki, K. (1972). *Ann. N.Y. Acad. Sci.* **202**, 297–307.

Lochhead, J. H. and Lochhead, M. S. (1941). *J. Morphol.* **68**, 593–632.

Lorand, L. (1972). *Ann. N.Y. Acad. Sci.* **202**, 6–30.

McKay, D. and Jenkin, C. R. (1970a). *Austr. J. exp. biol. med. Sci.* **48**, 139–150.

McKay, D. and Jenkin, C. R. (1970b). *Austr. J. exp. biol. med. Sci.* **48**, 609–617.

Madhyastha, M. N. and Rangneker, P. V. (1972). *Experientia* **28**, 580–581.

Marrec, M. (1944). *Bull. Inst. Oceanog.* **41**, 1–4 No. 867.

Martin, J. L. M., Van Wormhoudt, A. and Ceccaldi, H. J. (1977). *Comp. Biochem. Physiol.* **58A**, 193–195.

Matsumoto, K. and Tongu, Y. (1966). *Zool. Mag. Tokyo.* **75**, 203–206.

Maupas, E. (1899). *Archs Zool. exp. gén.* **27**, 563–628.

Mengeot, J. C., Bauchau, A. G., De Brouwer, M. B. and Passelecq-Gérin, E. (1976). *Comp. Biochem. Physiol.* **54A**, 145–148.

Mengeot, J. C., Bauchau, A. G., De Brouwer, M. B. and Passelecq-Gérin, E. (1977). *Comp. Biochem. Physiol.* **58A**, 393–403.

Metchnikoff, E. (1884). *Virchows Arch. Pathol. Anat. Physiol. Klin. Med.* **96**, 177–195.

Morrisson, P. R. and Morrisson, K. C. (1952). *Biol. Bull., Woods Hole* **103**, 395–406.

Nolf, P. (1909). *Archs Intern. Physiol.* **7**, 411–461.

Nyhlen, L. and Unestam, T. (1975). *J. Invertebr. Pathol.* **26**, 353–366.

Parish, C. R. (1977). *Nature* **267**, 711–713.

Paterson, W. D. and Stewart, J. E. (1974). *J. Fish. Res. Board Can.* **31**, 1051–1056.

Paterson, W. D., Stewart, J. E. and Zwicker, B. M. (1976). *J. Invertebr. Pathol.* **27**, 95–104.

Pixell-Goodrich, H. (1928). *Quart. Jl. Microsc. Sci.* **72**, 325–353.

Poinar, G. O. and Hess, R. T. (1977). *In* "Comparative Pathobiology", Vol. 3, pp. 135–154. Invertebrate Immune Responses. Plenum Press, New York.

Poisson, R. (1930). *Bull. Biol. France-Belgique* **64**, 288–331.

Rabin, H. (1970). *J. Reticuloendoth. Soc.* **7**, 195–207.

Ravindranath, M. H. (1974). *J. Morphol.* **144**, 11–22.

Ravindranath, M. H. (1975). *Biol. Bull., Woods Hole* **149**, 226–236.

Ravindranath, M. H. (1977a). *Cytologia* **42**, 743–751.

Ravindranath, M. H. (1977b). *Biol. Bull., Woods Hole* **152**, 415–423.

Sawyer, T. K. (1969). *Proc. Nat. Shellfish. Assoc.* **59**, 60–64.

Schapiro, H. C. (1975). *Amer. Zool.* **15**, 13–19.

Schapiro, H. C., Steenbergen, J. F. and Fitzgerald, Z. A. (1977). *In* "Comparative Pathobiology", Vol. 3, 127–133. Invertebrate Immune Responses. Plenum Press, New York.

Scharrer, B. (1972). *Z. Zellforsch. mikrosk. Anat.* **129**, 301–319.

Schoffeniels, E. and Gilles, R. (1970). *In* "Chemical Zoology", Vol. 5, pp. 255–286. Academic Press, New York and London.

Sewell, M. T. (1955). *Quart. Jl. Microsc. Sci.* **96**, 73–83.
Shivers, R. R. (1977). *Tissue and Cell.* **9**, 43–56.
Smith, V. J. and Ratcliffe, N. A. (1978). *J. Mar. Biol. Ass. U.K.* **58**, 367–379.
Smith, V. J. and Ratcliffe, N. A. (1980a). *J. Invertebr. Pathol.* **35**, 65–74.
Smith, V. J. and Ratcliffe, N. A. (1980b). *J. Mar. Biol. Ass. U.K.* **60**, 89–102.
Solangi, M. A. and Lightner, D. V. (1976). *J. Invertebr. Pathol.* **27**, 77–86.
Stang-Voss, C. (1971). *Z. Zellforsch. mikrosk. Anat.* **122**, 68–75.
Stewart, J. E. and Dingle, J. R. (1968). *J. Fish. Res. Board. Can.* **25**, 607–610.
Stewart, J. E., Dingle, J. R. and Odense, P. H. (1966). *Can. J. Biochem.* **44**, 1447–1459.
Stutman, L. J. and Dolliver, M. (1968). *Amer. Zool.* **8**, 481–489.
Tait, J. (1911). *J. Mar. Biol. Assoc. U.K.* **9**, 191–198.
Tait, J. and Gunn, J. D. (1918). *Quart. Jl. exp. Physiol.* **12**, 35–80.
Toney, M. E. jr. (1958). *Growth* **22**, 35–50.
Tyson, C. J. and Jenkin, C. R. (1973). *Austr. J. exp. biol. med. Sci.* **51**, 609–688.
Tyson, C. J. and Jenkin, C. R. (1974). *Austr. J. exp. biol. med. Sci.* **52**, 341–348.
Unestam, T. (1976). *J. Invertebr. Pathol.* **27**, 391–393.
Unestam, T. and Ajaxon, R. (1976). *J. Invertebr. Pathol.* **27**, 287–295.
Unestam, T. and Beskow, S. (1976). *J. Invertebr. Pathol.* **27**, 297–305.
Unestam, T. and Nylund, J. E. (1972). *J. Invertebr. Pathol.* **19**, 94–106.
Unestam, T. and Söderhäll, K. (1977). *Nature* **267**, 45–46.
Unestam, T. and Weiss, D. W. (1970). *J. Gen. Microbiol.* **60**, 77–90.
Vago, C. (1966). *Nature* **209**, 1290.
Vendrely, R., Ghidalia, N., Coirault, Y., Montmory, C., Brouard, M. O. and Prou-Wartelle, O. (1977). *C.R. Acad. Sci. Paris* **285D**, 1069–1072.
Vivares, C. P. (1972–73). *Vie et Milieu* **23**, 191–218.
Vranckx, R. (1978). Contribution à l'étude de la biosynthèse des protéines de la carapace d'un crustacé décapode: Analyse immunochimique des variations des protéines de l'hémalymphe et des téguments d'*Astacus leptodactylus* au cours du cycle de mue. *Thèse Univ. Paris VI.* 108 pp.
Vranckx, R. and Durliat, M. (1977). *C.R. Acad. Sci. Paris.* **285D**, 1045–1047.
Williams, A. J. and Lutz, P. L. (1975a). *J. Mar. Biol. Ass. U.K.* **55**, 667–670.
Williams, A. J. and Lutz, P. L. (1975b). *J. Mar. Biol. Ass. U.K.* **55**, 671–674.
Wood, P. J. and Karpawich, P. P. (1972). *Comp. Biochem. Physiol.* **42B**, 41–48.
Wood, P. J. and Visentin, L. P. (1967). *J. Morphol.* **123**, 559–568.
Wood, P. J., Podlewski, J. and Shenk, T. E. (1971). *J. Morphol.* **134**, 479–488.
Yeager, J. F. and Tauber, O. E. (1935). *Biol. Bull., Woods Hole* **69**, 66–70.

13. Insects

A. F. ROWLEY AND N. A. RATCLIFFE

Department of Zoology, University College of Swansea, Singleton Park, Swansea, SA2 8PP, U.K.

CONTENTS

I. Introduction

Insects, in terms of numbers of species, are the most successful group of invertebrates. Like other arthropods, they are protected by a heavily armoured exoskeleton which defends against mechanical damage and excess water loss. They also have an open circulatory system with the haemolymph in direct contact with the internal organs and containing various inorganic ions, amino acids, sugars, organic acids, lipids and organic phosphates (Florkin and Jeauniaux, 1974). Within this fluid are a variable number of blood cells called haemocytes, which either circulate freely or are attached to the various organs. Unlike many other animals, the insects do not usually rely on their circulatory system to transport oxygen since this is achieved by a unique system of tubes called tracheae which ramify the body.

The haemocytes have been the subject of many hundreds of scientific papers since they were first described by Swammerdam (1737), and have a number of distinct functions some of which are still poorly understood.

II. Structure of the circulatory system

The circulatory system has been described in detail in many entomological texts (e.g. Wigglesworth, 1965; Richards and Davies, 1977), as well as in a more specialized treatise (Jones, 1977).

Basically, the circulatory system is an open space or haemocoel in which blood movement is maintained by muscular pumps in the dorsal vessel. The dorsal vessel can be divided into three regions: (1) the posterior region, (2) the heart, which has valve openings called ostia in each segment and (3) the anterior region, which is often referred to as the aorta (Figs 1, 2).

The complexity of the heart differs dramatically from one insect species to another. For example, in nymphs of agrionid dragonflies it consists of a single chamber, while in many dictyopterans the heart is more highly developed, extending throughout the abdomen and hind-part of the thorax (Nutting, 1951) (Fig. 2a). The heart is not usually connected to any other "arteries" or "veins" although in cockroaches, vessels termed lateral

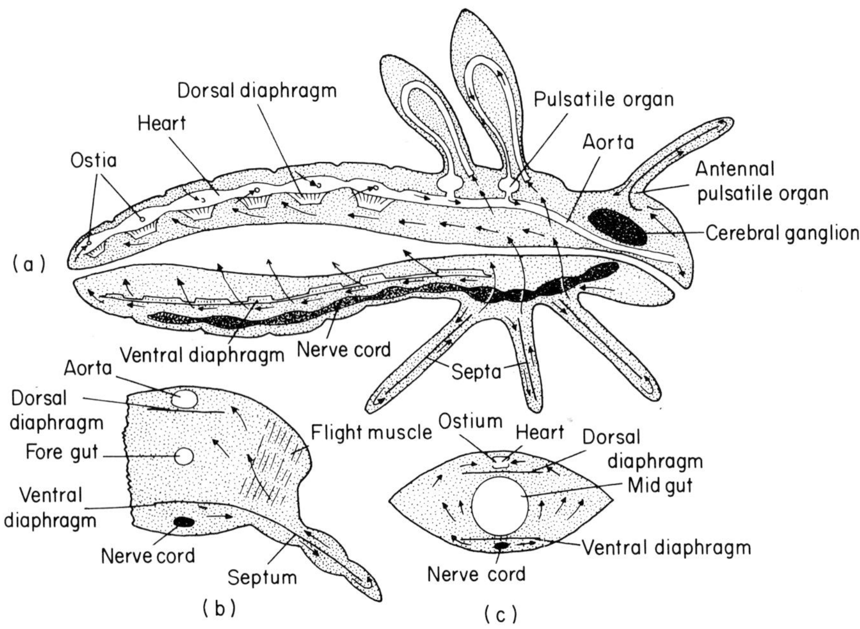

Fig. 1. (a) Schematic drawing of an insect with a fully developed circulatory system. (b) Transverse section through the thoracic region. (c) Transverse section through the abdominal region of Fig. 1a. Arrows indicate direction of circulation. (Redrawn from Wigglesworth, 1965.)

segmental vessels are present through which the blood flows out of the heart and into the haemocoel (Fig. 2b) (Nutting, 1951).

The heart is a muscular organ which is attached to the epidermis of the dorsal integument by a variety of muscles and fine strands of connective tissue. During expansion (diastole), blood enters the heart through the incurrent ostia and is propelled forward by waves of contraction. Most of the blood leaves the heart either through the excurrent ostia or via the aorta and out into the head region. In some insects, the ostia have developed into flap-like structures which only allow forward movement of blood through the heart (Wigglesworth, 1965).

Although most insect hearts' maintain their contractions when removed from the body, indicating a degree of myogenic control, the rate and amplitude of the beat is probably under nervous control (Wigglesworth, 1965). The heart rate is also affected by other factors such as temperature, deprivation of food, light and various drugs and hormones (Jones, 1977). In the cockroach, *Periplaneta americana*, extracts of the corpora cardiaca accelerate the heart rate (Davey, 1961a,b). The hormone(s) produced by the corpora cardiaca stimulate the pericardial cells which lie close to the heart (see section on haemocyte structure and classification) to produce a substance similar to serotonin or 5-hydroxytryptamine which directly accelerates the heart beat.

In addition to the dorsal vessel, some insects also have heart-like structures, called pulsatile organs or accessory hearts, which are found in various regions of the body including in the thorax near the wings, in the antennae and in the legs (Fig. 1). These organs are thought to assist circulation in peripheral regions and in those areas which need a constant blood supply, such as the wings.

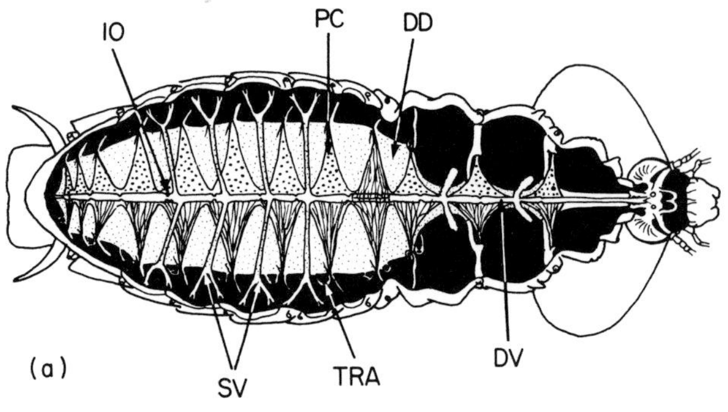

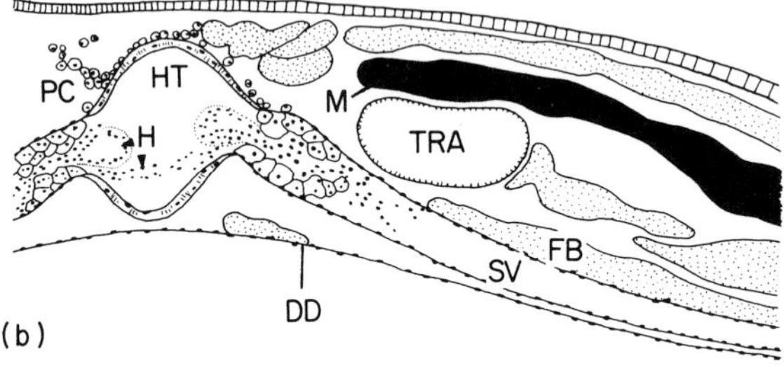

Fig. 2. (a) Ventral dissection of *Blaberus trapezoideus* showing the dorsal vessel (DV) and the associated segmental vessels (SV). Incurrent ostia (IO) pericardial cells (PC), dorsal diaphragm (DD) and trachea (TRA). (Redrawn from Nutting, 1951.) (b) Transverse section through the cockroach *Blaberus craniifer* showing the location of the heart (HT), segmental vessel (SV), haemocytes (H) and pericardial cells (PC). Fat body (FB), muscles (M), trachea (TRA), dorsal diaphragm (DD). Redrawn from Nutting (1951).

Blood flow is also directed by two septa, termed the dorsal and ventral diaphragms (Figs 1, 2). The dorsal diaphragm lies beneath the heart and is attached to the terga. Above it is the pericardial sinus which is in direct contact with the heart via the ostia. The ventral diaphragm is very extensive in some insects and is capable of undulatory movements which help to move the blood from the anterior to the posterior regions of the body and into the perineural sinus.

III. Structure and classification of haemocytes

Insect blood cells (haemocytes) are generally colourless cells, most of which float around freely in the haemolymph. Periodically, they may settle out of circulation and attach to various organs. Other groups of fixed cells which are sometimes confused with sessile haemocytes are the pericardial cells and oenocytes (see section on fixed haemocytes and other cells).

As in most other invertebrates, it has been extremely difficult, until recently, to establish a concise classification scheme for insect haemocytes. This has been mainly due to the many inconsistencies in nomenclature, experimental techniques and in the use of insects in different developmental stages. For example, various microscopical methods have been employed to study haemocyte structure including stained smears (e.g. Åkesson, 1954; Arnold, 1972), phase contrast microscopy (e.g. Jones, 1954a, 1959, 1962, 1965; Maier, 1969; Baerwald and Boush, 1970a; Price and Ratcliffe, 1974), transmission electron microscopy (e.g. Crossley, 1964; Beaulaton, 1968; Harpaz *et al.*, 1969; Hoffman, 1969a; Baerwald and Boush, 1970b; Lai-Fook, 1970, 1973; Stang-Voss, 1970; Akai and Sato, 1971, 1979; Devauchelle, 1971; Hagopian, 1971; Moran, 1971; Scharrer, 1972; Vecchi *et al.*, 1972; Neuwirth, 1973; Zachary and Hoffman, 1973; François, 1974; Ratcliffe and Price, 1974; Rowley and Ratcliffe, 1976a,b; Beaulaton and Monpeyssin, 1976, 1977; Schmit and Ratcliffe, 1978), scanning electron microscopy (e.g. Akai and Sato, 1971, 1979; Arnold, 1972; Olson and Carlson, 1974), various histochemical methods (Ashhurst and Richards, 1964a; Costin, 1975; Monpeyssin and Beaulaton, 1977; Schmit *et al.*, 1977), and freeze fracture (Baerwald, 1974, 1979), but only rarely have the results from different methods been compared. Some authors, possibly anticipating the problems involved, made no attempt to classify the cells found (e.g. Moran, 1971; Scharrer, 1972). Undoubtedly, one of the most useful methods is phase contrast microscopy in which unfixed, living cells can be examined for relatively long periods *in vitro*. This technique coupled with transmission electron microscopy, forms a useful combination for characterization of the cell types (Ratcliffe and Price, 1974).

Hollande (1911), proposed a useful classification scheme which recognized six categories of haemocytes, including, proleucocytes, phagocytes, granular leucocytes, oenocytoids, spherule cells and adipohaemocytes. Subsequently, many later workers introduced their own terminologies with the result that over 70 different names were ascribed to just a handful of haemocyte types (see review by Gupta, 1969). For example, the phagocytic haemocytes of the wax-moth, *Galleria mellonella*, have been termed leukocytes, lymphocytes and spherule cells (Cameron, 1934), Type A and B cells (Iwasaki, 1927), plasmatocytoids and adipohaemocytes (Werner and Jones, 1969) and macroplasmatocytes and microplasmatocytes (Rabinovitch and De Stefano, 1970). The inconsistency in terminology is still a problem to be overcome by insect haematologists (see, however, Gupta, 1979).

One of the best and most widely used classification schemes is that proposed by Jones in 1962. This scheme is based mainly on the phase contrast appearance of a number of species from six insect orders. Jones proposed nine different cell-types, the prohaemocytes, plasmatocytes, granular cells, cystocytes, spherule cells, oenocytoids, adipohaemocytes, podocytes and vermiform cells. More recently, Price and Ratcliffe (1974), examined the blood cells of 28 different species from 15 insect orders in an attempt to produce a simplified classification system which would be valid for a large number of different orders. They based their scheme on the previous Jones (1962) classification and described six common cell types, the prohaemocytes, plasmatocytes, granular cells, cystocytes, spherule cells and oenocytoids (Tables I, II). The podocytes and vermiform cells, described by Jones (1962), were included in the plasmatocyte category, since they are probably specialized types of these cells. Likewise, the adipohaemocytes were not recognized as a separate cell type as they may be modified granular cells (Neuwirth, 1973) or fat body cells (Wigglesworth, 1956).

A. Prohaemocytes

The prohaemocytes are thought to be the basic "stem-type" cell from which all others develop (see haemocyte inter-relationships). They have previously been called proleucocytoids and proleucocytes (Hollande, 1911; Yeager, 1945; Wigglesworth, 1959) (see Table I).

Under the light microscope, the prohaemocytes are small, round or slightly elliptical cells, 6–13 μm in diameter with a high nuclear : cytoplasmic ratio (Fig. 3). The thin rim of cytoplasm is usually homogeneous or occasionally contains a few granule-like inclusions (Price and Ratcliffe, 1974).

Ultrastructurally, prohaemocytes are identified by their lack of differentiation. The cytoplasm has little rough endoplasmic reticulum (RER) or

TABLE I. List of various haemocyte synonyms.

Classification scheme	Prohaemocytes	Plasmatocytes	Authors equivalent classes to: Granular cells	Cystocytes	Spherule cells	Oenocytoids
Hollande (1911)	proleucocytes	phagocytes	granular leucocytes adipoleucocytes[a]		spherule cells	oenocytoids
Metalnikov (1924)	lymphocytes proleucocytes	←leucocytes→	←leucocytes→		cell sphéruleuses	
Cameron (1934)	lymphocytes	leucocytes	leucocytes?		spherule cells	oenocytes
Yeager (1945)	proleucocytoids	plasmatocytes podocytes[b] vermiform cells[b]	chromophilic cells?	cystocytes	spheroidocytes	oenocyte-like cells
Wigglesworth (1959)	proleucocytes	phagocytic amoebocytes			phagocytic amoebocytes?	oenocytoids
Jones (1962) and Arnold (1974)	prohemocytes	plasmatocytes podocytes[b] vermiform cells[b]	granular hemocytes adipohemocytes[a]	cystocytes	spherule cells	oenocytoids
Brehélin *et al*. (1978)	prohemocytes	plasmatocytes granulocytes?[c] thrombocytoids[b] podocytes[b]	granulocytes	coagulocytes	spherule cells	oenocytoids
Gupta (1979)	prohemocytes	plasmatocytes	granulocytes	coagulocytes	spherulocytes	oenocytoids

[a] Some workers class adipohaemocytes as granular cells.
[b] In some instances these may be classified with the plasmatocytes.
[c] See text.

TABLE II. A summary of the morphological characteristics of insect haemocytes.

Feature	Prohaemocyte	Plasmatocyte	Granular cell	Cystocyte	Spherule cell	Oenocytoid
Size (μm)[a]	6–13	10–15	8–20	8–15	3–16	12–30
Shape	round to oval	round to spindle shaped (variable *in vitro*)	round to oval	round	round to spindle shaped	round to oval
Rough endoplasmic reticulum	little or none, not distended	moderate and not distended	extensive and distended near Golgi complexes	variable, sometimes distended	moderate and distended	little and distended
Golgi complexes	absent or few, poorly developed	moderate and reasonably well-developed	many and actively secreting	moderate and actively secreting	moderate	few/absent and very poorly developed
Granular/spherular inclusions	occasional	none or moderate/large numbers	many, with variable substructure	many, with variable substructure	large spherular inclusions with variable substructure	
Lysosome-like bodies	—	+	+	+	?	—
Vacuoles containing debris	—	+	+	+	—	—
Stability and reactions *in vitro*	highly stable, some produce small protoplasmic extensions	stable, put out protoplasmic extensions and spread out	unstable, occasionally form protoplasmic extensions	highly unstable, nucleus becomes refractile *in vitro*	highly stable, occasionally form protoplasmic extensions	highly stable, no protoplasmic extensions
Other characteristic features	high nuclear: cytoplasmic ratio	capable of amoeboid movement		high nuclear: cytoplasmic ratio	spherules distend cell membrane	eccentric nucleus microtubules in nucleus and cytoplasm

[a] Based on values from Price and Ratcliffe, (1974).

Golgi complexes and encloses many free ribosomes and a few mitochondria (Fig. 4) (Devauchelle, 1971; Ratcliffe and Price, 1974; Rowley, 1977a). The nucleus often contains prominent blocks of both hetero- and eu-chromatin, features often seen in other undifferentiated cells such as unstimulated vertebrate lymphocytes (Cline, 1975).

As with most other haemocyte types, the proportion of prohaemocytes compared with other cell types varies throughout the life cycle but is rarely more than 5% (Jones, 1962), and, as would be expected in a stem cell, is sometimes greatest in early instars (Arvy and Lhoste, 1946). Prohaemocytes are thought to be actively mitotic cells which give rise to plasmatocytes by direct differentiation (see section on origin and formation of haemocytes and, haemocyte inter-relationships).

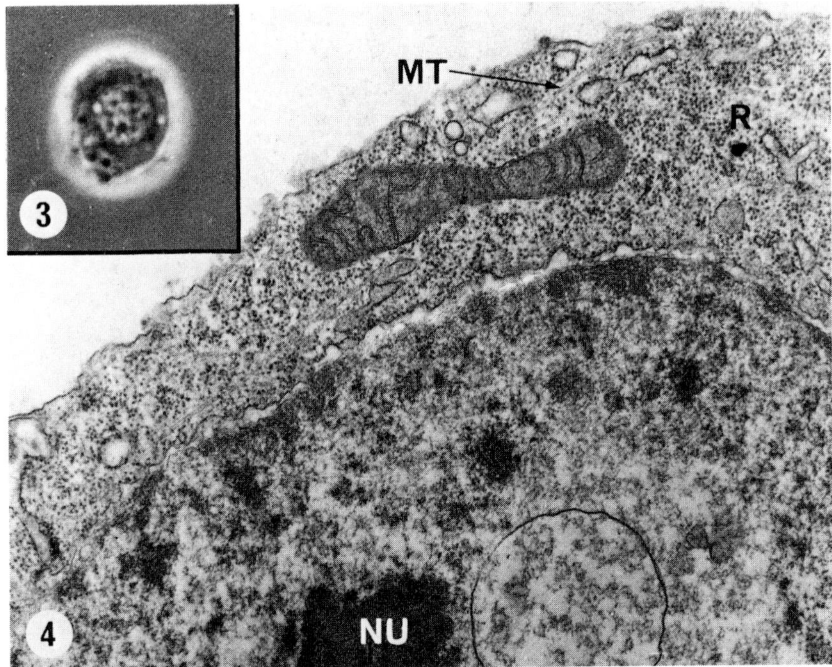

Fig. 3. Phase contrast micrograph of a *Galleria mellonella* prohaemocyte. Note large nuclear:cytoplasmic ratio. ×1600.

Fig. 4. Electron micrograph of a part of a prohaemocyte of *G. mellonella*. Characteristic features include the prominent nucleolus (NU), many free ribosomes (R). Microtubules (MT). ×23 000.

B. Plasmatocytes

The plasmatocytes are larger cells than the prohaemocytes and have been called macro-nucleocytes, amoebocytes, phagocytes, leucocytes and macrophages by some authors (Table I) (Ratcliffe and Rowley, 1979b). *In vivo*, they are usually spindle-shaped (Arnold, 1974; Price and Ratcliffe, 1974), while *in vitro*, they attach to glass slides by the formation of protoplasmic extensions and become amoeboid (Baerwald and Boush, 1970a; Cherbas, 1973). In their native state, these cells are highly refractile with little cytoplasmic detail visible, however, during spreading *in vitro*, the cytoplasmic contents progressively become more clearly defined (Fig. 5). The cytoplasm of the plasmatocytes may contain phase-dark granules of various shapes and sizes (Baerwald and Boush, 1970b; Arnold, 1974; Rowley and Ratcliffe, 1976a) or be agranular (Neuwirth, 1973; Price and Ratcliffe, 1974; Rowley, 1977a) as in most lepidopterans (Figs 6–10). This variation in the

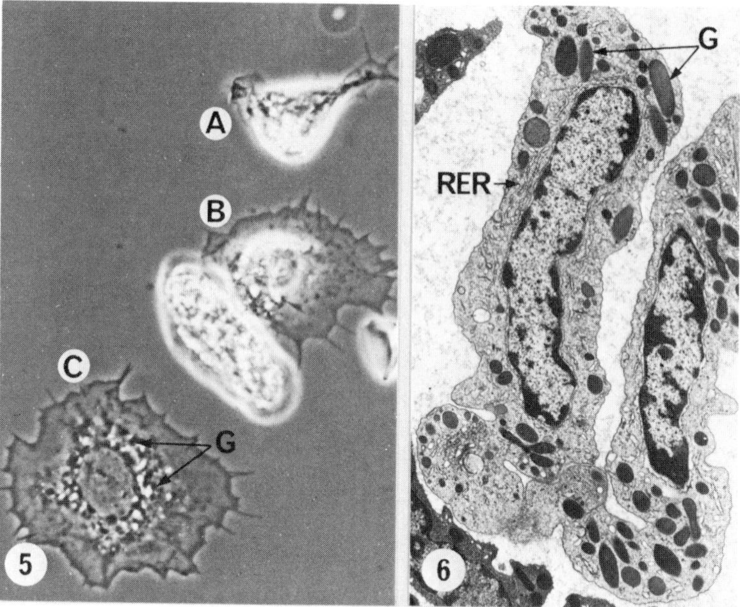

Fig. 5. Successive stages in spreading of *Periplaneta americana* plasmatocytes (A,B,C) with the loss of refractiveness and unmasking of cytoplasmic detail. Granules (G). Phase contrast. ×800.

Fig. 6. Electron micrograph of two plasmatocytes from *P. americana*. Note the cytoplasmic granules (G) and rough endoplasmic reticulum (RER). ×5400.

degree of granulation has led to a certain amount of confusion in the literature (e.g. Brehélin *et al.*, 1975; Ravindranath, 1978) where granular plasmatocytes and granular cells have sometimes been confused. Indeed, ultrastructurally, the granule-containing plasmatocytes may be difficult to distinguish from granular cells and this problem is exacerbated by the presence of these two cell types in a common lineage (see section on haemocyte inter-relationships).

The granule structure in the plasmatocytes varies from species to species. Often, they are amorphous and electron-dense, as in the plasmatocytes of *Calliphora erythrocephala* (Zachary and Hoffmann, 1973; Rowley and Ratcliffe, 1976a), *Melolontha melolontha* (Devauchelle, 1971) and *Periplaneta americana* (Fig. 6) (Ratcliffe and Price, 1974; Rowley, 1977a). Other species may contain both amorphous granules and granules with a distinct microtubular substructure (Ratcliffe and Price, 1974; Schmit and Ratcliffe, 1978) (Fig. 8). In granule-containing plasmatocytes, the Golgi complexes are usually reasonably well-developed and the stages in granule formation may be clearly visible (Fig. 9). Immature granules, which form directly from the Golgi, are often larger and their contents rather more

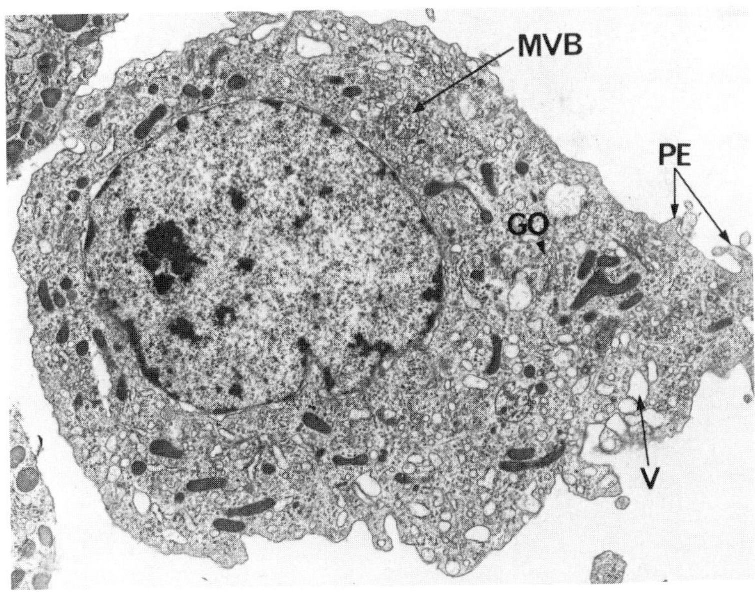

Fig. 7. Electron micrograph of a *G. mellonella* agranular plasmatocyte. Note the cytoplasm contains many vacuoles (V), a multivesicular body (MVB) and a reasonably well-developed Golgi (GO). Protoplasmic extensions (PE). ×7250.

dispersed and flocculent, as compared with the mature forms (Fig. 9). Cytochemically, the plasmatocyte granules also vary. For example, in *C. erythrocephala* (Crossley, 1975; Rowley, 1977a) and *Clitumnus extradentatus* (Rowley and Ratcliffe, unpublished), they are lysosomal and acid phosphatase positive (Fig. 10), while in *P. americana*, they are apparently non-lysosomal (Rowley and Ratcliffe, unpublished). The granules also usually contain acid mucopolysaccharide-like substances (Hoffmann, 1967; Costin, 1975).

The cytoplasm also encloses a moderate amount of RER, free ribosomes, multivesicular bodies, various forms of debris, which is probably mainly phagocytic in origin, vacuoles and mitochondria (Figs 6, 7, 9, 10). At the cell periphery, small protoplasmic extensions are usually formed and a variable number of pinocytotic vesicles may be present.

Cells such as vermiform cells and podocytes (=thrombocytoids of Zachary and Hoffmann (1973) =filamentous plasmatocytes of Rowley and Ratcliffe, 1976a) are included in this group as they are probably highly

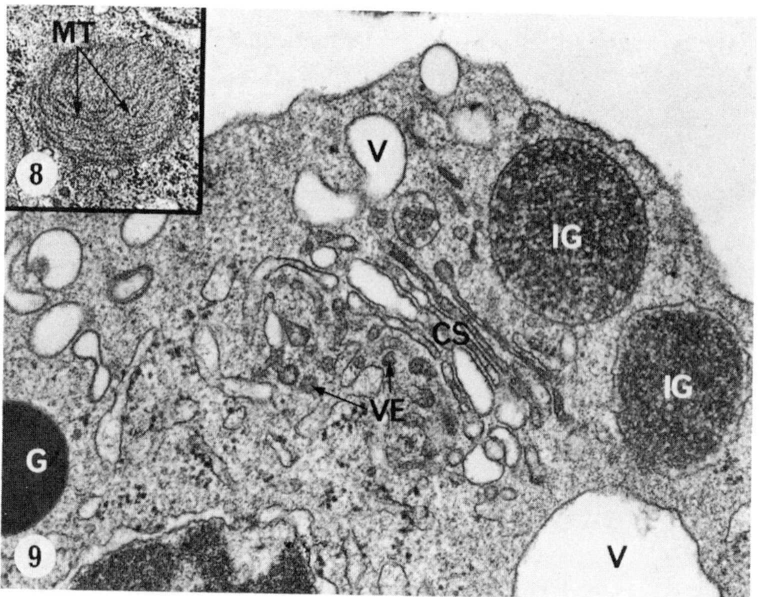

Fig. 8. Granule with a microtubular (MT) substructure present in a plasmatocyte of *Clitumnus extradentatus*. × 25 000.

Fig. 9. Detail of part of a *P. americana* plasmatocyte showing a well-developed Golgi complex composed of vesicles (VE) and cisternae (CS) and immature granules (IG) formed at the active face. Note also the vacuoles (V) and a mature more electron-dense granule (G). × 34 000.

specialized types of plasmatocytes. In *C. erythrocephala*, the podocytes are similar to typical plasmatocytes in that they readily form protoplasmic extensions and ingest bacteria (Rowley and Ratcliffe, 1976a), but unlike true plasmatocytes have the ability to fragment (Zachary and Hoffmann, 1973). The vermiform cells, as described by Jones (1962, 1977), are highly elongate and uncommon.

As with other haemocyte types, the percentage of plasmatocytes varies from insect to insect, even within the same species, as well as during the life cycle of any individual. However, in most insects the plasmatocytes account for between 30–60% of the total circulating haemocyte population, although in some cases, such as *Zooptermopsis nevadensis* they may form as much as 90% of the cells (Schmit, 1979).

The plasmatocytes have been shown to be involved in phagocytosis (Wittig, 1965a,b, 1966; Salt, 1970; Ratcliffe and Rowley, 1975), encapsulation (Salt, 1970; Schmit and Ratcliffe, 1977, 1978), basement membrane formation (Wigglesworth, 1956, 1973), wound repair (Lai-Fook, 1970; Bohn, 1975; Rowley and Ratcliffe, 1978), nodule formation (Ratcliffe and Gagen, 1976, 1977) and metamorphosis (Whitten, 1964) (see functions of haemocytes).

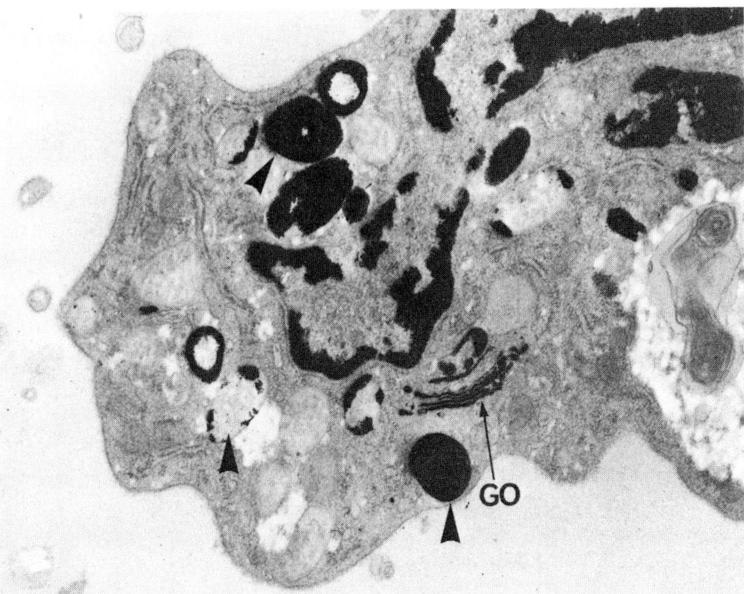

Fig. 10. Part of a plasmatocyte of *C. extradentatus* showing the presence of the enzyme acid phosphatase in the granules (unlabelled arrows) and the Golgi cisternae (GO). × 20 000.

C. Granular cells

Granular cells are round or oval, 8–20 μm in diameter with a central nucleus (Fig. 11) and have been termed adipohaemocytes, cystocytes and granular leucocytes by some authors (Table I). They are packed with granules, and, in contrast to plasmatocytes, do not spread extensively *in vitro* and only rarely form protoplasmic extensions (Price and Ratcliffe, 1974). Granular cells usually rapidly degranulate *in vitro* leaving clear vacuoles in the cytoplasm (Fig. 11) (Rowley and Ratcliffe, 1976b; Rowley, 1977b). This process appears to be involved in haemolymph coagulation as well as other cellular defence reactions (see section on haemocyte functions).

Ultrastructurally, the granular cells of many lepidopterans are easily distinguished from agranular plasmatocytes (Akai and Sato, 1973;

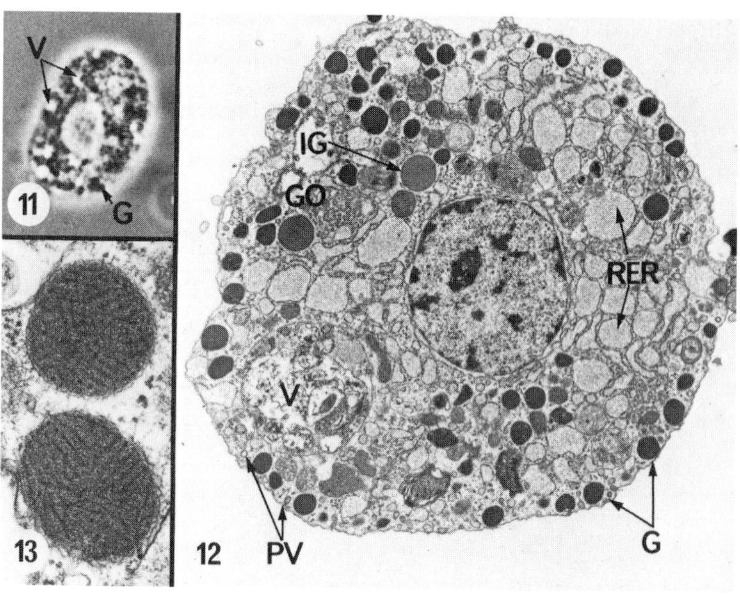

Fig. 11. Phase contrast micrograph of a *G. mellonella* granular cell with prominent phase-dark granules (G), and vacuoles (V) which have been formed during granule discharge *in vitro*. × 1300.

Fig. 12. A typical granular cell of *G. mellonella*. Note the dilated rough endoplasmic reticulum (RER), Golgi (GO), mature amorphous electron-dense granules (G) and an immature less electron-dense, microtubule-containing granule (IG). Vacuole containing debris (V), pinocytotic vesicles (PV). × 7000.

Fig. 13. Detail showing the microtubule-containing granules of a *G. mellonella* granular cell. × 39 500.

Neuwirth, 1973; Rowley and Ratcliffe, 1976b). However, in most other orders, the distinction between these two cell types may not be readily apparent (Ratcliffe and Price, 1974), and this, as mentioned above, may reflect a close inter-relationship between these cells (see section on haemocyte inter-relationships).

The cytoplasm of granular cells contains a large number of membrane-bound granules (Figs 12–14) and, as in the plasmatocytes, these may be electron-dense and unstructured, or less electron-dense, with a microtubular substructure. In *G. mellonella*, the immature granules formed by the Golgi complex always have a microtubular substructure (Neuwirth, 1973; Rowley and Ratcliffe, 1976b) which is probably lost during condensation to form the mature granules. Conversely, during degranulation, the microtubular substructure reappears prior to discharge from the cell (Rowley and Ratcliffe, 1976b). Neuwirth (1973) reported that the granules of *G. mellonella* granular cells are non-lysosomal and like those of the plasmatocytes contain acid mucopolysaccharides. However, in *C. extradentatus* some granules are

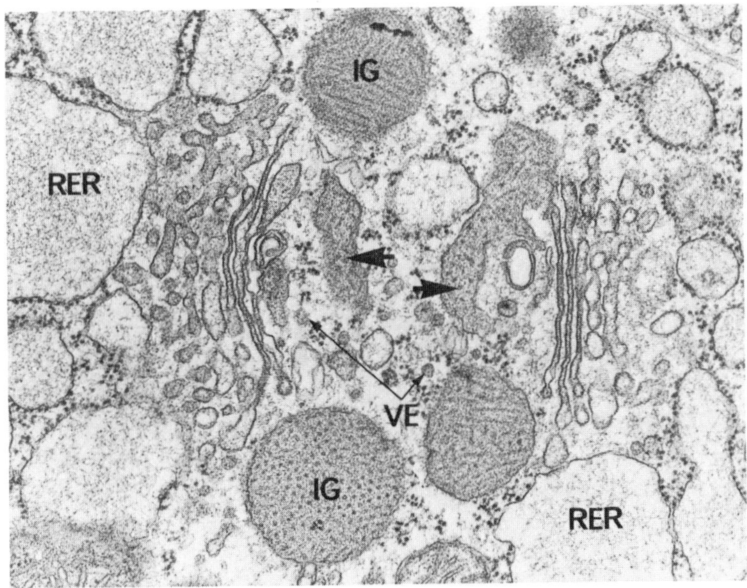

Fig. 14. Portion of a *G. mellonella* granular cell showing the formation of microtubule-containing granules (IG). Note the numerous vesicles (VE) and cisternae of the Golgi complex, the swollen cisternae of the rough endoplasmic reticulum (RER), and the condensation of material with a microtubular substructure (unlabelled arrows) from the Golgi. (From Rowley and Ratcliffe, 1976b.) × 34 000.

occasionally acid phosphatase positive (Rowley, unpublished). Unlike the plasmatocytes, however, the endoplasmic reticulum in the granular cells is often extensively swollen, particularly around the Golgi complexes, presumably as a result of the large amount of material synthesized by the ribosomes which passes through the RER into the Golgi (Fig. 14). The Golgi complexes are usually extremely well-developed consisting of several cisternae and numerous vesicles. The cytoplasm also contains a variable number of mitochondria, vacuoles and vesicles (Fig. 12). The cell outline is usually very smooth with few protoplasmic extensions, and pinocytotic vesicles frequently occur in the peripheral cytoplasm.

Several authors, including Akai (1969, 1971), Lai-Fook (1973) and Neuwirth (1973), believe that the adipohaemocytes described by Jones (1962) and other authors are in fact a mature form of the granular cells, filled with lipid-like inclusions, while Wigglesworth (1956) is of the opinion that they may be fat body cells. The so-called adipohaemocytes of Pipa and Woolever (1965) look very unlike granular cells and more like degenerating plasmatocytes.

Granular cells make up 30–60% of the total haemocyte population and are readily found in most insect species (Price and Ratcliffe, 1974). The known functions of these cells include phagocytosis (Neuwirth, 1974), nodule formation (Ratcliffe and Gagen, 1976, 1977), encapsulation (Schmit and Ratciffe, 1977), melanin formation (Schmit *et al.*, 1977), coagulation (Rowley and Ratcliffe, 1976b), wound repair (Rowley and Ratcliffe, 1978) and hormone transport (Takeda, 1977) (see section on functions of haemocytes).

D. Cystocytes

The cystocytes are round cells, 8–15 μm in diameter with a high nuclear:cytoplasmic ratio and have been termed granular haemocytes, explosive corpuscles and coagulocytes by other workers (see Grégoire, 1970) (Table I). *In vitro*, these cells are highly fragile and quickly degenerate (Figs 15, 16). These changes involve the rapid degranulation and apparent loss of cytoplasmic contents and an increase in the refractivity of the nucleus (Figs 15, 16). At the same time, flocculent material forms around the degenerating cell and builds up to form an "islet of coagulation" (Grégoire, 1955a,b, 1957) (Fig. 15). In the cockroach, *P. americana*, this material is composed of precipitated plasma proteins (Siakotos, 1960a,b).

Ultrastructurally, there is some variation in their morphology and in section they may be difficult to distinguish from granular cells and plasmatocytes. We have found that in *C. extradentatus* (Rowley, 1977b) and

P. americana (Rowley and Ratcliffe, unpublished), the cytoplasm contains little or no RER but small numbers of polyribosomes and smooth endoplasmic reticulum are present as well as a variable number of granules (Fig. 17). Again, like the plasmatocytes and granular cells, both unstructured and structured granules are found in these cells. One useful characteristic features is the swelling of the perinuclear space (Fig. 17) (Goffinet and Grégoire, 1975).

Cystocytes are commonly observed in most insect orders except the Diptera, Hymenoptera, Lepidoptera and Thysanura (Price and Ratcliffe, 1974) and account for between 30–60 % of the total haemocyte population.

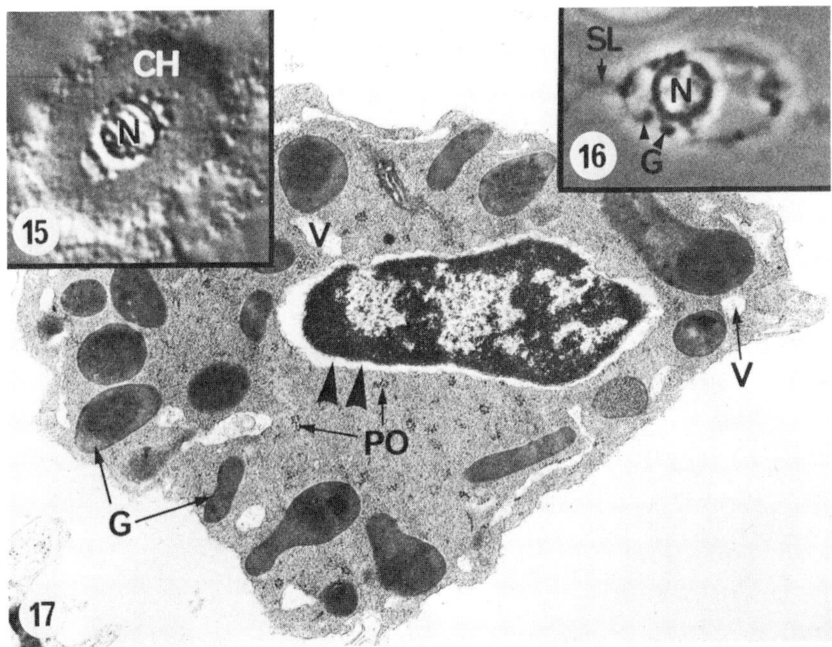

Fig. 15. Nomarski interference micrograph of a degenerated cystocyte from *C. extradentatus* after approximately 10 min *in vitro*. Note the refractile nucleus (N) and a surrounding zone of coagulated haemolymph (CH). ×1100.

Fig. 16. Phase contrast micrograph of a degenerated cystocyte from *Tenebrio molitor*. Note the prominent nucleus (N) patchy cytoplasm containing a few granules (G) and strand-like material (SL) around the cell. ×1900.

Fig. 17. Electron micrograph of a *C. extradentatus* cystocyte with many granules (G), polyribosomes (PO), vacuoles (V) and a swollen perinuclear cisterna (unlabelled arrows). (From Rowley, 1977b.) ×20 000.

In the Lepidoptera, their role in coagulation seems to be fulfilled by the granular cells, which they may be equivalent to, while the Diptera, podocytes (specialized plasmatocytes) seem to be involved in haemostasis. Apart from their functions in haemolymph coagulation, cystocytes also take part in encapsulation, nodule formation (Ratcliffe *et al.*, 1976a,b) and phagocytosis (Brehélin *et al.*, 1978).

E. Spherule cells

The spherule cells are spindle-shaped or oval cells, 8–16 μm in diameter

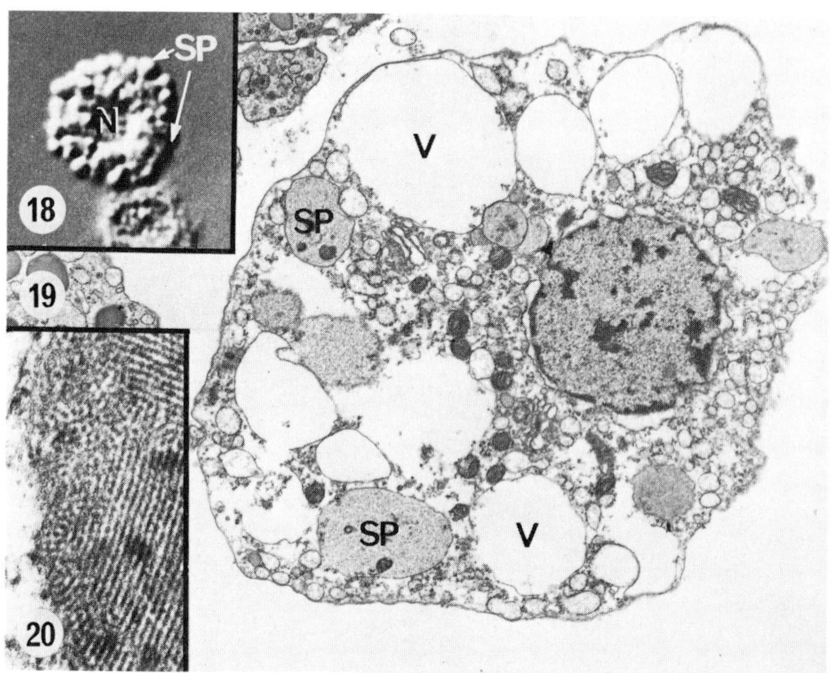

Fig. 18. Nomarski interference micrograph of a *G. mellonella* spherule cell. Note the prominent spherules (SP) which distend the cell. Nucleus (N). ×1400.

Fig. 19. Electron micrograph of a spherule cell of *G. mellonella* containing large spherules (SP) which fill the cytoplasm and distend the cell periphery. The vacuoles (V) are probably caused by spherule lysis/extraction during fixation and processing. ×10 000.

Fig. 20. Electron micrograph showing the crystalline substructure of a spherule in a spherule cell of *G. mellonella*. ×90 000.

and are usually filled with spherular inclusions which range from 1·5–3·0 μm in diameter (Fig. 18). They have been called spherulocytes, adipohaemocytes, coarsely granular cells, eruptive cells and eleocytes by other authors (see Ratcliffe and Rowley, 1979a,b) (Table I). With phase contrast microscopy, the spherules are highly refractile, and due to their size and number sometimes obscure the nucleus and distend the cell periphery (Fig. 18). The spherule cells have been reported to put out fine pseudopodia in some insects (Price, 1974) but this does not generally occur.

Ultrastructurally, the spherule cells are easily identified by the large inclusions which fill the cytoplasm and distend the cell membrane (Fig. 19). These membrane-bound spherules have a very variable structure. For example, in the Egyptian cottonworm, *Spodoptera littoralis*, Harpaz *et al.* (1969) found that the spherules (called spherulites) had a crystal-like lattice often arranged in concentric layers (Fig. 21). In *Antheraea pernyi* (Beaulaton and Monpeyssin, 1977) and *G. mellonella* (Fig. 20) (Neuwirth, 1973) a crystalline substructure is also present in the inclusions, while in

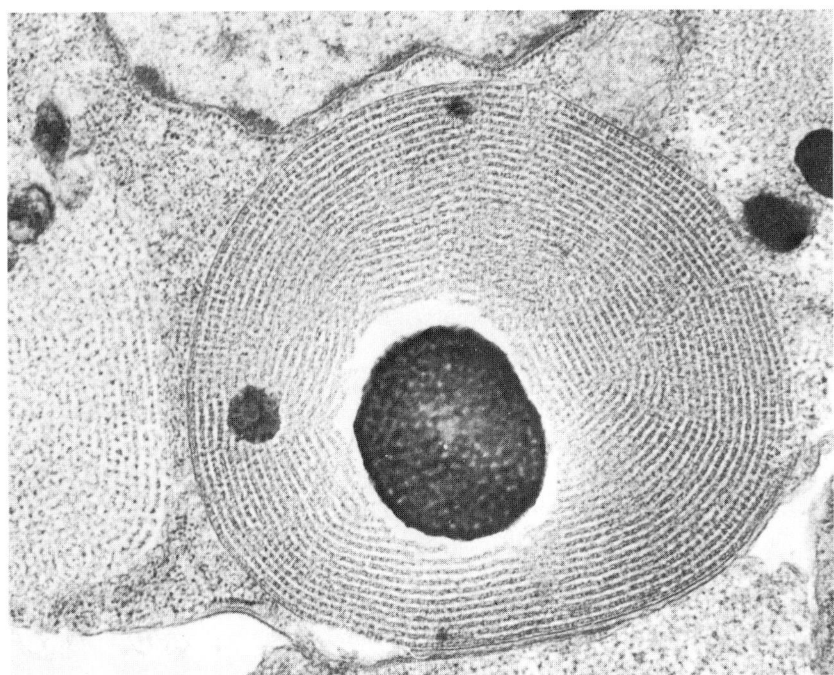

Fig. 21. Part of a spherule cell of *Spodoptera littoralis* showing the structure of a spherule (spherulite). (Courtesy of Professor I. Harpaz, from Harpaz *et al.*, 1969.) × 32 000.

Sphodromantis bioculata the centres of the spherules are composed of cross-linked microtubules (Ratcliffe and Price, 1974). In contrast, in *C. extradentatus* (Schmit and Ratcliffe, 1978) and *M. melolontha* (Brehélin *et al.*, 1978) the spherules are electron-dense and unstructured.

In most spherule cells, the spherules account for approximately 90% of the cytoplasm (Fig. 19) and rarely are active Golgi complexes present. These may well have regressed after the formation of the spherules. The rest of the cytoplasm contains mitochondria, a little distended RER, free ribosomes and a variety of vacuoles and vesicles (Fig. 19). Some reports (Lai-Fook and Neuwirth, 1972) indicate that the spherules are poorly preserved by fixatives such as glutaraldehyde, and this may well explain the presence of large vacuoles often found in spherule cells (Fig. 19). Similar observations have been noted using phase contrast microscopy, in which commonly used fixatives were seen to lyse the spherules (Jones, 1977). Finally, Gupta and Sutherland (1967) suggested that the spherule cells of some cockroaches contain spherules which themselves had the capacity to form plasmatocytes. This observation has not been substantiated and seems most unlikely.

The percentage of spherule cells present is usually relatively low (<5%), however, they are widely distributed within the species examined by Price and Ratcliffe (1974). The functions of spherule cells are uncertain, they have, however, been implicated in silk production in *Bombyx mori* (Nittono, 1960).

F. Oenocytoids

Oenocytoids are round to oval shaped cells and are easily identifiable in the light microscope due to their large size (up to 30 μm in diameter) and their relatively homogeneous cytoplasm (Fig. 22). The nucleus is often eccentric and accounts for only 20–40% of the cell volume. In *G. mellonella*, the cytoplasm contains a few indistinct rod-like filaments (Fig. 22). These cells are very stable *in vitro*, rarely if ever change their shape and do not put out protoplasmic extensions.

Ultrastructurally, the oenocytoids are also highly characteristic with a cytoplasm containing, apart from numerous ribosomes, only a few of the usually encountered organelles such as RER, which in *G. mellonella* is associated with the poorly-developed Golgi complexes (Figs 23, 24). Generally, any mitochondria present are found either in the close vicinity of the nucleus or at the cell periphery (Fig. 23). In *B. mori* and *Calpodes ethlius*, the major feature of the cytoplasm is a number of fibres which either form whorls or rod-like structures (Akai and Sato, 1973; Lai-Fook, 1973). In *G. mellonella*, no fibres are present but instead bundles of microtubules extend throughout the cytoplasm and nucleus (Figs 23–25). In some instances, these microtubules are absent and this is probably due to fixation at low temperatures which brings about microtubule breakdown (Stebbings and Hyams, 1979).

The crystal cells reported in some Diptera (Rizki and Rizki, 1959; Nappi and Streams, 1969; Brehélin *et al.*, 1978) may be a special type of oenocytoid since they contain large crystalline bodies in a cytoplasm otherwise devoid of organelles (Fig. 26).

The oenocytoids are not widely distributed cells and are mainly confined to the Lepidoptera (Price and Ratcliffe, 1974). They usually account for only 1–2% of the total haemocyte population. Their functions are uncertain but they may be involved in melanization processes and reactions to parasites (Rizki and Rizki, 1959; Schmit *et al.*, 1977).

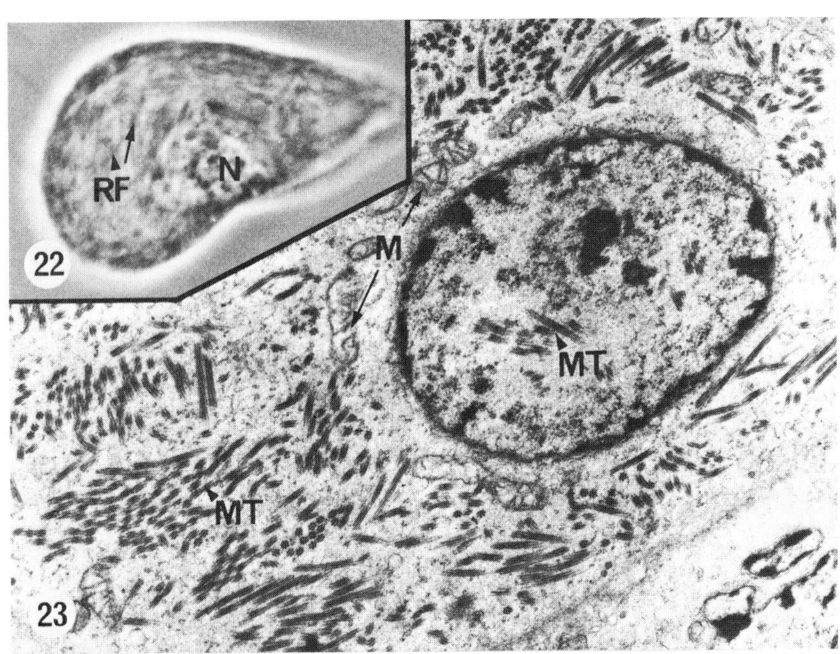

Fig. 22. Phase contrast micrograph of an oenocytoid from *G. mellonella*. Note the eccentric nucleus (N) and rod-like filaments (RF) in the cytoplasm. ×1500.

Fig. 23. Electron micrograph of an oenocytoid of *G. mellonella*. Note the bundles of microtubules (MT) in the nucleus and cytoplasm and the ring of mitochondria (M) around the nucleus. ×11 000.

G. Haemocyte inter-relationships

Basically two schools of thought exist on the inter-relationships of haemocytes. Arnold (1972), believes that in some cockroaches the different cell types are probably formed on separate developmental lines from the prohaemocytes. However, most other insect haematologists (e.g. Beaulaton, 1968; Lai-Fook, 1973; Neuwirth, 1973; Zachary and Hoffmann, 1973) believe that the different cell types are only the stages in the development of one or two basic cell lines (unitarian hypothesis of Scharrer, 1972). In reality, both of these views may well be partially correct.

In the unitarian hypothesis we would expect to find a number of intermediate cells with characteristic features of two or more cell types. This, in fact, seems to be the situation in many species (e.g. Beaulaton, 1968; Lai-Fook, 1973; Neuwirth, 1973).

In *G. mellonella* Neuwirth (1973) found many intermediates between prohaemocytes and plasmatocytes, and plasmatocytes and granular cells and we have also seen similar cells (Rowley and Ratcliffe, unpublished). Intermediates between plasmatocytes and granular cells are characterized by variable amounts of swollen RER, protoplasmic extensions and a few granules (*ca.* 10/section), often with a microtubular substructure (Fig. 27).

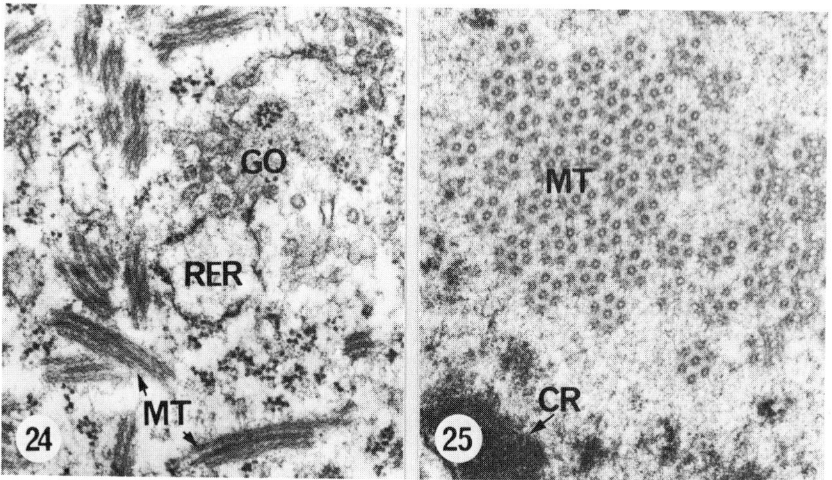

Fig. 24. Detail of part of the cytoplasm of an oenocytoid of *G. mellonella* showing a poorly developed Golgi complex (GO) associated with swollen, sparse, rough endoplasmic reticulum (RER). Microtubules (MT). × 39 500.

Fig. 25. Electron micrograph of part of the nucleus of an oenocytoid of *G. mellonella* showing bundles of microtubules (MT) in cross-section. Chromatin (CR). × 58 000.

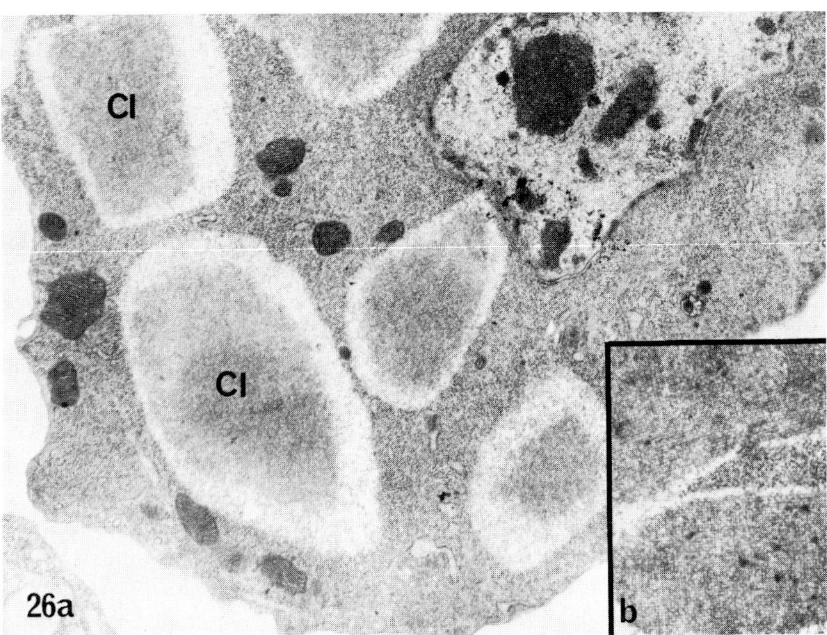

Fig. 26. (a) Electron micrograph of a crystal cell (=oenocytoid?) of *Drosophila melanogaster*. Crystal-like inclusions (CI). ×14 000. (b) Higher power electron micrograph showing the substructure in a crystal. (Courtesy Dr M. Brehélin, from Brehélin *et al.*, 1978.) ×22 000.

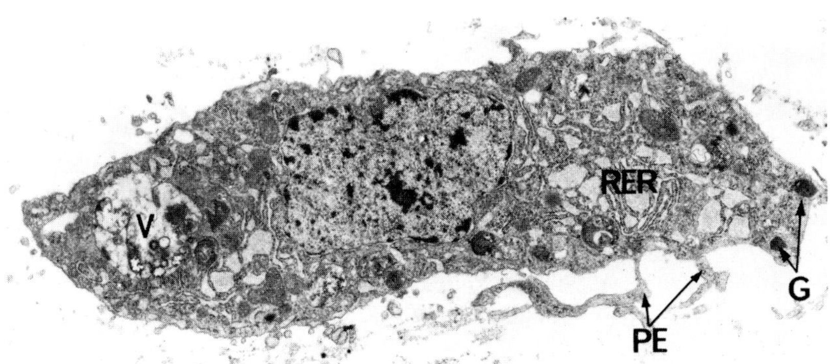

Fig. 27. Low power electron micrograph of a cell from *G. mellonella* intermediate between a granular cell and plasmatocyte. Only a few granules (G) are present. Note the swollen rough endoplasmic reticulum (RER), vacuoles containing debris (V) and protoplasmic extensions (PE). ×6700.

These cells are clearly distinct from typical "mature" granular cells which contain many granular inclusions (up to 100/section) and well-developed RER and Golgi complexes (Fig. 12). We found, however, little evidence for any inter-relationship between the granular cells and the spherule cells, particularly as their inclusions are structurally so dissimilar (compare Figs 13 and 20).

These morphological results corroborate the work of Shrivastava and Richards (1965), in which autoradiographic techniques were used to study the development of the various haemocyte types in the larval life of *G. mellonella*. They found a developmental series passing from prohaemocytes → plasmatocytes → granular cells (they termed these adipohaemocytes). This differentiation took about three days to complete and the cells disappeared within another three days indicating a life span of some six days. Further autoradiographic studies would clearly be useful.

Some workers have used changes in the haemogramme as a source of information for establishing the inter-relationships of haemocytes, but any conclusions will be complicated by the many variable factors found in the *in vivo* state. To our knowledge no *in vitro* study has shown any indication of haemocyte differentiation in culture. A hormonal control mechanism responsible for cell differentiation *in vivo* may thus be present, which would be missing *in vitro*.

H. Fixed haemocytes and other cells

Most of the information given above concerns free haemocytes. Not all haemocytes, however, are found in circulation and in *Rhodnius prolixus*, for example, most of the haemocytes are thought to be attached to various tissues (unpublished observations given in Wigglesworth, 1959). It seems likely that many insects contain a variable number of fixed haemocytes and that these cells provide a reservoir which can be mobilized at times of stress such as during microbial infections or wounding and subsequent haemorrhage (Shapiro, 1968). Jones and Tauber (1951) found that after heat fixation of *Tenebrio molitor* larvae (a process which apparently causes fixed cells to become free) the number of circulating cells approximately doubled as compared with the unfixed controls. Similar results have been found by Walters (personal communication) with *G. mellonella* larvae after acetic acid vapour treatment. Here the total haemocyte count rose from $2{\cdot}6 \times 10^4$ cells/ml to $1{\cdot}6 \times 10^5$ cells/ml. Most of this difference was caused by the mobilization of fixed plasmatocytes.

The fixed haemocytes do not appear to represent a distinct population of cells from those found in circulation. However, there are some permanently fixed cells which do exist and these include the nephrocytes (including the pericardial cells) and oenocytes. Whether these cells are true blood cells is unclear, but Wigglesworth (1970) has likened the pericardial cells to the vertebrate reticuloendothelial system.

1. Nephrocytes

These cells are found in many insect species and include the pericardial cells (=dorsal nephrocytes, Hollande, 1922), ventral nephrocytes (Metalnikov, 1902), garland cells (Chapman, 1969) and the diaphragm cells (Edwards and Challice, 1960).

The most commonly described cells are the pericardial cells which are found in the dorsal sinus attached to the heart and alary muscles (Fig. 2) (Crossley, 1972; Jones, 1977). These cells have been widely studied in both the light (Hollande, 1922) and electron microscopes (Kessel, 1961, 1962; Bowers, 1964; Hoffmann, 1966; Crossley, 1972; Brehélin, 1977).

Morphologically, pericardial cells vary from species to species. They are usually round to ovoid, often pigmented and contain a variable number of granules (Hollande, 1922; Jones, 1954b; Kessel, 1962; Brehélin, 1977) (Fig. 28). Ultrastructurally, these cells are very complex as shown by a study of the pericardial cells of *Calliphora erythrocephala* (Crossley, 1972). They are composed of several distinct regions, including an outer cortex characterized by a series of deep infoldings of the plasma membrane with associated

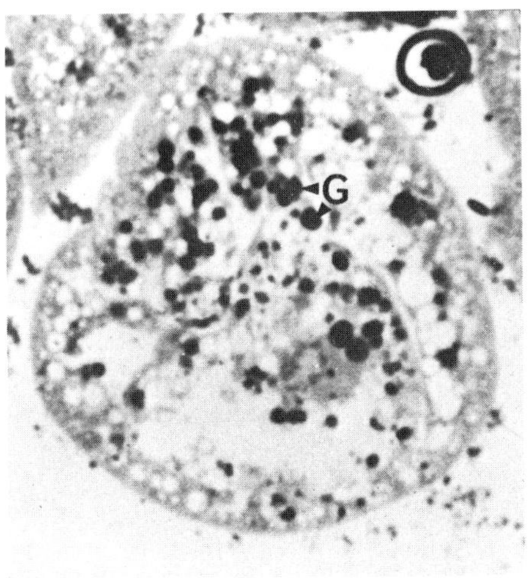

Fig. 28. Thick plastic section of a pericardial cell from *Schistocerca gregaria*. Granules (G). ×1100.

pinocytotic vesicles, and immediately below this a "transitional zone" containing mitochondria and small electron-dense vesicles/vacuoles. The transitional zone merges into an area of large electron-dense vacuoles which further into the cell body is transformed into a region containing large amounts of RER, Golgi and glycogen rosettes (Crossley, 1972).

Various authors (e.g. Hollande, 1922; Wigglesworth, 1943; Hoffmann, 1966; Crossley, 1972) have shown that the pericardial cells readily pinocytose colloidal particles such as dyes and tracer substances, but it seems unlikely that they are phagocytic (see, however, Cameron, 1934). This particle uptake is aided by their large surface area, formed by the infoldings of the cell membrane (Crossley, 1972), and reflects their main function which is the removal of toxic or waste substances from the haemolymph (Hollande, 1922). Wigglesworth (1943, 1970) has also shown that the pericardial cells of *Rhodnius prolixus* are involved in the removal and detoxification of waste products associated with the haemoglobin from the blood meal. More recently, Crossley (1972) reported that the pericardial cells of *C. erythrocephala* are involved in the formation of lysozyme which has an important antibacterial role (Chadwick, 1977).

2. *Oenocytes*

This is probably an unfortunate name for these cells as they are easily confused with the oenocytoids which are a distinct population of true haemocytes. The oenocytes are often large cells and in *C. ethlius* are up to 200 μm in diameter (Locke, 1969). They are found in a variety of sites, including close to the epidermis (Locke, 1969) or associated with the spiracles or fat body (Wigglesworth, 1965). Oenocytes characteristically contain an acidophilic cytoplasm (Richards, 1951; Wigglesworth, 1965) and may be binucleate.

In *C. ethlius*, the oenocytes are characteristically packed with large amounts of tubular smooth endoplasmic reticulum and also contain autophagic vacuoles, microbodies, RER, Golgi complexes and mitochondria (Locke, 1969). The oenocytes of other insect species are ultrastructurally similar to those of *C. ethlius* (Fig. 29) (Evans, 1967; Gnatzy, 1970; Romer, 1972, 1974). These ultrastructural characteristics are noticeably different to those of the oenocytoids which are mainly devoid of such organelles (Fig. 23).

The functional significance of oenocytes is not well understood, but it has been suggested that they are involved in the formation of the moulting hormone, ecdysone (Locke, 1969), or of cuticular wax (Evans, 1967). Certainly, ultrastructurally, they are similar to steroid hormone synthesizing cells, such as those in the vertebrate corpus luteum (Bjersing, 1967).

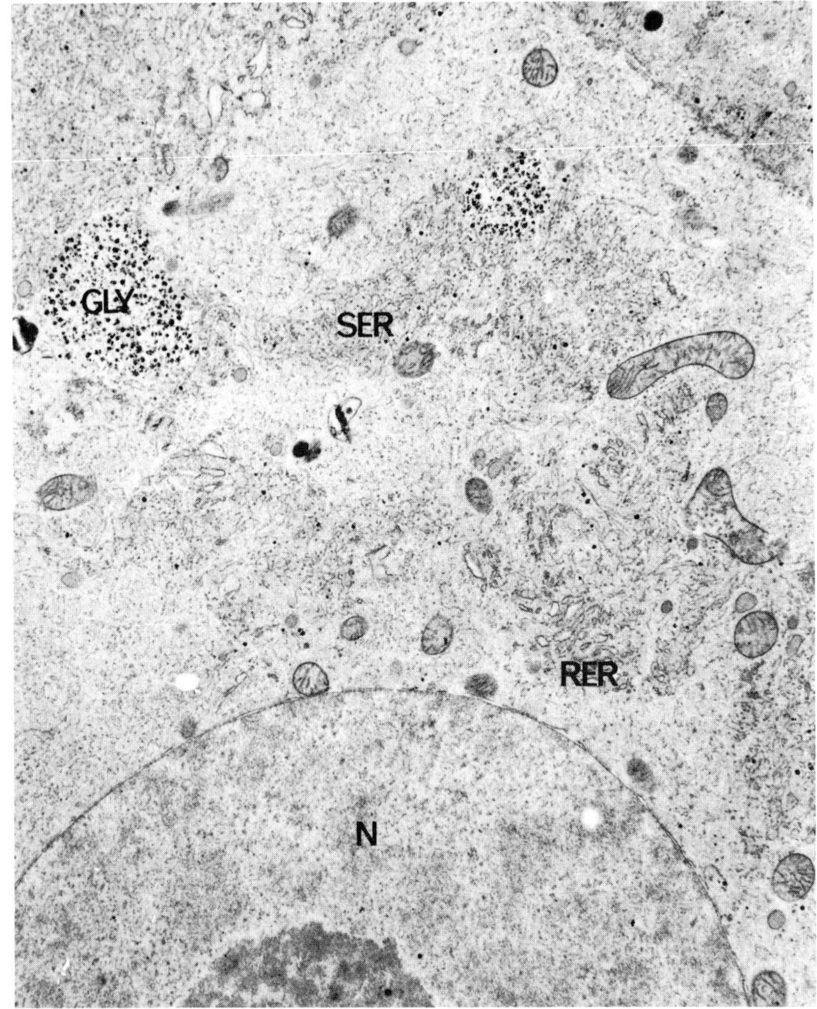

Fig. 29. Electron micrograph showing the structure of a typical oenocyte from *Gryllus bimaculatus*. Note the smooth (SER) and rough (RER) endoplasmic reticulum, glycogen deposits (GLY) and nucleus (N). (Courtesy Professor F. Romer, from Romer, 1972.) $\times$ 12 000.

Furthermore, in some insects, the oenocytes enlarge and appear more active just prior to moulting as would be expected if they were synthesizing moulting hormone or cuticular wax. They also increase in numbers during cuticular wound healing (Gray, personal communication).

Other reports indicate that like the fat body cells and nephrocytes, the oenocytes may also be important in the detoxification process. Clark and Dahm (1973) fed *Musca domestica* with phenobarbitol and found that, as in the mammalian liver, the oenocytes showed marked ultrastructural changes which may have been associated with detoxification.

IV. Origin and formation of haemocytes

This can be divided into the embryological and postembryological origins, and these are discussed separately.

A. Embryological origin

All cells of the circulatory system, including the haemocytes differentiate from mesodermal cells (Jones, 1977). Recently, this has been carefully studied in *Oncopeltus fasciatus*, by Dorn (1978). He found that during embryogenesis the haemocytes quickly segregate along the entire length of the mesoderm. The haemocytes produced are undifferentiated and are morphologically similar to prohaemocytes (Fig. 30). Mitoses are rarely seen in these cells and no distinct embryological haemopoietic organ has been observed. Later in embryogenesis, these cells appear to differentiate into plasmatocyte-like cells with an increased amount of RER and noticeable phagocytic activity. At no times are either differentiated granular cells or oenocytoids seen (Dorn, 1978).

B. Post-embryological origin

The post-embryological formation of haemocytes has recently been extensively reviewed by Jones (1970).

Basically, two methods of haemocyte formation (haemopoiesis or haemocytopoiesis) have been suggested. Firstly, by the mitotic division of circulating haemocytes and secondly, by the formation of haemocytes in distinct haemopoietic organs (Jones, 1970, 1977).

1. Mitotic division

Mitotic division of circulating haemocytes has often been recorded (see Jones, 1970). The mitotic indices (= % mitosis) are rarely higher than 1%, as recorded in *G. mellonella* (Jones, 1967b; Jones and Liu, 1968), *Prodenia eridania* (Yeager, 1945) and *Rhodnius prolixus* (Jones, 1967a). In *Drosophila melanogaster* larvae, however, Rizki (1957) found a mitotic rate of nearly 5%.

Confusion exists about which haemocyte types are capable of mitosis. Most workers have shown that the prohaemocytes and the plasmatocytes can actively divide (Jones, 1970), and Shapiro (1968) found that in *G. mellonella* the granular cells are also capable of mitosis. Arnold and Hinks (1976) reported that in *Euxoa declarata*, prohaemocytes, granular cells and

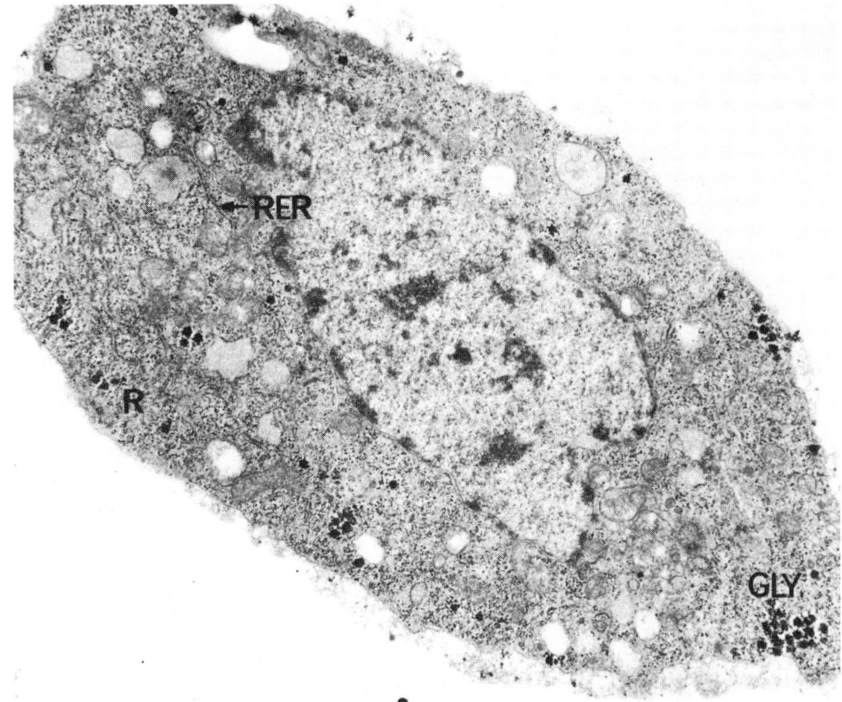

Fig. 30. Electron micrograph of a newly segregated prohaemocyte-like cell of a 57 h old *Oncopeltus fasciatus* embryo. Note the numerous free ribosomes (R), little rough endoplasmic reticulum (RER) and glycogen deposits (GLY). (Courtesy Dr A. Dorn, from Dorn, 1978.) ×12 800.

spherule cells are often seen in various stages of division, while plasmatocytes are only occasionally involved.

The low mitotic rate usually recorded may indicate that mitosis alone is not the only process involved in haemocyte production. However, in *G. mellonella*, Jones and Liu (1968) showed that even a 1% mitotic rate is sufficient to allow for the maintenance of cell numbers during larval life and so preclude the need for any haemopoietic organ.

2. *Haemopoietic organs*

Haemopoietic organs have been found in a large number of different insects and are present in various parts of the body. In lepidopteran larvae, they are often associated with imaginal wing discs in the thorax (Arvy, 1952; Nittono *et al.*, 1964; Akai and Sato, 1971; Hinks and Arnold, 1977; Monpeyssin and Beaulaton, 1978), while in some dipterans they are found in the posterior segments of the abdomen (Arvy, 1953; Zachary and Hoffmann, 1973). In *Gryllus bimaculatus* and *L. migratoria*, well-developed haemopoietic organs are present in the abdomen attached to the dorsal diaphragm where they have been termed "phagocytic organs" (Nutting, 1951) due to their ability to accumulate various dyes.

Hoffmann (1970a), graded insect haemopoietic organs into three types which he believed represented possible evolutionary stages in their development. The first type is composed of dissociated masses of haemocytes, including cells undergoing mitosis. Such accumulations may correspond to the "haemocyte reservoirs" described by Jones (1977) and may be purely transitional, caused by haemocytes temporarily aggregating together. The accumulations of haemocytes in the posterior regions of *Musca domestica* (Nappi, 1974) may represent this type of haemopoietic organ. Hoffmann's second category include groups of cells forming a diffuse tissue with little signs of differentiation into distinct regions and unbounded by either a limiting membrane or a connective tissue sheath. Examples of this type of haemopoietic organ include those of *L. migratoria* (Hoffmann, 1970a) and *C. erythrocephala* (Zachary and Hoffmann, 1973). In *L. migratoria* (Hoffmann, 1970a, 1973; Hoffmann *et al.*, 1974), *C. erythrocephala* (Zachary and Hoffmann, 1973) and *Melolontha melolontha* (Brehélin, 1973), the haemopoietic organs contain cells, called reticular cells, which are thought to be similar to the reticular cells of vertebrate lymphatic tissue. The cells are loosely aggregated into vast networks which divide and form haemopoietic foci which mature to form the haemocytes. Like vertebrate reticular cells, they are phagocytic (Hoffmann *et al.*, 1974) and serve to help keep the haemocoel clear of infectious agents (see section on functions of haemocytes—phagocytosis).

The third type of haemopoietic organ is more highly developed, showing some signs of differentiation into various zones and is bounded by a limiting membrane. This type of organ has been reported in *B. mori* (Akai and Sato, 1971), *Aglia tau*, *Antheraea pernyi* (Figs 31, 32) and *Manduca sexta* (Monpeyssin and Beaulaton, 1978) and *G. bimaculatus* (Hoffmann, 1970a). In *A. pernyi* these organs are composed of stem cells, arranged in islets and surrounded by a connective tissue sheath (Monpeyssin and Beaulaton, 1978). In some of these islets, the cells are held together by intercellular junctions (Fig. 32). The cells are morphologically similar to the prohaemocytes (see Fig. 4), with a thin rim of undifferentiated cytoplasm filled with many free ribosomes, little RER, poorly developed Golgi complexes and a few mitochondria (Fig. 32). In some of these islets, cells similar to plasmatocytes and immature granular cells are also present and have probably differentiated from prohaemocytes. As the cells are formed in the islets they apparently loose their connections and are released from the organ through gaps in the connective tissue sheath. Monpeyssin and Beaulaton (1978) also found that both oenocytoids and spherule cells differentiate in specific islets of haemopoietic organs. Similarly, in *B. mori*, Akai and Sato (1971) described "cysts" (=islets?) of differentiating haemocytes containing stem-like cells.

The importance of the haemopoietic organs in haemocyte production has been demonstrated by irradiating these organs (Hoffmann, 1972; Zachary and Hoffmann, 1973), ligaturing around the haemopoietic tissue (Hinks and Arnold, 1977) or by surgical removal (Beaulaton, 1978). These modifications generally cause a great drop in the number of circulating haemocytes and indicate the role of these organs in the formation of large numbers of haemocytes.

C. The relative importance of mitosis and haemopoiesis in maintaining haemocyte numbers

As mentioned above, Jones and Liu (1968, 1969) showed that mitosis alone could account for the maintenance of haemocyte numbers, at least under normal conditions. Presumably after the formation of haemocytes from the mesodermal elements these cells divide and differentiate during the rest of the life of the insect. Other authors have stressed the importance of the haemopoietic organs alone (e.g. Hoffmann, 1973) in maintaining the normal haemogramme and rarely mention the role of mitosis. In reality, both processes probably operate, depending on the species examined and the stage in the life cycle. In *Euxoa declarata* it has been found that the granular cells and spherule cells are derived from circulating cells by mitosis

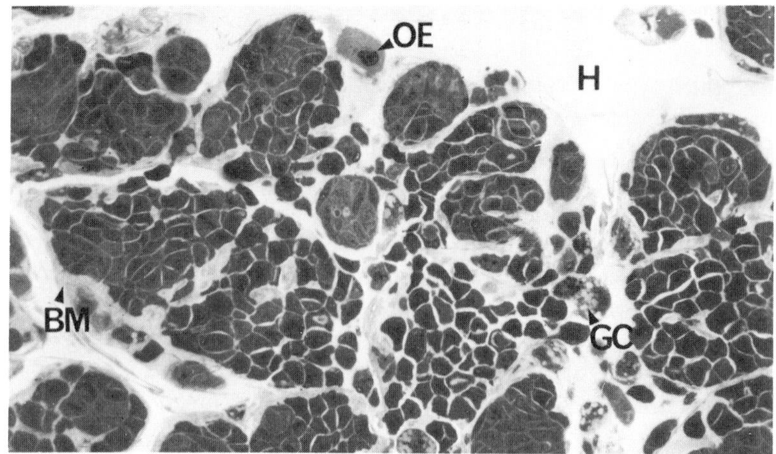

Fig. 31. Light micrograph of part of the haemopoietic tissue of *Antheraea pernyi* showing many islets surrounded by a basement membrane sheath (BM). An oenocytoid (OE) and a granular cell (GC) can be seen in the process of release into the haemocoel (H). (From Monpeyssin and Beaulaton, 1978.) $\times 370$.

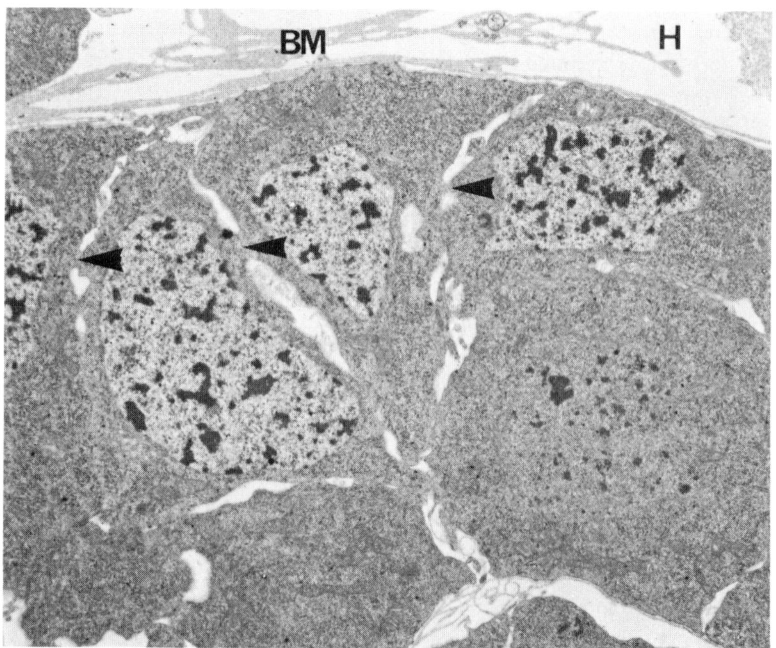

Fig. 32. Electron micrograph of part of a compact islet from the haemopoietic tissue of *A. pernyi* showing undifferentiated (prohaemocyte-like) cells. Note the numerous gap junctions (unlabelled arrows) holding the cells together. Basement membrane (BM), haemocoel (H). (Courtesy Drs M. Monpeyssin and J. Beaulaton, from Monpeyssin and Beaulaton, 1978.) $\times 6800$.

while the haemopoietic organs form prohaemocytes, plasmatocytes and oenocytoids which differentiate within the organ (Arnold and Hinks, 1976; Hinks and Arnold, 1977). However, the prohaemocytes also divide in the haemolymph to form other prohaemocytes or plasmatocytes. These studies show the close developmental relationship between the prohaemocytes and the plasmatocytes (see section on haemocyte inter-relationships), but also, surprisingly, indicates that the granular cells are on a separate lineage to these former cell types. In contrast, in *B. mori* (Akai and Sato, 1971) and *Antheraea pernyi* (Monpeyssin and Beaulaton, 1978), all the cell types are formed within the haemopoietic organ and the prohaemocytes, plasmatocytes and granular cells are all found in similar regions of the organ, indicating a common ancestory.

D. Control of haemopoiesis

It has been suggested that both haemocyte formation and maintenance of haemocyte numbers is under endocrine control (Hoffmann and Joly, 1969; Hoffmann and Perolini, 1969; Hoffmann, 1970b). In adult *L. migratoria*, the corpora allata are necessary for both the production and differentiation of the haemocytes (Hoffmann, 1970b). Removal of the corpora cardiaca also reduces the rate of differentiation of granular cells and cytocytes from the plasmatocytes. Furthermore, in final instar nymphs of *L. migratoria*, the production and differentiation of haemocytes appears to be under the control of the prothoracic gland. The hormones involved have not been identified but they may well act directly on the haemopoietic organs.

The mobilization of haemocytes during wound healing and encapsulation may also be under endocrine control (Nappi, 1975a; Rowley and Ratcliffe, 1978; Ratcliffe and Rowley, 1979a) (see section on functions of haemocytes—wound healing and encapsulation).

V. Functions of haemocytes

The role of insect haemocytes in cellular defence reactions has, over the years, received a great deal of attention while other functions such as hormone transport and nutrient storage have been neglected.

The cellular defence reactions of insects consists of at least five processes; phagocytosis, nodule formation, encapsulation, haemolymph coagulation and wound healing which have recently been reviewed (Ratcliffe and Rowley, 1979a). The latter two functions are not usually included in discussions of the defence reactions, but are considered here as they are involved in sealing off wounds caused by predators, mechanical damage, etc. and thus stop the influx of potential pathogens from the environment. It is when these initial defences fail that phagocytosis, nodule formation and/or encapsulation reactions are elicited.

A. *Phagocytosis*

Phagocytosis was first studied in invertebrates by Metchnikoff (1884) and his observation led to our present day understanding of the role of this process in killing invading microorganisms in vertebrates. Many early workers, including Metalnikov (1908, 1924, 1927), Metalnikov and Chorine (1928), Hollande (1930), Chorine (1931) and Cameron (1934) found that after injecting relatively large doses of bacteria or other test particles into the haemocoel these came to lie within the haemocytes. Many different particles are ingested by insect blood cells, including inert substances such as particulate dyes, India ink, polystyrene spheres, as well as biological agents such as viruses, bacteria, fungi, protozoa and vertebrate erythrocytes (Salt, 1970). During metamorphosis, phagocytic haemocytes also ingest cell and tissue debris (Perez, 1910; Whitten, 1964).

In vivo experiments, can give valuable if somewhat limited information as to the importance of phagocytosis as a defence reaction. For example, Bettini *et al.* (1951) found that prior injection of erythrocytes into *P. americana* caused a reduction in the ability of the insects to resist subsequent infection. The results of such "phagocytic blockade" experiments are often used as evidence to indicate the importance of phagocytosis in the cellular defence reactions. However, such treatments may also interfere with other cellular defences such as nodule formation, or even the synthesis of humoral substances which have been shown to be important in microbial control (Chadwick, 1975; Boman *et al.*, 1979).

The best way of analysing the effectiveness of phagocytosis is by the use of *in vitro* techniques, similar to those developed for vertebrate phagocytes (e.g. Van Furth and Van Zwet, 1973). Many early attempts to examine phagocytosis *in vitro* had limited success (e.g. Åkesson, 1954; Jones, 1956; Whitten, 1964), which may have resulted from a number of factors, including the choice of test particle, culture medium deficiencies, or even the inability to distinguish intra- from extracellular particles (Rowley, 1977a).

Recently, phagocytosis has been successfully studied *in vitro* using different techniques (Gilliam and Shimanuki, 1967a; Lüthy *et al.*, 1970; Rabinovitch and De Stefano, 1970; Anderson *et al.*, 1973a,b; Anderson, 1976a,b; Ratcliffe and Rowley, 1974, 1975; Rowley and Ratcliffe, 1980). Generally, one of two main methods are used, either the cells are incubated and suspended with the test particles in a suitable saline or culture medium on a roller drum (Anderson *et al.*, 1973a; Ratcliffe and Rowley, 1975), or, the haemocytes are allowed to attach to glass coverslips or Petri dishes and form monolayers which are then overlaid with test particles (Rabinovitch and De Stefano, 1970; Ratcliffe, 1975; Rowley and Ratcliffe, 1976c, 1980). Both of these methods have inherent advantages and disadvantages. For example, many haemocytes tend to clump together or attach to surfaces in suspension culture, so making recovery from the tubes difficult (Ratcliffe and Rowley, 1975). Furthermore, examination of haemocytes in the electron microscope or the assessment of the degree of killing of test particles is difficult with haemocyte monolayers and usually involves the removal of the cells from the glass or plastic substrate, either by chemical or mechanical means which inevitably results in some cell damage.

Most workers have shown that the plasmatocytes are the major phagocytic cell type both *in vivo* and *in vitro* (Wittig, 1965a,b; Werner and Jones, 1969; Ryan and Nicholas, 1972; Anderson *et al.*, 1973a; Ratcliffe and Rowley, 1974, 1975) and the granular cells (Neuwirth, 1974) and cystocytes (Brehélin *et al.*, 1978) are also phagocytic in some species. In some of the older literature, the phagocytic cell types have been given many different names such as amoebocytes, leukocytes, phagocytes, macroplasmatocytes and spherule cells, but most of these probably correspond to the plasmatocyte type (see Ratcliffe and Rowley, 1979a).

Phagocytosis is a dynamic process which is composed of a number of different stages. The first stage, as shown with vertebrate phagocytes, is chemotaxis, i.e. the unidirectional movement of phagocytes towards the "foreign object" to be engulfed. During the second stage, the particle becomes attached to the outside of the blood cell. This may be brought about by the direct interaction between receptors on the cell membrane and the particle surface, or, with the aid of factors free in the blood called opsonins. In the third stage, the particle is ingested by the formation of pseudopodia and comes to lie in the cell within a phagocytic vacuole (phagosome). Finally, in many instances, the particle, if microbial in nature, may be killed and digested with the aid of lysosomal enzymes and specific killing factors. The indigestible remnants may be voided from the cell by exocytosis or stored as pigment bodies etc. These different stages are described below for insect phagocytes and are compared with similar processes in vertebrate phagocytes such as polymorphonuclear (PMN) leucocytes and monocytes/macrophages.

1. Chemotaxis

Vertebrate PMN leucocytes and macrophages have been shown to migrate towards various infectious agents (Wilkinson, 1976), and this migration is usually mediated by factors found in the serum such as immunoglobulin and complement. In insects, the role of chemotaxis in phagocytosis is unclear. Salt (1970), could find no evidence for its presence based on his work with encapsulation of parasites, and Jones (1956), failed to demonstrate any movement of the plasmatocytes of *Sarcophaga bullata* towards foreign particles *in vitro*. However, although Gagen and Ratcliffe (unpublished, reviewed in Ratcliffe and Rowley, 1979a) working with short-term cultures were also unable to demonstrate the migration of *G. mellonella* or *P. brassicae* plasmatocytes towards bacteria, they did show the unidirectional movement of these cells towards bacterial/granular cell complexes (see section on nodule formation). Likewise, Vey *et al.* (1968) and Vey (1969) found that the haemocytes of *G. mellonella* are attracted to *Aspergillus flavus* conidia *in vitro*. Furthermore, there is some considerable evidence for chemotaxis involving plasmatocytes in other cellular defence reactions such as nodule formation, encapsulation and wound healing (Nappi, 1973, 1975b; Ratcliffe and Gagen, 1976, 1977; Ratcliffe *et al.*, 1976a; Rowley and Ratcliffe, 1978).

2. Attachment

In vertebrates, the attachment of particles prior to phagocytosis is at least partially dependent on recognition factors (opsonins) found free in the serum which coat the foreign object and help in its binding to the phagocyte's surface receptors. In invertebrates, other than insects, opsonic activity has been found associated with the naturally-occurring bacterial and erythrocyte agglutinins present in various body fluids (Tripp, 1966; Tripp and Kent, 1967; Prowse and Tait, 1969; McKay and Jenkin, 1970; Tyson and Jenkin, 1973, 1974; Paterson and Stewart, 1974; Anderson and Good, 1976; Hardy *et al.*, 1977; Sminia *et al.*, 1979), but in insects, although such factors exist (Bernheimer, 1952; Gilliam and Jeter, 1970; Scott, 1971a,b, 1972; Ratcliffe and Rowley, 1980) there is little evidence that they function as opsonins (Scott, 1971b; Rowley and Ratcliffe, 1980) (see below, however). For example, in our own experiments with the erythrocyte agglutinins found in the haemolymph of *P. americana* and *C. extradentatus*, erythrocytes coated with agglutinin are not ingested at a significantly faster rate than uncoated red cells (Ratcliffe *et al.*, 1976a; Rowley and Ratcliffe, 1980). However, more recently we have found a factor present in the haemolymph of *P. americana*, which is non-agglutinating and causes an increase in the uptake of a *B. cereus* isolate, and therefore has opsonin-like activity in this insect (Ratcliffe and Rowley, 1980).

The nature of the receptors on the cell membrane of the plasmatocytes and granular cells is unknown but the experiments of Scott (1971b) and Anderson (1976a,b, 1977) at least point to their existence.

3. *Ingestion*

The method of ingestion of particles by insect phagocytes has only recently been studied (Leutenegger, 1967; Ratcliffe and Rowley, 1974, 1975; Rowley and Ratcliffe, 1976a) and, basically, the results of these experiments are similar to those with vertebrate phagocytes. Pseudopodia produced at the cell surface, surround the particle (Fig. 33) and eventually fuse, either with other protoplasmic extensions or with the cell surface to enclose the particle in a phagocytic vacuole. This phagocytic vacuole is usually very tightly opposed to the outside of the ingested material, and this has probably led some workers to believe that particles may actually lie directly in the cytoplasm (see Salt, 1970). Subsequently, the phagosomes are drawn further into the cell body where interaction with other organelles may occur (Figs 34–37).

The ingestion phase, unlike the attachment stage, is an energy dependent process. Anderson *et al.* (1973b) and Anderson (1974) showed that in *Blaberus craniifer*, the uptake of latex spheres is accompanied by stimulated glycogen breakdown, glucose consumption and lactate production, indicating

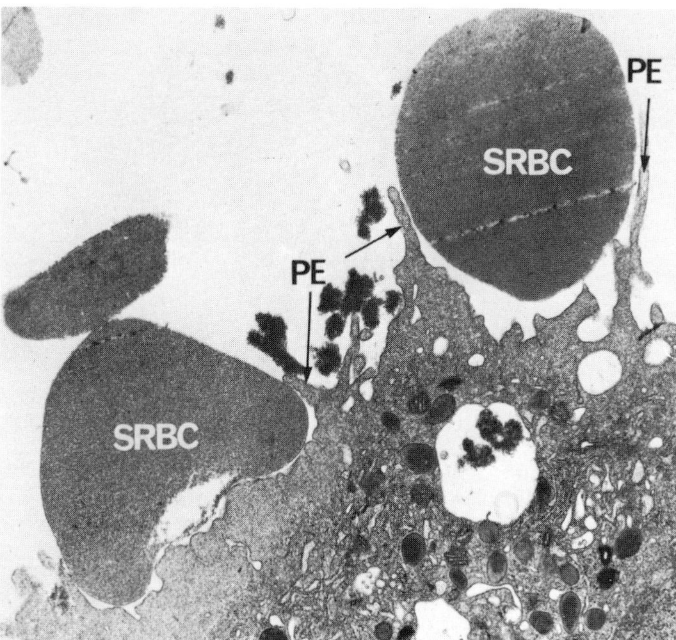

Fig. 33. Electron micrograph showing the ingestion of sheep erythrocytes (SRBC) by a plasmatocyte of *C. extradentatus*. Protoplasmic extensions (PE). ×11 500.

that energy for phagocytosis is produced via the glycolytic pathway. However, unlike mammalian phagocytes, during ingestion, the *B. craniifer* plasmatocytes show no increase in the activity of the hexose monophosphate pathway (Anderson *et al.*, 1973b).

4. *Intracellular events*

Many workers have shown that microorganisms are readily ingested by insect haemocytes (e.g. Cameron, 1934), but few have been able to clearly demonstrate their destruction within these cells. Early reports showed that intracellular bacteria became swollen and lost their distinct structure

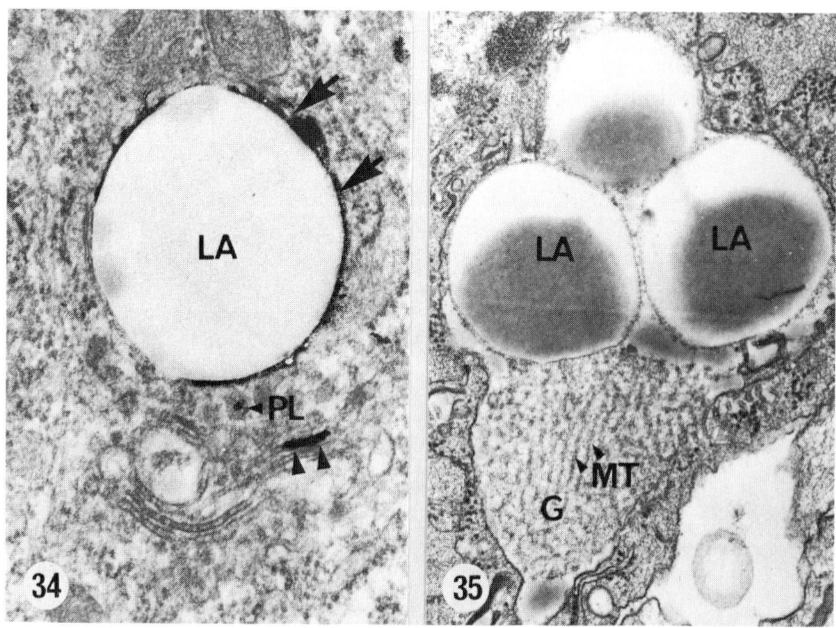

Fig. 34. Showing the distribution of acid phosphatase activity after incubation of latex beads (LA) with the plasmatocytes of *G. mellonella* for 24 h. Enzyme activity is marked by dense lead deposits. The partial halo of enzyme activity (large unlabelled arrows) in the phagosome indicates that lysosomal fusion has already occurred. Note enzyme activity in the Golgi complex (small unlabelled arrows) and primary lysosome (PL). (From Rowley and Ratcliffe, 1979.) ×45 000.

Fig. 35. Discharge of a granule (G) into a phagosome containing latex beads (LA) in the cytoplasm of a *P. americana* plasmatocyte. Note the microtubular remnants (MT) present in the granule. (From Ratcliffe and Rowley, 1979a.) ×38 000.

indicating digestion within the phagocytes (Hollande, 1930). However, some bacteria such as *Mycobacterium tuberculosis* in *G. mellonella* plasmatocytes (Cameron, 1934) and *Bacillus thuringiensis* in *Pseudaletia unipunctata* plasmatocytes and granular cells (Wittig, 1965b, 1966) remain viable. Furthermore, known pathogens such as *Pseudomonas aeruginosa* lyse the plasmatocytes of many insects, including *G. mellonella* (Madziora-Barusiewicz and Lysenko, 1971), which probably accounts for their pathogenicity.

Recently, two techniques have been used to examine the fate of microorganisms within insect haemocytes. First, bacteria and haemocytes are incubated together and the loss of microbial viability calculated by standard plate counting (Anderson *et al.*, 1973a). Secondly, haemocytes which have ingested microorganisms are fixed and examined in the electron microscope (Rowley and Ratcliffe, 1976a,c, 1979; Kawanishi *et al.*, 1978).

Anderson *et al.* (1973a) found that incubation of various bacterial species

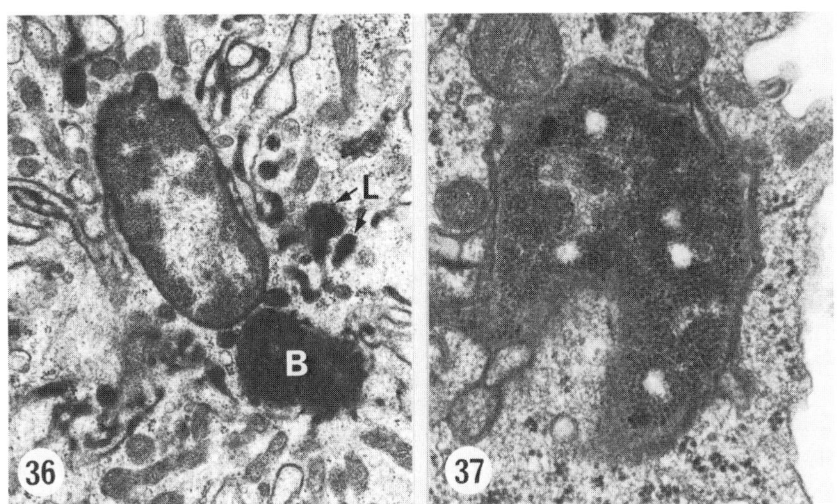

Figs 36 and 37. Interaction between lysosome-like bodies and *Escherichia coli* in the plasmatocytes of *Calliphora erythrocephala*. Fig. 36. Accumulation of lysosomes (L) and membranous structures around intracellular bacteria after 15 min incubation of haemocytes with test particles. Fusion of lysosomes with bacteria has probably occurred, resulting in an increased electron-density of one microorganism (B). (From Rowley and Ratcliffe, 1976a.) ×21 000. Fig. 37. Showing the change in the appearance of an intracellular bacterium after 120 min incubation. The bacterium has become pleomorphic and is probably breaking down. (From Rowley and Ratcliffe, 1976a.) ×45 500.

with the haemocytes of *B. craniifer* in an *in vitro* roller tube suspension culture system led to their phagocytosis and subsequent killing. Of the ten bacterial species tested, six were killed within the plasmatocytes. In the case of *Staphylococcus aureus* 502A, over 50% of the test particles were killed after 60 min incubation. Unfortunately, this is the only study which directly demonstrates the loss of bacterial viability within insect haemocytes.

In our own morphological and cytochemical studies with the haemocytes of *C. erythrocephala*, *Clitumnus extradentatus*, *G. mellonella* and *P. americana* we have concentrated on the intracellular events following the ingestion of bacteria or inert particles *in vitro* (Rowley and Ratcliffe, 1976a,c, 1979; Ratcliffe and Rowley, 1979a). If *G. mellonella* haemocyte cultures, consisting primarily of plasmatocytes, are challenged with live *E. coli*, *Klebsiella aerogenes*, *S. aureus* 502A and *Sarcina lutea*, only the *S. lutea* are killed and the other species, although ingested, multiply within the cells and are eventually released back into the culture medium (Rowley and Ratcliffe, unpublished). Limited lysosomal fusion with phagosomes containing *E. coli* and some bacterial breakdown is also noted, but this is insufficient to control their multiplication. In *G. mellonella* cultures, we have also studied lysosomal interaction with the phagosomes by acid phosphatase cytochemistry using sterile latex spheres as inert test particles. This cytochemical technique shows that after 24 h incubation, less than 5% of the intracellular latex beads are surrounded by a "halo" of acid phosphatase reaction product which is confined within the phagosomes, indicating that limited lysosomal fusion has occurred (Rowley and Ratcliffe, 1979). Usually, small primary lysosomes are found adjacent to these phagosomes, some of which are probably about to fuse and discharge their contents around the latex (Fig. 34). The limited response of *G. mellonella* plasmatocytes to intracellular particles probably indicates the role of humoral substances or other cellular defence reactions, such as nodule formation, in overcoming invading microorganisms in this insect. In *P. americana*, not only does fusion of small primary lysosomes with the phagosomes enclosing latex beads occur, but the larger granules in the plasmatocytes of this species also fuse and discharge their contents (Fig. 35). Landureau and Grellet (1975), also working with *P. americana* plasmatocytes in culture, have suggested that the granules contain chitinase which is an enzyme similar to lysozyme and involved in the digestion of bacterial cell walls.

In *C. erythrocephala*, initial experiments indicate that the haemocytes are more competent at disposing of intracellular bacteria than those of *G. mellonella*. The filamentous plasmatocytes (thrombocytoids and podocytes of some other workers) rapidly ingest *E. coli* and after only 15 min incubation this leads to the accumulation of lysosomes around the intracellular bacteria (Fig. 36). After 1–2 h incubation, the bacteria appear swollen and this probably indicates their breakdown within the cells (Fig. 37).

Little information is available as to how insect haemocytes kill intracellular microorganisms. Vertebrate PMN leucocytes have a comprehensive antimicrobial armoury, including lactoferrin, cationic proteins, lysozyme, myeloperoxidase—H_2O_2—halide systems and superoxide anion (O_2^-) (Klebanoff, 1972, 1975) as well as many digestive enzymes present in the lysosomes. Anderson *et al.* (1973b) were unable to find any evidence for the existence of the myeloperoxidose—H_2O_2—halide system in the plasmatocytes of *B. craniifer* and, furthermore, nitroblue tetrazolium reduction, a characteristic reaction of mammalian leucocytes associated with H_2O_2 production, is also mainly absent (see Chapter 17). Recently, lysozyme-like activity has been demonstrated in the haemocytes of *Spodoptera eridania* (Anderson and Cook, 1979).

B. Nodule formation

Nodules are multicellular structures consisting of a central core of necrotic often melanized haemocytes and associated infectious agents, such as bacteria protozoa or fungi, surrounded by an outer sheath or capsule of flattened blood cells (Fig. 38). Nodules have been recovered from the haemocoel of natural field populations of insects (Bucher, 1959; Huger, 1960; Henry, 1967; Bywater and Ratcliffe, unpublished), and also form in laboratory reared insects in response to injections of bacteria (e.g. Metalnikov, 1908, 1924, 1927; Metalnikov and Chorine, 1929; Hollande, 1930; Cameron, 1934; Toumanoff, 1949; Wittig, 1965a,b; Kurstak *et al.*, 1969; Gagen and Ratcliffe, 1976; Ratcliffe *et al.*, 1976a,b; Ratcliffe and Gagen, 1976, 1977), fungi (e.g. Ermin, 1939; Vey, 1968; Vey *et al.*, 1968, 1973; Vey and Vago, 1969, 1971; Vey and Fargues, 1977), protozoa (e.g. Evans and Elias, 1970; Ratcliffe and Rowley, 1979a), as well as inert particles such as ink (Marshall, 1966) and erythrocytes (Ryan and Nicholas, 1972).

Until recently, nodule formation was thought to be merely a mixture of phagocytosis and encapsulation in which haemocytes containing phagocytosed particles clumped together, degenerated and became surrounded by a multicellular capsule composed of plasmatocytes (see section of encapsulation). However, Gagen and Ratcliffe (1976), and Ratcliffe and Gagen (1976, 1977), found that in *G. mellonella* and *P. brassicae* the first stage in nodule formation occurs almost immediately after the injection of large doses of bacteria into the haemocoel, with the formation of clumps of microorganisms and haemocytes (Fig. 39). Subsequent ultrastructural studies showed that the bacteria are entrapped in material released from the granular cells (Figs 39, 40) and that the clumps are almost entirely composed of granular cells with only a limited involvement of phagocytosis or other cell types (Ratcliffe and Gagen, 1977). The material released from the granular cells is derived from the granules and is discharged by exocytosis (Fig. 40). Within 5 min of injection, the clumps of haemocytes and bacteria compact and the material around the granular cells begins to melanize (Fig. 39). Some 2–4 h later, plasmatocytes attach to the now necrotic mass of granular cells and bacteria and begin to form the characteristic multicellular capsule described by many authors, e.g. Grimstone *et al.* (1967) (see section on encapsulation) (Fig. 39).

The attachment of plasmatocytes to the necrotic core is probably mediated by factors released from interaction of the bacteria with the degenerating granular cells. Gagen and Ratcliffe (unpublished, reported in

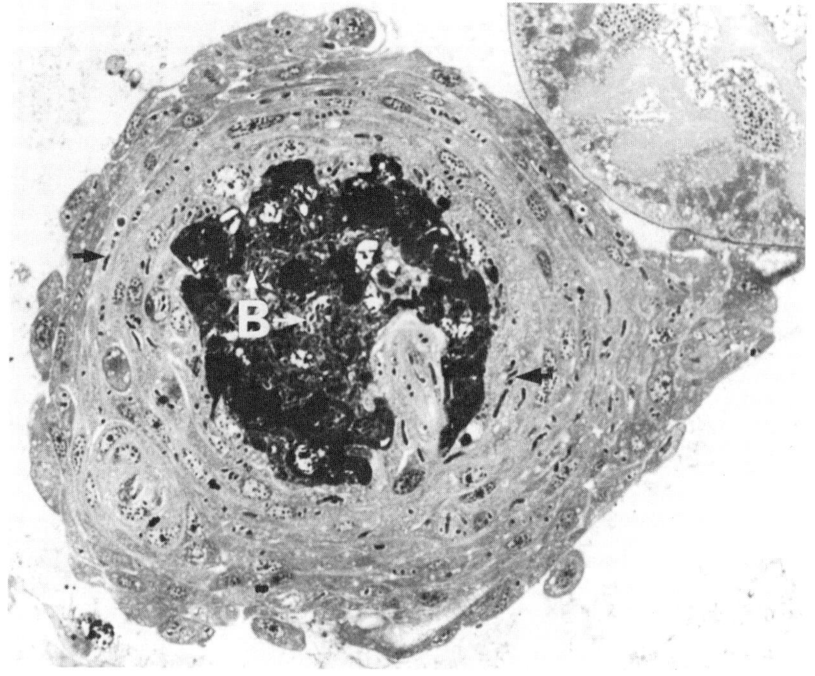

Fig. 38. Fully developed nodule formed in *Pieris brassicae* 24 h after the injection of *Bacillus cereus*. Note the typical melanized core containing bacteria (B) and the multilayered sheath of plasmatocytes, some of which enclose a few intracellular bacteria (unlabelled arrows). (From Ratcliffe and Gagen, 1976.) × 500.

Ratcliffe and Rowley, 1979a), found evidence that these clumps produce chemotactic factors which cause the specific immigration of plasmatocytes towards them (see also section on phagocytosis and encapsulation).

In preliminary work with three other species, *Clitumnus extradentatus*, *Schistocerca gregaria* and *Tenebrio molitor*, we have found that nodule formation after bacterial injection follows the general pattern outlined above (Ratcliffe and Rowley, 1979a). In these species, nodule formation is also extremely rapid, with clumps of bacteria and haemocytes recoverable after only 5 min post-injection (Fig. 41). In *C. extradentatus*, both the granular cells and cystocytes are involved in this clumping reaction, while in *S. gregaria* and *T. molitor* only the cystocytes discharge their granules to entrap the bacteria. By 1 h post-injection, some phagocytosis of the bacteria by plasmatocytes occurs in all three species, but it is important to stress that this takes place after completion of the initial clumping reaction. By 24 h post-injection, distinct, mature nodules have been formed and these are composed of the characteristic melanized core surrounded by a multi-layered capsule (Fig. 42).

Whether the bacteria are normally actively killed in the nodules is unknown although it has been shown that some can survive in such structures throughout the life of the insect (Cameron, 1934). Furthermore, how some bacteria avoid sequestration in nodules is also uncertain. Ratcliffe and Gagen (1976) found that after injection of *Staphylococcus aureus* into *G. mellonella* some small nodules are formed but eventually the bacteria escape and multiply in the haemolymph to kill the insect. Similar results have been described by Kurstak *et al.* (1969) in which *Salmonella typhimurium* escapes nodule formation by means of its toxic lipopolysaccharides.

In summary, nodule formation is a biphasic process. The first stage occurs very quickly after infection and consists of microbial entrappment by factors produced by the interaction of bacteria with either granular cells and/or cystocytes. The second stage takes place some hours later and consists of the specific attachment and flattening of many plasmatocytes on to this core to form the typical multicellular sheath.

C. Encapsulation

This cellular defence reaction operates against foreign objects which are too large to be phagocytosed by single blood cells. Capsules are formed around both non-biological and biological agents after natural infection, or experimental implantation into the haemocoel. The non-biological agents include pieces of Araldite (Grimstone *et al.*, 1967; François, 1975; Hillen, 1977; Schmit and Ratcliffe, 1978; Schmit, 1979), nylon threads (Scott,

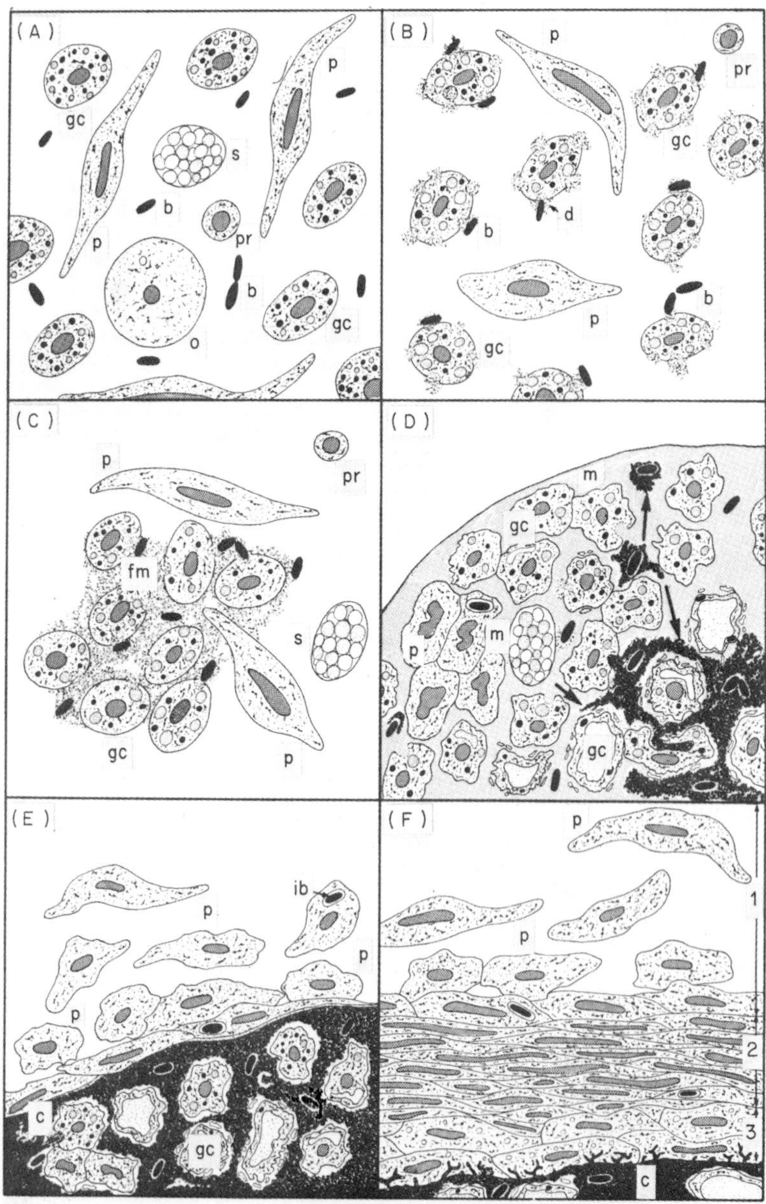

Fig. 39. Diagrammatic representation of main events during nodule formation in *G. mellonella*. (A) Haemocyte types free in the haemolymph immediately following

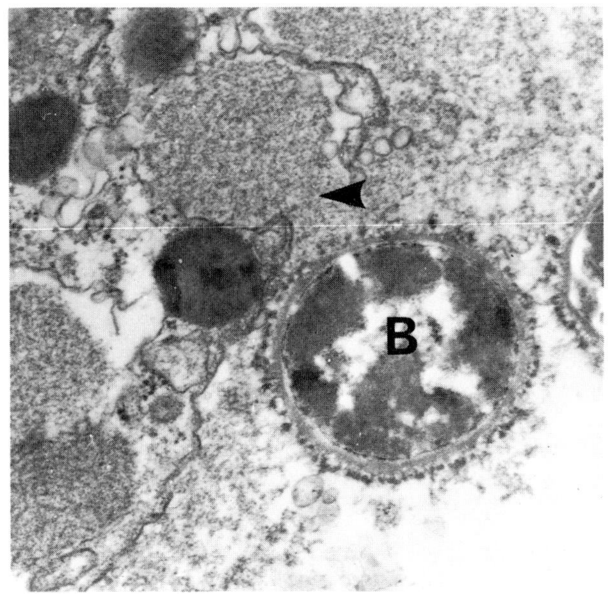

Fig. 40. Showing granule discharge (unlabelled arrow) from a granular cell of *G. mellonella* 1 min after the injection of *B. cereus* (B) into the haemocoel. Release of this material causes the bacteria and haemocytes to aggregate together. (From Ratcliffe and Gagen, 1977.) ×43 000.

---

injection of bacteria (b). Granular cell (gc); plasmatocyte (p); prohaemocyte (pr); spherule cell (s); oenocytoid (o). (B) Showing the initial stage in nodule formation. On random contact with the bacteria the granular cells have immediately discharged their contents (d) to entrap the bacteria. (C) By 1 m post-injection the granular cells, coated with discharged contents, have cohered to segregate the bacteria. Flocculent material (fm). (D) At 5–30 min the clumps have compacted and the matrix (m) is melanizing (unlabelled arrows) especially in the regions of the bacteria. (E) Showing the beginning of the second stage of nodule formation by the specific attachment of large numbers of plasmatocytes, some of which contain intracellular bacteria (ib), to the inner melanized core (c). (F) A mature nodule has formed by 12–24 h and the sheath is clearly divided into an outer region of newly attached cells (1), a middle region of extremely flattened cells (2) and an inner region of partially flattened cells containing melanized inclusions (3). (From Ratcliffe and Gagen, 1977.)

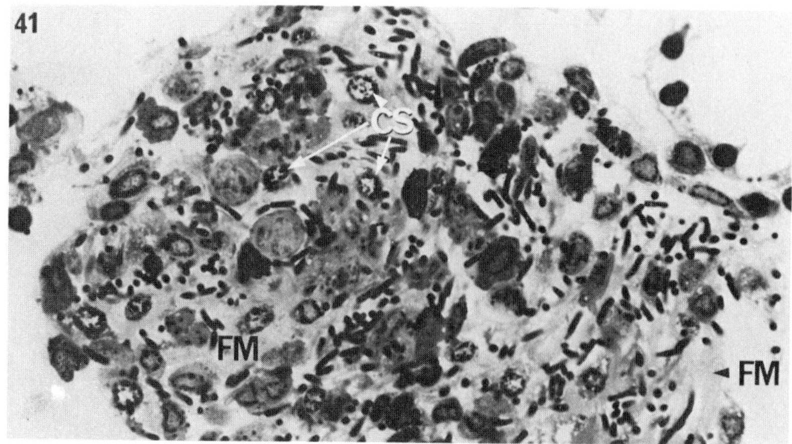

Fig. 41. Thick plastic section of a nodule in *Tenebrio molitor* formed 5 min after the injection of *B. cereus*. Most of the bacteria are embedded in a flocculent material (FM) which is formed by granule discharge from cystocytes (CS). ×800.

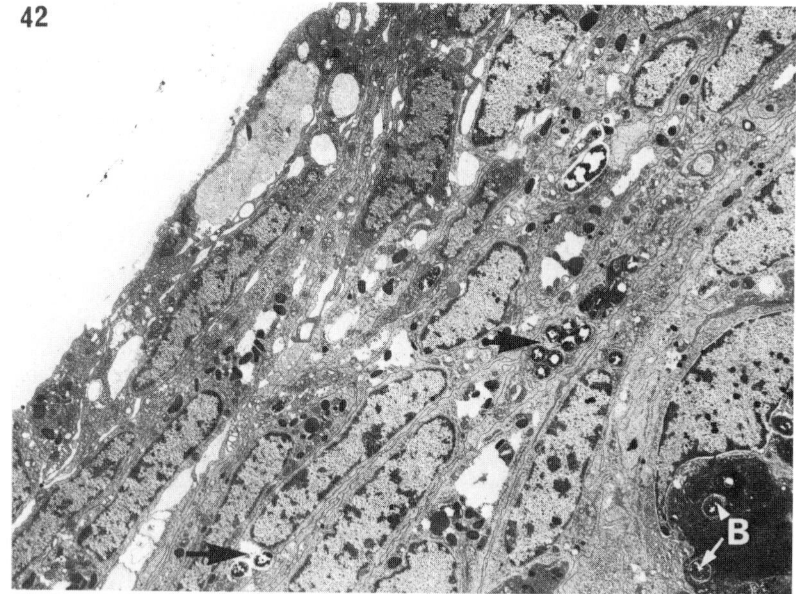

Fig. 42. Electron micrograph of a nodule from *C. extradentatus* formed 24 h after the injection of *B. cereus*. Note the central melanized core containing bacteria (B) which is surrounded by a sheath of flattened plasmatocytes some of which contain intracellular bacteria (unlabelled arrows). ×2600.

1971c; Sato *et al.*, 1976), large latex spheres (Lackie, 1976), glass (Salt, 1956, 1957) and cellophane fragments (Matz, 1965, 1977; Brehélin *et al.*, 1975; Zachary *et al.*, 1975). A wide range of biological agents are also encapsulated including fungi (Salt, 1970; Götz and Vey, 1974), acanthocephalans (Robinson and Strickland, 1969; Rotheram and Crompton, 1972; Ravindranath and Anataraman, 1977), cestodes (Lackie, 1976), nematodes (Poinar *et al.*, 1968; Poinar and Leutenegger, 1971; Poinar, 1974; Nappi and Stoffolano, 1971, 1972a,b; Misko, 1972; Nappi, 1974, 1975b), large protozoa (Ratcliffe and Rowley, 1979a), insect parasitoids (Salt, 1963, 1970, 1973, 1975; Kitano, 1969a,b, 1974; Nappi, 1970; Vinson, 1971, 1972, 1977) and various foreign tissues (Scott, 1971c; Schmit and Ratcliffe, 1977; Lackie, 1977, 1979).

Like nodules, mature capsules are composed of a multilayered sheath formed by plasmatocytes (Fig. 43). Grimstone *et al.* (1967), showed that in *Ephestia kühniella*, this sheath could be divided into 3 morphologically distinct regions; (1) an inner zone composed of degenerating haemocytes associated with a layer of melanin opposing the implant; (2) a middle layer consisting of tightly packed and flattened plasmatocytes; and (3) an outer irregular zone of newly attached plasmatocytes showing few morphological differences from those found in general circulation (Fig. 43). The plasmatocytes in the middle zone usually contained large numbers of cytolysosomes, microtubules underlying the cell membrane, and prominent desmosomes (François, 1975; Schmit and Ratcliffe, 1977).

Only a few studies have demonstrated how capsules are formed and, in particular, examined the early events in this process (Sato *et al.*, 1976; Schmit and Ratcliffe, 1977, 1978). The work of Schmit and Ratcliffe (1977) showed that encapsulation, like nodule formation, is a biphasic process (at least in the insects so far examined), in which rapid lysis of cystocytes and/or granular cells on the implant surface is followed by the attachment of plasmatocytes to form the outer sheath described above. Haemocyte lysis on the surface of the foreign body has also been described by Poinar *et al.* (1968) and Reik (1968), but only recently has the full significance of this process in initiating encapsulation been realized. Schmit and Ratcliffe (1977), found that in *G. mellonella* within 5 min of implanting a small piece of locust nerve cord, the granular cells lysed and coated the surface of the implant with a flocculent material (Fig. 44). Basically, this process is similar to the first stage of nodule formation and haemolymph coagulation (see relevant sections and Figs 45–48). Some 30 min later, the plasmatocytes attached to the implant, although only at sites where granular cell lysis had occurred. This suggests that factors from the granular cells may control the attraction and attachment of the plasmatocytes. The chemotactic attraction of plasmatocytes during encapsulation has previously been suggested by

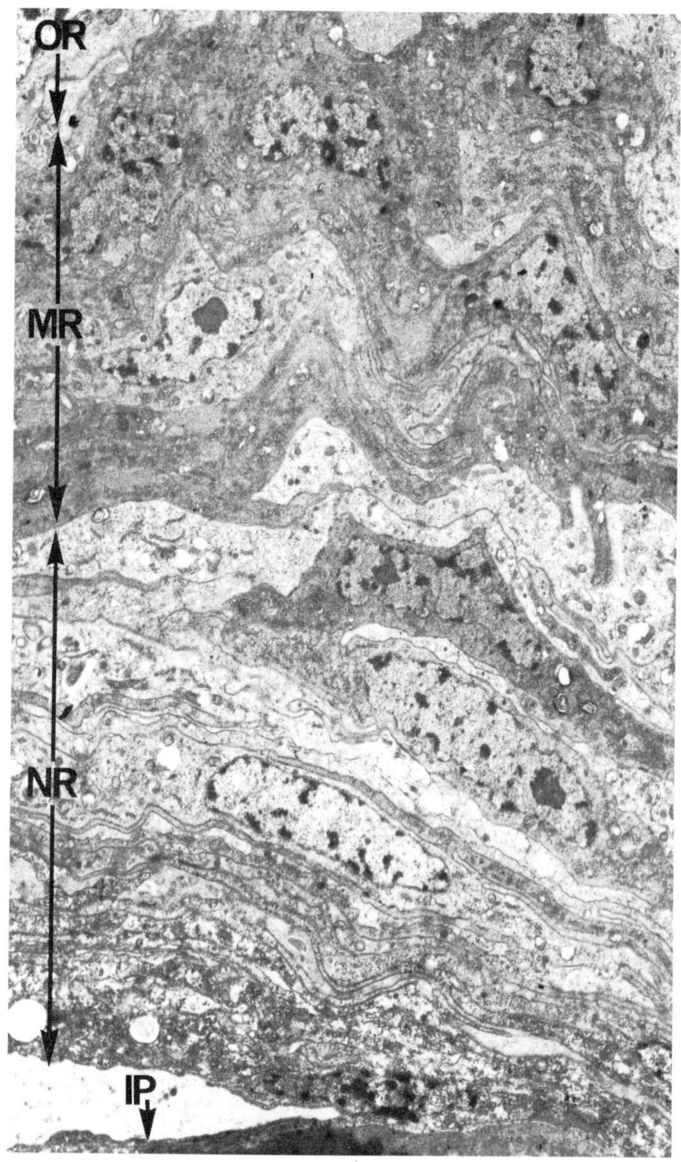

Fig. 43. 72 h capsule of *G. mellonella* showing the characteristic three regions: an inner necrotic region (NR), an electron-dense middle region of flattened plasmatocytes (MR) and an outer region (OR) of newly attached cells. Note implant (IP). (From Schmit and Ratcliffe, 1977.) $\times$ 11 000.

Nappi and Staffolano (1971, 1972a,b) and Nappi (1975b) had has been demonstrated during nodule formation by Gagen and Ratcliffe (unpublished).

The possible role of the endocrine system in controlling encapsulation has also been suggested (Nappi, 1974, 1975a,b). Lynn and Vinson (1977), however, could find no evidence for the participation of either ecdysone or juvenile hormone analogue in encapsulation, but this does not preclude the possibility of other hormones being involved. Furthermore, the first stage of granular cell lysis, is so rapid that it is probably not controlled by such mechanisms.

What causes the termination of encapsulation is also unclear, but the products of granular cell/cystocyte lysis may well progressively decrease in concentration as further layers of plasmatocytes wall-off the implant, until, finally, such factors no longer influence the behaviour of circulating haemocytes.

How, or whether encapsulation kills or prevents the development of parasites is generally unclear. It is probable though that as this process deals with such a large range of infectious agents that no specific killing mechanisms exist. Many authors, however, have suggested that active

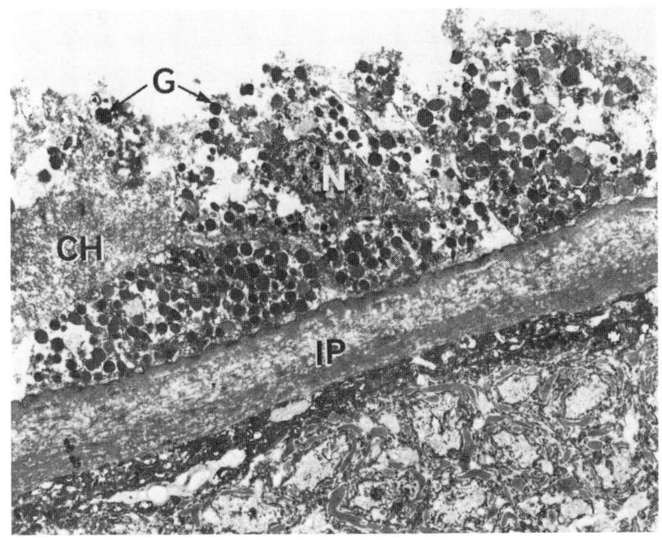

Fig. 44. The first stage of encapsulation in *G. mellonella* with granular cells lysing on the surface of locust nerve cord (IP) 5 min after implantation. The resultant debris consists of granules (G), isolated nuclei (N) and is associated with clot-formation (CH) caused by granule discharge. (From Schmit and Ratcliffe, 1977.) ×4400.

killing mechanisms are present and involve melanization and its toxic by-products (Taylor, 1969; Lipke, 1975; Nappi, 1975b; Cawthorn and Anderson, 1977; Ratcliffe and Rowley, 1979a) or, killing may be achieved simply by starvation and asphyxiation (Salt, 1963, 1970).

Mention must also be made of the habitual hymenopteran parasitoids which in their usual hosts manage to avoid the encapsulation process. This may be achieved either by the acquisition of a coat of resistant substance as the eggs pass through the calyx of the female parasitoid prior to oviposition (Salt, 1965; Rotheram, 1967, 1973a,b; Bedwin, 1970; Hillen, 1977), or, by the production of "anti-encapsulation factors" which actively suppress the host's immune response (Kitano, 1969a,b, 1974; Kitano and Nakatsuji, 1978; Nappi and Streams, 1969; Nappi, 1975b; Osman, 1978).

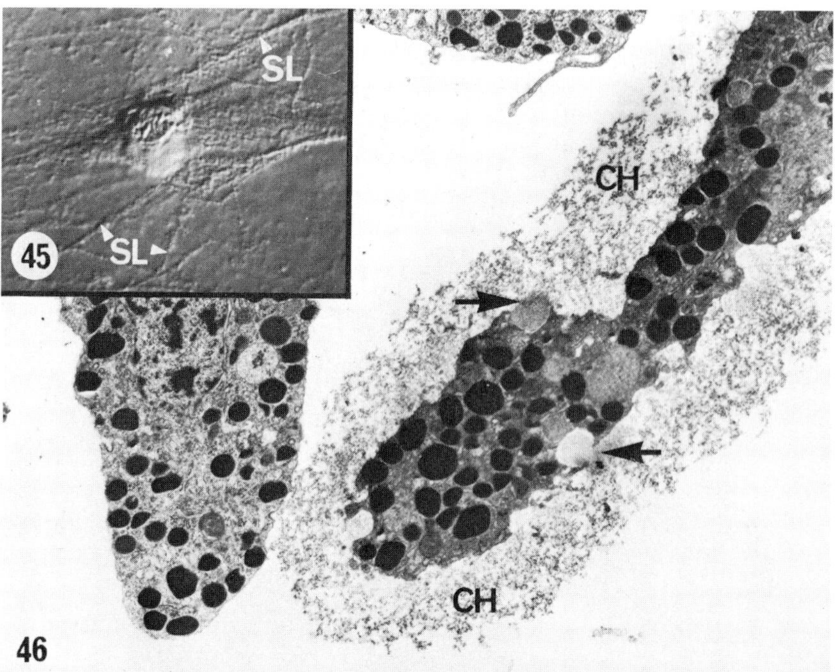

Fig. 45. Phase contrast micrograph of a cystocyte of *C. extradentatus* after 15 min *in vitro*. Note the strand-like material (SL) which connects other cells out of the frame. ×900.

Fig. 46. Electron micrograph of a granular cell of *G. mellonella* showing granule discharge (unlabelled arrows) and coagulation (CH) in the surrounding haemolymph. Note that in the other granular cell where release has not occurred the zone of coagulated haemolymph is wanting. (From Rowley and Ratcliffe, 1976b.) ×7200.

D. Haemolymph coagulation

Haemolymph coagulation is a widespread phenomenon within the arthropods. It occurs after wounding or other physical damage and is very efficient at preventing excess blood loss and hindering the entry of microorganisms. In insects, the degree of coagulation has been found to differ markedly from species to species. For example, in bee larvae, haemolymph coagulation is apparently absent (Gilliam and Shimanuki, 1967b, 1970), while in many orthopterans and dictyopterans it occurs within a few seconds of bleeding.

Haemocytes are directly involved in blood clotting (Beard, 1950; Grégoire, 1951, 1953, 1954, 1955a,b, 1959, 1970, 1974; Brehélin, 1979) by

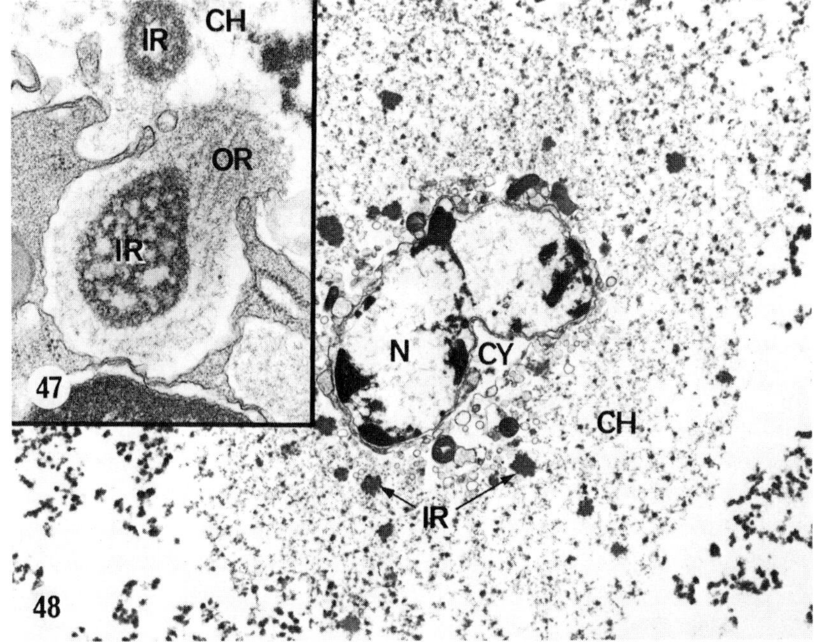

Fig. 47. Showing an early stage in granule discharge from a cystocyte of *C. extradentatus* after 30 sec *in vitro*. The diffuse outer region (OR) of the granule interacts with haemolymph components to form a coagulum (CH). The inner region (IR) of the granules remains intact after release. (From Rowley, 1977b.) ×29 000.

Fig. 48. Showing a highly degenerated cystocyte of *C. extradentatus* after 2 min *in vitro*. Note the pycnotic nucleus (N) empty cytoplasm (CY) and zone of coagulated haemolymph (CH) containing the inner regions (IR) of released granules. ×6500.

two distinct methods. In the majority of insects, true coagulation occurs and is brought about by the release of materials from the haemocytes which cause the formation of a gel, while in a few species, such as *Calliphora*, no gelation occurs and blood loss is controlled by the clumping and interdigitation of haemocytes (Crossley, 1975). True haemolymph coagulation involves cystocytes and occasionally granular cells (Rowley and Ratcliffe, 1976b; Rowley, 1977b); while the second, non-gelation process is mediated by fragmentation and agglutination of podocytes/thrombocytoids (specialized plasmatocytes). In those species with this type of clotting, cystocyte-like cells are wanting.

The role of the cystocytes and granular cells in blood clotting has been most readily observed using phase contrast microscopy. Obviously, with the rapidity of this process some of the early changes occurring within the cystocytes have been missed. This problem can, however, be partially overcome by cooling the insect prior to the bleeding, as this slows down the coagulation process (Price and Ratcliffe, 1974). The first change observed during clotting under the light microscope is the release of granules from the cystocytes leaving vacuoles in the cytoplasm. Concomitantly, the nucleus becomes much brighter under phase optics and the chromatin condenses to form the characteristic cartwheel shape (Grégoire, 1970). Next, the outline of the cell becomes indistinct and in most cases a cloud of precipitated plasma proteins is formed around the cystocytes ("islets of coagulation" of Grégoire, 1970) (Fig. 15). In some insects, as well as the islets of coagulation, adjacent cystocytes are interconnected by strand-like material which may be cytoplasmic in origin or formed from the newly clotted blood (Fig. 45). These stages are normally complete within 2–3 min and few further changes occur.

In *G. mellonella*, cystocytes are wanting and the granular cells bring about haemolymph clotting. Distinct islets of coagulation are not formed and the coagulation produced is very fine with many of the cells interconnected by strand-like material (Rowley and Ratcliffe, 1976b).

Haemolymph coagulation has also been studied using the electron microscope (Hoffmann and Stoekel, 1968; Moran, 1971; Goffinet and Grégoire, 1975; Rowley and Ratcliffe, 1976b; Neuwirth and Lai-Fook, 1977; Rowley, 1977b). Hoffmann and Stoekel (1968), first described the ultrastructural changes in *L. migratoria* cystocytes during the course of haemolymph coagulation. They found that the RER becomes dilated, the mitochondria more electron-dense, some of the granules are discharged from the cells, and the chromatin is more prominent. They concluded that although granule discharge is involved in coagulation, it does not appear to initiate it. This view was based on the observation that cell membrane rupture and coagulation occur before granule release. In contrast, in *C. extradentatus* and *G. mellonella* granule release appears to initiate coagulation (Rowley and Ratcliffe, 1976b; Rowley, 1977b). In *G. mellonella*, granule discharge from the granular cells is the first distinct stage in coagulation. During this process, the granules lose their electron-dense, unstructured nature and become less electron-dense with large numbers of microtubules visible within the granule matrix. As a result of granule discharge, a zone of coarsely flocculent material (coagulated haemolymph) forms around these cells (Fig. 46). This zone is absent from cells which have not undergone discharge, indicating that the process is essential for haemolymph coagulation (Rowley and Ratcliffe, 1976b).

In *C. extradentatus*, both the granular cells and cystocytes appear to be involved in haemolymph coagulation (Rowley, 1977b) and like *G. mellonella* this process is initiated by granule discharge. In the cystocytes, immediately after granule release the peripheral region of this material appears to interact with components in the haemolymph to form a coagulum (Fig. 47). These cells then become swollen and quickly degenerate (Fig. 48). Other workers, including Stang-Voss (1970) and Moran (1971), have also indicated the role of the granules in haemolymph coagulation, but Goffinet and Grégoire (1975) failed to find any evidence for their participation in this process in *Carausius morosus*.

Little is known about the biochemical changes occurring to the haemolymph during clotting, or, how the cystocytes/granular cells bring about the necessary changes in blood chemistry. Siakotos (1960a,b) showed that in *P. americana*, haemolymph clotting primarily involves lipoproteins. Using electrophoretic techniques, he compared the bands formed from unclotted and clotted blood and found that two new lipoproteins are formed during coagulation. One of these is the actual coagulum and the other is probably another product of the clotting process. This study, however, gives no indication of what stimulus triggers off the clotting process. From our own work, it seems likely to be a change in the cell membrane configurations of the cystocytes/granular cells which causes the granules to migrate to the cell periphery and fuse with the outer membrane and hence release their contents. Perhaps this is caused by alteration in environmental factors such as pH or oxygen tension which occur during bleeding, or may involve more complex mechanisms, for example, paralleling those operating during histamine release from vertebrate mast cells (Gomperts, 1976).

Finally, the possible role of endotoxin in haemolymph coagulation is unknown but it has been shown to cause rapid agglutination and coagulation in the King crab, *Limulus polyphemus* (Levin and Bang, 1964; Levin, 1967) (see Chapter 11). Furthermore, biochemical analysis of the contents of the cystocyte/granular cell granules as carried out in other arthropods (Murer *et al.*, 1975; Mengeot *et al.*, 1977) should help confirm their role in haemolymph coagulation.

E. Wound healing

Insects are covered by a toughened cuticle which is very resistant to mechanical and chemical damage. However, occasionally, this layer is penetrated either by natural abrasion, or predators and parasites. A number of researchers have examined the events during wound healing after first experimentally damaging the insect either through the alimentary canal (Day, 1952; Day and Bennetts, 1953), or the cuticle (Ries, 1932; Wigglesworth, 1937; Braemer, 1956; Locke, 1966; Lai-Fook, 1968, 1970; Aiouaz, 1975; Rowley and Ratcliffe, 1978).

In most insects, the cellular events during wound healing can be divided into four stages; (1) the sealing of the wound by haemolymph coagulation; (2) the migration of haemocytes into the wound-site; (3) the migration of epidermal cells underlying the wound-site to form a new intact layer; and finally, (4) the formation of a new cuticle by the reformed epidermis. The involvement of the haemocytes in wound healing is biphasic with the first phase involving the granular cells/cystocytes in an immediate clotting reaction (see section on haemolymph coagulation) while the second phase is the migration of plasmatocytes into the wound-site (Rowley and Ratcliffe, 1978). This biphasic nature is very similar to that seen during nodule formation and encapsulation (see relevant sections) and again indicates the similarities of many of the processes involved in the cellular defences.

The first stage, i.e. haemolymph coagulation, is apparently absent in some insects such as *R. prolixus* (Wigglesworth, 1937), *Aedes aegypti* and *Orosius argentatus* (Day and Bennetts, 1953) but is clearly involved in others (Day, 1952; Rowley and Ratcliffe, 1978). However, the "cuticulin-like" membrane described by Wigglesworth (1937) as being formed after wounding in *R. prolixus* has been shown by Lai-Fook (1968, 1970) to be a sort of coagulum. Other factors, such as extrusion of fat body through cuticular wounds and muscle contraction in gut wounds (Day and Bennetts, 1953), may well also help to stop the initial bleeding.

The second stage, i.e. the specific migration of plasmatocytes into the wound-site occurs 6–12 h after wounding in *G. mellonella* (Rowley and Ratcliffe, 1978), indicating that these cells have to be first mobilized from other sites within the insect (see section on encapsulation and nodule formation). By this time, the initial coagulum has hardened and melanized, presumably as a result of release of activating agents from the granular cells which elicit melanization (Schmit *et al.*, 1977), and no doubt this process is important in preventing further blood loss and infection. What role this second phase of haemocyte involvement has in wound healing is unclear. It has been suggested that haemocytes may help in the formation of a new cuticle, either by the transportation of necessary nutrients or by the control of epidermal regeneration (Bohn, 1975, 1976, 1977a,b,c). Wigglesworth (1937) first suggested that products from broken down cells at the wound-site (granular cells/cystocytes?) control the accumulation of the epidermal cells across the wound-site to form a complete new layer, capable of producing a new cuticle. Bohn (1975), however, demonstrated by using a novel *in vitro* system that the migration of epidermal cells only occurs in the presence of haemocytes (mainly plasmatocytes), that may produce some factor(s) which controls the rearrangement of the epidermal cells into a complete new layer. Certainly in our own histological studies, the plasmatocytes appear to form a "template" over which the epidermal cells migrate (Rowley and Ratcliffe, 1978). Later *in vitro* studies by Bohn (1977a,b,c) suggested that the plasmatocytes release a "conditioning factor" which causes the epidermal cells to attach and flatten over various substrates. The factor may be associated with the plasmatocyte granules which have been shown to be released *in vitro* under various conditions (see section on phagocytosis). Chemically, the conditioning factor has not been fully analysed, but it is broken down by some proteolytic enzymes and may be associated with carbohydrate (Bohn, 1977c).

One other possible role for the large numbers of plasmatocytes at the wound-site is in the reformation of the basement membrane underlying the epidermis (see section on connective tissue formation).

F. Hormone transport

The interaction between haemocytes and hormones is probably very complex and as yet is not well-understood. Wigglesworth (1955), first suggested that haemocytes were involved in the transportation of hormones between the corpus cardiacum and the thoracic glands. These hormones include thoracotrophic hormone, which stimulates the thoracic glands to produce ecdysone. More recently, Takeda (1977) found that in the slug-moth, *Monema flavescens*, just before the termination of diapause, granular haemocytes specifically gather around the pars intercerebralis, which is the site of release of thoracotrophic hormone in this insect. These haemocytes were found to contain material which stained similarly to the neurosecretion formed by the pars intercerebralis. Later, similar cells were observed around the prothoracic gland indicating that they may have migrated from one organ to another. Only the granular cells contain this hormone-like material with no activity present in the plasmatocytes, spherule cells or oenocytoids.

Goltzené and Hoffmann (1974), also suggested that the haemocytes formed in the haemopoietic tissue of *L. migratoria* are necessary for the transportation of hormones from the corpora allata to the developing oocyte. Whether these haemocytes actually physically transport these hormones or produce substances involved in their synthesis is unclear. However, X-irradiation of the haemopoietic tissue in some way slows down the development of the oocyte. Interestingly, Landureau and Szöllösi (1974) and Landureau (1977) found that factors (hormones?) produced by the plasmatocytes of *P. americana* in culture stimulate the maturation of the sperm cells, indicating that haemocytes may not only transport hormones but may actually produce them or their associated molecules.

In summary, haemocytes probably play an important role in the transportation of hormones to target tissues and this may involve specific migration of these cells (chemotaxis?). Transport of the hormones within the haemocytes may well provide a method of precisely controlling the amount of hormones released at the target tissues and may also protect these substances from accidental metabolism at other sites in the circulatory system.

G. Connective tissue synthesis

It has often been suggested that haemocytes are responsible for the formation of some types of connective tissue (Lazarenko, 1925; Wigglesworth, 1956, 1973, 1979; Beaulaton, 1968; Percy, 1978). Most commonly noted is the association between the basement membrane underlying the epidermal layer of the integument and certain haemocyte types. Wigglesworth (1956), showed that the granular plasmatocytes of *R. prolixus* are often intimately associated with various connective tissues and that the granular inclusions discharged from these cells appear to form this tissue. Later studies, utilizing electron microscopy (Wigglesworth, 1973), confirmed that the release of granules from the plasmatocytes is the principal mechanism of basement membrane formation. These granules have a microtubular substructure characteristic of the granular cells and cystocytes of other species (Figs 13, 14) and this release is very much like that seen during nodule formation, encapsulation and haemolymph coagulation. Indeed, Wigglesworth (1973) believes that during parasite encapsulation a connective tissue layer is laid down by the haemocytes and this is probably similar to the material in the cores and between the cells of nodules and capsules.

More recently, Percy (1978) showed in the cabbage looper, *Trichoplusia ni*, that granular cells are present around the basement membrane of the sex pheromone gland. This basement membrane is typically bi-layered with an inner amorphous zone and an outer zone containing parallel arrays of fibrils, which may be similar to collagen fibres found in the connective tissue of other insects (Ashhurst, 1968). Percy (1978), believes that at least the fibrillar part of the basement membrane is secreted by the granular cells as the granules discharging around the membrane also have a fibrillar (microtubular?) structure. The agranular plasmatocytes, although sometimes found attached to the basement membrane, do not appear to be involved in its formation.

Not all workers agree as to the role of the haemocytes in connective tissue formation. For example, Ashhurst and Richards (1964b,c) and Ashhurst (1968) could find no evidence for the participation of the blood cells of *G. mellonella* in the formation of the fibrous connective tissue around the dorsal nerve cord. Here, this material is formed by the so-called sheath cells which underlie the neural lamella.

Finally, in a recent review (Ashhurst, 1979) stated that there is no indisputable evidence for the production of any of the components of connective tissue by insect haemocytes.

H. Storage and secretion

Haemocytes store many different materials including proteins, lipids and carbohydrates (Yeager and Munson, 1941; Wigglesworth, 1965; Crossley, 1979), either in distinct granules or in the rest of the cytoplasm. In some other invertebrates, blood cells have been shown to be very important in the storage of metabolites (see Chapters 3, 4) but this has never been clearly demonstrated in insects.

Specific examples of secretion of various substances by insect haemocytes have already been described in the sections on the cellular defences and connective tissue formation. However, one important haemocyte function which has not been discussed, is their role in the production of melanin either in the blood or cuticle. Release of the enzyme phenoloxidase (tyrosinase) from certain haemocytes causes the haemolymph to melanize (Pye and Yendol, 1972), and this process is probably important in the cellular defences (see section on nodule formation and encapsulation). Schmit *et al.* (1977), showed that in *G. mellonella* two cell types are involved in melanin production, the granular cells and oenocytoids. Presumably, when the granular cells break down, during nodule formation and encapsulation, phenoloxidase is also released and this accounts for the melanization which occurs during these processes. Dennell (1947) also suggested that the haemocytes are involved in cuticle tanning.

The haemocytes may also synthesize many of the major components of the haemolymph (Wigglesworth, 1965) and this may include humoral "immune" factors (Boman *et al.*, 1979), and heteroagglutinins believed to be important in the recognition of foreignness (Amirante, 1976, 1978). These humoral factors include enzymes such as lysozyme which has the ability to digest part of the cell wall of mainly Gram positive bacteria. Landureau *et al.* (1972) and Bernier *et al.* (1974) showed that the plasmatocytes of *P. americana* in culture produce the enzyme chitinase, which has similar properties to lysozyme. Anderson and Cook (1979), recently reported the presence of lysozyme-like activity in the haemocytes and cell-free haemolymph of *Spodoptera eridania* which was inducible by the injection of various foreign materials. When maintained *in vitro*, the haemocytes released this enzyme but unlike those of molluscs (see review of Cheng, 1975) phagocytic stimulation failed to increase extracellular lysozyme levels.

Using immunofluorescent methods, Amirante (1976, 1978) demonstrated that the granular cells and spherule cells of *Leucophaea maderae* are responsible for the synthesis of two distinct heteroagglutinins which may be involved in the recognition and binding of foreign particles to the haemocyte surface (see section on phagocytosis).

I. Metamorphosis

In some insects, the haemocytes have been shown to be important in phagocytosing cell debris during the tissue remodelling which occurs at pupation (Perez, 1910; Åkesson, 1954; Whitten, 1964; Crossley, 1965). This is particularly clear in some dipterans in which towards pupation the plasmatocytes increase in number and progressively become filled with lysosomes and debris (Crossley, 1964, 1975; Rowley and Ratcliffe, unpublished). This debris fills the cytoplasm and has caused such plasmatocytes to be wrongly identified as spherule cells (Åkesson, 1954) due to the spherular nature of this material.

VI. Summary and concluding remarks

Insects have an open circulatory system which bathes most of the internal organs and ramifies the appendages. The blood (haemolymph) contains a large number of colourless cells called haemocytes which either float freely in the circulation or are attached to the various organs. Insect haemocytes have been extensively studied, particularly in the last twenty years with the development of new microscopical techniques including transmission and scanning electron microscopy. As a result, insect haematologists are now in the enviable position of having a relatively simple, widely accepted classification scheme for these cells. This scheme recognizes six basic cell "types"; the prohaemocytes, plasmatocytes, granular cells, cystocytes, spherule cells and oenocytoids as well as two or three unusual, and often relatively rare, additional categories; the podocytes, crystal cells and adipohaemocytes, which are probably best considered as variations of the basic types.

There is, however, still some controversy about the site of formation, differentiation and inter-relationships of the various cell types. For example, many authors have studied the haemogramme in insects throughout the life cycle in an attempt to determine the relative importance of the haemopoietic tissue versus the mitotic division of freely circulating blood cells in the maintenance of cell numbers. At present, no clear picture has emerged and, furthermore, the factors controlling the production and differentiation of the various haemocyte types are unknown. It would be of great interest to evaluate the role (if any) of hormones in the control of haemocyte multiplication and differentiation.

Insect haemocytes are involved in many different processes, including immunosurveillance, wound healing, haemolymph coagulation, hormone transport and, possibly, connective tissue formation. Many important questions, however, are still unanswered, for example, how do the phagocytic haemocytes recognize, react to and kill microorganisms and how do these killing factors compare with those produced by mammalian phagocytes? Many other functions of haemocytes are also poorly researched and warrant careful analysis, in particular, their possible roles in hormone and nutrient transport/production and storage at particular times in the life of the insect.

Acknowledgements

We are indebted to the following scientists: Dr J. Beaulaton, Dr M. Brehélin, Dr A. Dorn, Mr S. J. Gagen, Prof. I. Harpaz, Prof. W. Nutting, Dr A. R. Schmit, Miss J. Walters and Prof. Sir Vincent Wigglesworth, who have provided both published and unpublished material for this chapter. Thanks also go to Prof. E. W. Knight-Jones in whose department this work was carried out and to Mrs M. Colley and Mr P. Llewellyn for technical assistance and Mrs D. Bowditch and Miss L. Millett for typing the manuscript. This work was supported by grants from the Royal Society and the Science Research Council (grant Nos B/RG. 5924.3, GR.A.2286.0 and GR/B/1014.4).

References

Aiouaz, M. (1975). *Bull. Soc. Étude. Sci. Anjou N.S.* **9**, 15–21.

Akai, H. (1969). *Jap. J. appl. Ent. Zool.* **13**, 17–21.

Akai, H. (1971). *Cell (Japan)* **3**, 36–45.

Akai, H. and Sato, S. (1971). *J. Insect Physiol.* **17**, 1665–1676.

Akai, H. and Sato, S. (1973). *Int. J. Insect Morphol. Embryol.* **2**, 207–231.

Akai, H. and Sato, S. (1979). *In* "Insect Hemocytes, Development, Forms, Functions, and Techniques" (A. P. Gupta, Ed.), pp. 129–154. Cambridge University Press, Cambridge.

Åkesson, B. (1954). *Ark. Zool.* **6**, 203–211.

Amirante, G. A. (1976). *Experientia* **32**, 526–528.

Amirante, G. A. (1978). *Devl. Comp. Immunol.* **2**, 735–740.

Anderson, R. S. (1974). *In* "Contemporary Topics in Immunobiology" (E. L. Cooper, Ed.), Vol. 4, pp. 47–54. Plenum Press, New York.

Anderson, R. S. (1976a). *In* "Phylogeny of Thymus and Bone Marrow-Bursa Cells" (R. K. Wright and E. L. Cooper, Eds), pp. 27–34. Elsevier/North Holland, Amsterdam.

Anderson, R. S. (1976b). *In* "Proc. 1st Int. Colloq. Invert. Pathol" (T. Angus, P. Faulkner and A. Rosenfield, Eds), pp. 215–219. Queens University, Queens University Printing Department.

Anderson, R. S. (1977). *Cell. Immunol.* **29**, 331–336.

Anderson, R. S. and Cook, M. L. (1979). *J. Invertebr. Pathol.* **33**, 197–203.

Anderson, R. S. and Good, R. A. (1976). *J. Invertebr. Pathol.* **27**, 57–64.

Anderson, R. S., Holmes, B. and Good, R. A. (1973a). *J. Invertebr. Pathol.* **22**, 127–135.

Anderson, R. S., Holmes, B. and Good, R. A. (1973b). *Comp. Biochem. Physiol.* **46B**, 595–602.

Arnold, J. W. (1972). *Can. Ent.* **104**, 309–348.

Arnold, J. W. (1974). *In* "The Physiology of Insecta" (M. Rockstein, Ed.), 2nd edn, Vol. 5, pp. 201–254. Academic Press, New York.

Arnold, J. W. and Hinks, C. F. (1976). *Can. J. Zool.* **54**, 1003–1012.

Arvy, L. (1952). *C. r. hebd. Seanc. Acad. Sci. Paris*, **235**, 1539–1541.

Arvy, L. (1953). *Bull. Soc. Zool. Fr.* **78**, 158–171.

Arvy, L. and Lhoste, J. (1946). *Bull. Soc. Zool. Fr.* **70**, 144–148.

Ashhurst, D. E. (1968). *A. Rev. Ent.* **13**, 45–74.

Ashhurst, D. E. (1979). *In* "Insect Hemocytes, Development, Forms, Functions, and Techniques" (A. P. Gupta, Ed.), pp. 319–330. Cambridge University Press, Cambridge.

Ashhurst, D. E. and Richards, A. G. (1964a). *J. Morph.* **114**, 247–254.

Ashhurst, D. E. and Richards, A. G. (1964b). *J. Morph.* **114**, 237–246.

Ashhurst, D. E. and Richards, A. G. (1964c). *J. Morph.* **114**, 225–236.

Baerwald, R. J. (1974). *Cell. Tiss. Res.* **151**, 385–394.

Baerwald, R. J. (1979). *In* "Insect Hemocytes, Development, Forms, Functions, and Techniques" (A. P. Gupta, Ed.). pp. 155–188. Cambridge University Press, Cambridge.

Baerwald, R. J. and Boush, G. M. (1970a). *Exp. Cell Res.* **63**, 208–213.

Baerwald, R. J. and Boush, G. M. (1970b). *J. Ultrastruct. Res.* **31**, 151–161.

Beard, R. L. (1950). *Physiol. Zool.* **23**, 47–57.

Beaulaton, J. (1968). *J. Ultrastruct. Res.* **23**, 474–498.

Beaulaton, J. (1978). *C. r. hebd. Seanc. Acad. Sci., Paris, D.* **287**, 713–716.

Beaulaton, J. and Monpeyssin, M. (1976). *J. Ultrastruct. Res.* **55**, 143–156.

Beaulaton, J. and Monpeyssin, M. (1977). *Biol. Cellulaire* **28**, 13–18.

Bedwin, O. R. (1970). The particulate basis of the resistance of a parasitoid to its host. Ph.D. Thesis, University of Cambridge.

Bernheimer, A. W. (1952). *Science, N.Y.* **115**, 150–151.

Bernier, I., Landureau, J. C., Grellet, P. and Jollès, P. (1974). *Comp. Biochem. Physiol.* **47B**, 41–44.

Bettini, S. D., Sarkaria, S. and Patton, R. L. (1951). *Science, N.Y.* **113**, 9–10.

Bjersing, L. (1967). *Z. Zellforsch. mikrosk. Anat.* **82**, 173–186.

Bohn, H. (1975). *J. Insect Physiol.* **21**, 1283–1293.

Bohn, H. (1976). *In* "Insect Development" (P. Lawrence, Ed.), pp. 170–185. Blackwell, London.

Bohn, H. (1977a). *J. Insect Physiol.* **23**, 185–194.

Bohn, H. (1977b). *In Vitro* **13**, 100–107.

Bohn, H. (1977c). *J. Insect Physiol.* **23**, 1063–1073.

Boman, H. G., Faye, I., Pye, A. and Rasmuson, T. (1979). *In* "Comparative Pathobiology" (L. Bulla and T. C. Cheng, Eds), Vol. 4. Plenum Press, New York and London.

Bowers, B. (1964). *Protoplasma* **60**, 352–367.

Braemer, H. (1956). *Wilhelm Roux Arch. Entw Mech. Org.* **148**, 362–390.

Brehélin, M. (1973). *Experientia* **29**, 1539–1540.

Brehélin, M. (1977). Etude morphologique et fonctionnelle des hémocytes d'insectes. Ph.D. thesis, University of Strasbourg, France.

Brehélin, M. (1979). *Experientia* **35**, 270–271.

Brehélin, M., Hoffmann, J. A., Matz, G. and Porte, A. (1975). *Cell Tiss. Res.* **160**, 283–289.

Brehélin, M., Zachary, D. and Hoffmann, J. A. (1978). *Cell Tiss. Res.* **195**, 45–57.

Bucher, G. E. (1959). *J. Insect Path.* **1**, 391–405.

Cameron, G. R. (1934). *J. Path. Bact.* **38**, 441–466.

Cawthorn, R. J. and Anderson, R. C. (1977). *Can. J. Zool.* **55**, 368–375.

Chadwick, J. S. (1975). *In* "Invertebrate Immunity" (K. Maramorosch and R. E. Shope, Eds), pp. 241–271. Academic Press, New York and London.

Chadwick, J. S. (1977). *In* "Comparative Pathobiology" (L. Bulla and T. C. Cheng, Eds), Vol. III. Plenum Press, New York and London.

Chapman, R. F. (1969). "The Insects: Structure and Function". English University Press, London.

Cheng, T. C. (1975). *Ann. N.Y. Acad. Sci.* **266**, 343–379.

Cherbas, L. (1973). *J. Insect Physiol.* **19**, 2011–2023.

Chorine, V. (1931). *Bull. biol. Fr. Belg.* **65**, 291–393.

Clark, M. K. and Dahm, P. A. (1973). *J. Cell Biol.* **56**, 870–875.

Cline, M. J. (1975). "The White Cell". Harvard University Press, Cambridge, Mass.

Costin, N. M. (1975). *Histochem. J.* **7**, 21–43.

Crossley, A. C. S. (1964). *J. exp. Zool.* **157**, 375–398.

Crossley, A. C. S. (1965). *J. Embryol. exp. Morph.* **14**, 89–110.

Crossley, A. C. S. (1972). *Tissue and Cell* **4**, 529–560.

Crossley, A. C. S. (1975). *Adv. Insect Physiol.* **11**, 117–222.

Crossley, A. C. S. (1979). *In* "Insect Hemocytes, Development, Forms, Functions, and Techniques" (A. P. Gupta, Ed.), pp. 423–473. Cambridge University Press, Cambridge.

Davey, K. G. (1961a). *Gen. Comp. Endocr.* **1**, 24–29.
Davey, K. G. (1961b). *J. Insect Physiol.* **8**, 205–208.
Day, M. F. (1952). *Aust. J. Scient. Res* (*B*) **5**, 282–289.
Day, M. F. and Bennetts, M. J. (1953). *Aust. J. biol. Sci.* **6**, 580–585.
Dennell, R. (1947). *Proc. R. Soc. B.* **136**, 94–109.
Devauchelle, G. (1971). *J. Ultrastruct. Res.* **34**, 492–516.
Dorn, A. (1978). *Cell Tiss. Res.* **187**, 479–488.
Edwards, G. A. and Challice, C. E. (1960). *Ann. ent. Soc. Am.* **53**, 369–383.
Ermin, R. (1939). *Z. Zellforsch. mikrosk. Anat.* **29**, 613–669.
Evans, J. J. T. (1967). *Z. Zellforsch. mikrosk. Anat.* **81**, 49–61.
Evans, W. A. and Elias, R. G. (1970). *Acta Protozool.* **7**, 227–241.
Florkin, M. and Jeuniaux, C. (1974). *In* "The Physiology of Insecta" (M. Rockstein, Ed.), 2nd edn, Vol. V, pp. 255–307. Academic Press, New York and London.
François, J. (1974). *Pedobiologia* **14**, 157–162.
François, J. (1975). *J. Insect Physiol.* **21**, 1535–1546.
Gagen, S. J. and Ratcliffe, N. A. (1976). *J. Invertebr. Pathol.* **28**, 17–24.
Gilliam, M. and Jeter, W. S. (1970). *J. Invertebr. Pathol.* **16**, 69–70.
Gilliam, M. and Shimanuki, H. (1967a). *J. Invertebr. Pathol.* **9**, 387–389.
Gilliam, M. and Shimanuki, H. (1967b). *Am. Bee J.* **107**, 256.
Gilliam, M. and Shimanuki, H. (1970). *Experientia* **26**, 908–909.
Gnatzy, W. (1970). *Z. Zellforsch. mikrosk. Anat.* **110**, 401–413.
Goffinet, G. and Grégoire, Ch. (1975). *Archs. int. Physiol. Biochim.* **83**, 707–722.
Goltzené, F. and Hoffmann, J. A. (1974). *Gen. Comp. Endocrinol.* **22**, 489–498.
Gomperts, B. D. (1976). *In* "Receptors and Recognition" Series A (P. Cuatrecasas and M. F. Greaves, Eds), Vol. 2, pp. 43–102. Chapman and Hall, London.
Götz, P. and Vey, A. (1974). *Parasitology* **68**, 1–13.
Grégoire, Ch. (1951). *Blood* **6**, 1173–1198.
Grégoire, Ch. (1953). *Biol. Bull., Woods Hole* **104**, 372–393.
Grégoire, Ch. (1954). *Arch. int. Physiol.* **62**, 117–119.
Grégoire, Ch. (1955a). *Arch. Biol., Paris* **66**, 103–148.
Grégoire, Ch. (1955b). *Arch. Biol., Paris* **66**, 489–508.
Grégoire, Ch. (1959). *Explor. Parc. natn. Albert, deux. Ser. No.* **10**, 1–17.
Grégoire, Ch. (1970). *In* "The Haemostatic Mechanism in Man and Other Animals" (R. G. Macfarlane, Ed.), Symp. zool. Soc. Lond. 27, pp. 45–74. Academic Press, London.
Grégoire, Ch. (1974). *In* "The Physiology of Insecta" (M. Rockstein, Ed.), 2nd edn, Vol. 5, pp. 309–355. Academic Press, New York.
Grimstone, A. V., Rotheram, S. and Salt, G. (1967). *J. Cell Sci.* **2**, 281–292.
Gupta, A. P. (1969). *Cytologia* **34**, 300–344.
Gupta, A. P. (1979). "Insect Hemocytes: Development, Forms, Functions, and Techniques." Cambridge University Press, New York.
Gupta, A. P. and Sutherland, D. J. (1967). *Ann. ent. Soc. Am.* **60**, 557–564.
Hagopian, M. (1971). *J. Ultrastruct. Res.* **36**, 646–658.
Hardy, S. W., Fletcher, T. C. and Olafsen, J. A. (1977). *In* "Developmental Immunobiology" (J. B. Solomon and J. D. Horton, Eds), pp. 59–66. Elsevier/North Holland, Amsterdam.
Harpaz, I., Kislev, N. and Zelcer, A. (1969). *J. Invertebr. Pathol.* **14**, 175–185.
Henry, J. E. (1967). *J. Invertebr. Pathol.* **9**, 331–341.
Hillen, N. (1977). Experimental studies on the reactions of insect haemocytes to artificial implants and habitual parasitoids and on the initiation of wound healing in insects. Ph.D. Thesis, University of London.

Hinks, C. F. and Arnold, J. W. (1977). *Can. J. Zool.* **55**, 1740–1755.
Hoffmann, D., Brehélin, M. and Hoffmann, J. A. (1974). *J. Invertebr. Pathol.* **24**, 238–247.
Hoffmann, J. A. (1966). *C. r. hebd. Séanc. Acad. Sci. Paris* **262**, 1496–1471.
Hoffmann, J. A. (1967). *Archs Zool. exp. gén.* **108**, 251–291.
Hoffmann, J. A. (1969a). Etude des cellules sanguines chez *Locusta migratoria.* These, Université de Strasbourg, France.
Hoffmann, J. A. (1969b). *J. Insect. Physiol.* **15**, 1375–1384.
Hoffmann, J. A. (1970a). *Z. Zellforsch. mikrosk. Anat.* **106**, 451–472.
Hoffmann, J. A. (1970b). *Gen. Comp. Endocrinol.* **15**, 198–219.
Hoffmann, J. A. (1972). *J. Insect Physiol.* **18**, 1639–1652.
Hoffmann, J. A. (1973). *Experientia* **29**, 50–51.
Hoffmann, J. A. and Joly, L. (1969). *C. r. hebd. Séanc. Acad. Sci., Paris, D.* **268**, 1218–1220.
Hoffmann, J. A. and Perolini, M. (1969). *C. r. hebd. Séanc. Acad. Sci. Paris, D.* **268**, 2469–2471.
Hoffmann, J. A. and Stoekel, M. E. (1968). *C. r. hebd. Séanc. Soc. Biol.* **162**, 2257–2259.
Hollande, A. C. (1911). *Archs Zool. exp. gén.* **6**, 283–323.
Hollande, A. C. (1922). *Archs Anat. microsc.* **18**, 85–307.
Hollande, A. C. (1930). *Archs Zool. exp. gén.* **70**, 231–280.
Huger, A. (1960). *Z.P.J.L. Krankh. P.J.L. Path. P.J.L. Schutz.* **67**, 65–77.
Iwasaki, Y. (1927). *Archs Anat. microsc.* **23**, 319–346.
Jones, J. C. (1954a). *Ann. ent. Soc. Am.* **47**, 308–315.
Jones, J. C. (1954b). *J. Morph.* **94**, 71–123.
Jones, J. C. (1956). *J. Morph.* **99**, 233–257.
Jones, J. C. (1959). *Quart. Jl. microsc. Sci.* **100**, 17–23.
Jones, J. C. (1962). *Amer. Zool.* **2**, 209–246.
Jones, J. C. (1965). *Biol. Bull., Woods Hole* **129**, 282–294.
Jones, J. C. (1967a). *J. Insect Physiol.* **13**, 1133–1141.
Jones, J. C. (1967b). *Biol. Bull., Woods Hole* **132**, 211–221.
Jones, J. C. (1970). *In* "Regulation of Hematopoiesis" (A. S. Gordon, Ed.), Vol. 1, pp. 7–65. Appleton, New York.
Jones, J. C. (1977). "The Circulatory System of Insects". C. C. Thomas, Springfield, Illinois.
Jones, J. C. and Liu, D. P. (1968). *J. Insect Physiol.* **14**, 1053–1061.
Jones, J. C. and Liu, D. P. (1969). *J. Insect Physiol.* **15**, 1703–1708.
Jones, J. C. and Tauber, O. E. (1951). *Ann. ent. Soc. Am.* **44**, 539–543.
Kawanishi, C. Y., Splittstoesser, C. M. and Tashiro, H. (1978). *J. Invertebr. Pathol.* **31**, 91–102.
Kessel, R. G. (1961). *Expl. Cell. Res.* **22**, 108–119.
Kessel, R. G. (1962). *J. Morph.* **110**, 79–103.
Kitano, H. (1969a). *Appl. Ent. Zool.* **4**, 51–55.
Kitano, H. (1969b). *Bull. Tokyo Gekugei Univ.* **21**, 95–136.
Kitano, H. (1974). *J. Insect Physiol.* **20**, 315–327.
Kitano, H. and Nakatsuji, N. (1978). *J. Insect Physiol.* **24**, 261–271.
Klebanoff, S. J. (1972). *In* "Phagocytic Mechanisms in Health and Disease" (R. C. Williams and H. H. Fudenberg, Eds), pp. 3–21. Intercontinental Medical Book Corp., New York and London.
Klebanoff, S. J. (1975). *In* "The Phagocytic Cell in Host Resistance" (J. A. Bellanti and D. H. Dayton, Eds), pp. 45–57. Raven Press, New York.

Kurstak, E., Goring, I. and Vega, C. (1969). *Antonie von Leeuwenhoek* **35**, 45–51.
Lackie, A. M. (1976). *Parasitology* **73**, 97–107.
Lackie, A. M. (1977). *In* "Developmental Immunobiology" (J. B. Solomon and J. D. Horton, Eds), pp. 75–81. Elsevier/North Holland, Amsterdam.
Lackie, A. M. (1979). *Immunology* **36**, 909–914.
Lai-Fook, J. (1968). *J. Morphol.* **124**, 37–78.
Lai-Fook, J. (1970). *J. Morphol.* **130**, 297–314.
Lai-Fook, J. (1973). *J. Morphol.* **139**, 79–104.
Lai-Fook, J. and Neuwirth, M. (1972). *Can. J. Zool.* **50**, 1011–1013.
Landureau, J. C. (1977). *Publ. Lab. Zool. E.N.S.* **8**, 131–167.
Landureau, J. C. and Grellet, P. (1975). *J. Insect Physiol.* **21**, 137–151.
Landureau, J. C. and Szöllösi, A. (1974). *C. r. hebd. Séanc. Acad. Sci. Paris, D.* **278**, 3359–3362.
Landureau, J. C., Grellet, P. and Bernier, I. (1972). *C. r. hebd. Séanc. Acad. Sci. Paris, D.* **274**, 2200–2203.
Lazarenko, T. (1925). *Z. Zellforsch. mikrosk. Anat.* **3**, 409–499.
Leutenegger, R. (1967). *Virology* **32**, 109–116.
Levin, J. (1967). *Fedn. Proc. Fedn. Am. Socs. exp. Biol.* **26**, 1707–1712.
Levin, J. and Bang, F. B. (1964). *Bull. Johns Hopkins Hosp.* **115**, 265–274.
Lipke, H. (1975). *In* "Invertebrate Immunity" (K. Maramorosch and R. E. Shope, Eds), pp. 327–336. Academic Press, New York and London.
Locke, M. (1966). *J. Insect Physiol.* **12**, 389–395.
Locke, M. (1969). *Tissue and Cell* **1**, 103–154.
Lüthy, P., Wyss, Ch. and Ettlinger, L. (1970). *J. Invertebr. Pathol.* **16**, 325–330.
Lynn, D. C. and Vinson, S. B. (1977). *J. Invertebr. Pathol.* **29**, 50–55.
Madziara-Borusiewicz, K. and Lysenko, O. (1971). *J. Invertebr. Pathol.* **17**, 138–140.
Maier, W. (1969). *Z. Zellforsch. mikrosk. Anat.* **99**, 54–63.
Marschall, K. J. (1966). *Z. Morph Ökol. Tiere.* **58**, 182–246.
Matz, G. (1965). *Bull. Soc. zool. Fr.* **90**, 429–433.
Matz, G. (1977). *Annls. Parasit. hum. comp.* **52**, 68–69.
McKay, D. and Jenkin, C. R. (1970). *Aust. J. exp. Biol. med. Sci.* **48**, 139–150.
Mengeot, J. C., Bauchau, A. G., DeBrouwer, M. B. and Passelecq-Gérin, E. (1977). *Comp. Biochem. Physiol.* **58A**, 393–403.
Metalnikov, S. (1902). *Izv. imp. Akad, Nauk.* **17**, 49–58.
Metalnikov, S. (1908). *Archs Zool. exp. gén.* **8**, 489–588.
Metalnikov, S. (1924). *Annls. Inst. Pasteur, Paris* **38**, 787–826.
Metalnikov, S. (1927). *Monogr. Inst. Pasteur Masson.* Paris.
Metalnikov, S. and Chorine, V. (1928). *Int. Corn Borer Invest. Sci. Rep.* **1**, 41–69.
Metalnikov, S. and Chorine, V. (1929). *Int. Corn Borer Invest. Sci. Rep.* **2**, 22–38.
Metchnikoff, E. (1884). *Virchows Arch. path. Anat. Physiol.* **96**, 177–195.
Misko, I. S. (1972). The cellular defense mechanisms of *Periplaneta americana* (L.). Ph.D. Thesis, Australian National University.
Monpeyssin, M. and Beaulaton, J. (1977). *J. Insect Physiol.* **23**, 939–943.
Monpeyssin, M. and Beaulaton, J. (1978). *J. Ultrastruct. Res.* **64**, 35–45.
Moran, D. T. (1971). *Tissue and Cell* **3**, 413–422.
Murer, E. H., Levin, J. and Holme, R. (1975). *J. Cell Physiol.* **86**, 523–543.
Nappi, A. J. (1970). *J. Invertebr. Pathol.* **16**, 408–418.
Nappi, A. J. (1973). *Expl. Parasit.* **33**, 285–303.
Nappi, A. J. (1974). *In* "Contemporary Topics in Immunobiology, Vol. 4,

Invertebrate Immunology" (E. L. Cooper, Ed.), pp. 207–244. Plenum Press, New York and London.
Nappi, A. J. (1975a). *J. Parasit.* **61**, 373–376.
Nappi, A. J. (1975b). *In* "Invertebrate Immunity" (K. Maramorosch and R. E. Shope, Eds), pp. 273–326. Academic Press, New York, San Francisco and London.
Nappi, A. J. and Stoffolano, Jr. J. G. (1971). *Expl. Parasit.* **29**, 116–125.
Nappi, A. J. and Stoffolano, Jr, J. G. (1972a). *J. Insect Physiol.* **18**, 169–179.
Nappi, A. J. and Stoffolano, Jr. J. G. (1972b). *Parasitology* **65**, 295–302.
Nappi, A. J. and Streams, F. A. (1969). *J. Insect Physiol.* **15**, 1551–1566.
Neuwirth, M. (1973). *J. Morphol.* **139**, 105–124.
Neuwirth, M. (1974). *Can. J. Zool.* **52**, 783–784.
Neuwirth, M. and Lai-Fook, J. (1977). *Can. J. Zool.* **55**, 1767–1772.
Nittono, Y. (1960). *Bull. sericult. Exp. Stn. Japan* **16**, 171–266.
Nittono, Y., Tomabechi, S. and Onodera, N. (1964). *J. seric. Sci. Tokyo.* **33**, 43–45.
Nutting, W. L. (1951). *J. Morphol.* **89**, 501–597.
Olson, K. and Carlson, S. D. (1974). *Ann. ent. Soc. Am.* **67**, 61–65.
Osman, S. E. (1978). *Z. ParasitKde.* **57**, 89–100.
Paterson, W. D. and Stewart, J. E. (1974). *J. Fish. Res. Bd. Can.* **31**, 1051–1056.
Percy, J. (1978). *Can. J. Zool.* **56**, 238–245.
Perez, C. (1910). *Archs Zool. exp. gén.* **4**, 1–274.
Pipa, R. L. and Woolever, P. S. (1965). *Z. Zellforsch. mikrosk. Anat.* **68**, 80–101.
Poinar, Jr. G. O. (1974). *In* "Contemporary Topics in Immunobiology, Invertebrate Immunology" (E. L. Cooper, Ed.), Vol. 4, pp. 167–178. Plenum Press, New York and London.
Poinar, Jr. G. O. and Leutenegger, R. (1971). *J. Ultrastruct. Res.* **36**, 149–158.
Poinar, Jr. G. O., Leutenegger, R. and Götz, P. (1968). *J. Ultrastruct. Res.* **25**, 293–306.
Price, C. D. (1974). Studies on insect haemocytes. Ph.D. thesis, University of Wales.
Price, C. D. and Ratcliffe, N. A. (1974). *Z. Zellforsch. mikrosk. Anat.* **147**, 537–549.
Prowse, R. H. and Tait, N. N. (1969). *Immunology* **17**, 437–443.
Pye, A. E. and Yendol, W. G. (1972). *J. Invertebr. Pathol.* **19**, 166–170.
Rabinovitch, M. and DeStefano, M. (1970). *Expl. Cell Res.* **59**, 272–282.
Ratcliffe, N. A. (1975). *J. Invertebr. Pathol.* **26**, 217–223.
Ratcliffe, N. A. and Gagen, S. J. (1976). *J. Invertebr. Pathol.* **28**, 373–382.
Ratcliffe, N. A. and Gagen, S. J. (1977). *Tissue and Cell* **9**, 73–85.
Ratcliffe, N. A. and Price, C. D. (1974). *J. Morphol.* **144**, 485–498.
Ratcliffe, N. A. and Rowley, A. F. (1974). *Nature, Lond.* **252**, 391–392.
Ratcliffe, N. A. and Rowley, A. F. (1975). *J. Invertebr. Pathol.* **26**, 225–233.
Ratcliffe, N. A. and Rowley, A. F. (1979a). *In* "Insect Haemocytes, Development, Forms, Functions, and Techniques" (A. P. Gupta, Ed.), pp. 331–414. Cambridge University Press, Cambridge.
Ratcliffe, N. A. and Rowley, A. F. (1979b). *Devl. Comp. Immunol.* **3**, 189–221.
Ratcliffe, N. A. and Rowley, A. F. (1980). *Comp. Pathobiol.* (L. A. Bulla, Jr. and T. C. Cheng, Eds). Plenum Press, New York (in press).
Ratcliffe, N. A., Gagen, S. J., Rowley, A. F. and Schmit, A. R. (1976a). *In* "Proc. 1st Int. Colloq. Invert. Pathol" (T. Angus, P. Faulkner and A. Rosenfield, Eds), pp. 210–214. Queens University Printing Department.

Ratcliffe, N. A., Gagen, S. J., Rowley, A. F. and Schmit, A. (1976b). *In* "Proceedings of the Sixth European Congress on Electron Microscopy, Vol. II. Biological Sciences" (Y. Ben-Shaul, Ed.), pp. 295–297. Tal. International Pub. Co. Israel.
Ravindranath, M. H. (1978). *Devl. Comp. Immunol.* **2**, 581–594.
Ravindranath, M. H. and Anantaraman, S. (1977). *Z. ParasitKde.* **53**, 225–237.
Reik, L. (1968). Contacts between blood cells with special reference to the structure of the capsules formed about parasites. M.Sc. Dissertation, University of Cambridge.
Richards, A. G. (1951). "The Integument of Arthropods". University of Minnesota Press, Minnesota.
Richards, O. W. and Davies, R. G. (1977). "Imms' General Textbook of Entomology, Vol. 1, Structure, Physiology and Development". Chapman and Hall, London.
Ries, E. (1932). *Z. Morph. Ökol. Tiere* **25**, 184–234.
Rizki, M. T. M. (1957). *J. Morphol.* **100**, 437–458.
Rizki, M. T. M. and Rizki, R. M. (1959). *J. biophys. biochem. Cytol.* **5**, 235–239.
Robinson, E. S. and Strickland, B. C. (1969). *Expl. Parasit.* **26**, 384–392.
Romer, F. (1972). *Cytobiologie* **6**, 195–213.
Romer, F. (1974). *Cell Tiss. Res.* **151**, 27–46.
Rotheram, S. M. (1967). *Nature, Lond.* **214**, 700.
Rotheram, S. M. (1973a). *Proc. R. Soc. B.* **183**, 179–194.
Rotheram, S. M. (1973b). *Proc. R. Soc. B.* **183**, 195–204.
Rotheram, S. M. and Crompton, D. W. T. (1972). *Parasitology* **64**, 15–21.
Rowley, A. F. (1977a). Studies on insect cellular defences *in vitro*. Ph.D. Thesis, University of Wales.
Rowley, A. F. (1977b). *Cell Tiss. Res.* **182**, 513–524.
Rowley, A. F. and Ratcliffe, N. A. (1976a). *J. Ultrastruct. Res.* **55**, 193–202.
Rowley, A. F. and Ratcliffe, N. A. (1976b). *Tissue and Cell* **8**, 437–446.
Rowley, A. F. and Ratcliffe, N. A. (1976c). *In* "Proceedings of the Sixth European Congress on Electron Microscopy Vol. II Biological Sciences" (Y. Ben-Shaul, Ed.), pp. 301–303. Tal International Pub. Co. Israel.
Rowley, A. F. and Ratcliffe, N. A. (1978). *J. Morphol.* **157**, 181–200.
Rowley, A. F. and Ratcliffe, N. A. (1979). *Cell. Tiss. Res.* **199**, 127–137.
Rowley, A. F. and Ratcliffe, N. A. (1980). *Immunology* **40**, 483–492.
Ryan, M. and Nicholas, W. L. (1972). *J. Invertebr Pathol.* **19**, 299–307.
Salt, G. (1956). *Proc. R. Soc. B.* **146**, 93–108.
Salt, G. (1957). *Proc. R. Soc. B.* **147**, 167–184.
Salt, G. (1963). *Parasitology* **53**, 527–642.
Salt, G. (1965). *Proc. R. Soc. B.* **162**, 303–318.
Salt, G. (1970). "The Cellular Defence Reactions of Insects." Cambridge Monographs in Experimental Biology No. 16. Cambridge University Press, London and New York.
Salt, G. (1973). *Proc. R. Soc. B.* **183**, 337–350.
Salt, G. (1975). *Trans. R. ent. Soc. Lond.* **127**, 141–161.
Sato, S., Akai, H. and Sawada, H. (1976). *Annotnes zool. jap.* **49**, 177–188.
Scharrer, B. (1972). *Z. Zellforsch. mikrosk. Anat.* **129**. 301–319.
Schmit, A. R. (1979). Studies on encapsulation in insects. Ph.D. Thesis, University of Wales.
Schmit, A. R. and Ratcliffe, N. A. (1977). *J. Insect Physiol.* **23**, 175–184.
Schmit, A. R. and Ratcliffe, N. A. (1978). *J. Insect Physiol.* **24**, 511–521.

Schmit, A. R., Rowley, A. F. and Ratcliffe, N. A. (1977). *J. Invertebr. Pathol.* **29**, 232–234.
Shrivastava, S. C. and Richards, A. G. (1965). *Biol. Bull., Woods Hole* **128**, 337–345.
Scott, M. T. (1971a). *Archs Zool. exp. gén.* **112**, 73–80.
Scott, M. T. (1971b). *Immunology* **21**, 817–827.
Scott, M. T. (1971c). *Transplantation* **11**, 78–86.
Scott, M. T. (1972). *J. Invertebr. Pathol.* **19**, 66–71.
Shapiro, M. (1968). *J. Insect Physiol.* **14**, 1725–1733.
Siakotos, A. N. (1960a). *J. gen. Physiol.* **43**, 999–1013.
Siakotos, A. N. (1960b). *J. gen. Physiol.* **43**, 1015–1030.
Sminia, T., Van der Knaap, W. P. W. and Edelenbosch, P. (1979). *Devl. Comp. Immunol.* **3**, 37–44.
Stang-Voss, C. (1970). *Z. Zellforsch. mikrosk. Anat.* **103**, 589–605.
Stebbings, H. and Hyams, J. S. (1979). "Cell Motility." Longman, London and New York.
Swammerdam, J. (1737). "Bybel der Nature, historie der Insekten". Edite par Boerhaave.
Takeda, N. (1977). *J. Insect Physiol.* **23**, 1245–1254.
Taylor, R. L. (1969). *J. Invertebr. Pathol.* **14**, 427–428.
Toumanoff, C. (1949). *Revue can. Biol.* **8**, 343–369.
Tripp, M. R. (1966). *J. Invertebr. Pathol.* **8**, 478–484.
Tripp, M. R. and Kent, V. E. (1967). *In Vitro* **3**, 129–135.
Tyson, C. J. and Jenkin, C. R. (1973). *Aust. J. exp. Biol. med. Sci.* **51**, 609–615.
Tyson, C. J. and Jenkin, C. R. (1974). *Aust. J. exp. Biol. med. Sci.* **52**, 341–348.
Van Furth, R. and Van Zwet, T. L. (1973). *In* "Handbook of Experimental Immunology" (D. M. Weir, Ed.), 2nd edn, pp. 36.1–36.24. Blackwell Scientific Publications, Oxford.
Vecchi, M. A., Bragaglia, M. M. and Wille, H. (1972). *Mitt. schweiz. ent. Ges.* **44**, 209–232.
Vey, A. (1968). *Annls. Épiphyt.* (*Paris*) **19**, 695–702.
Vey, A. (1969). *Ann. Zool. Écol. anim.* **1**, 93–100.
Vey, A. and Fargues, J. (1977). *J. Invertebr. Pathol.* **30**, 207–215.
Vey, A. and Vago, C. (1969). *Ann. Zool. Écol. anim.* **1**, 121–126.
Vey, A. and Vago, C. (1971). *Annls. Inst. Pasteur, Paris* **121**, 527–532.
Vey, A., Quiot, J. M. and Vago, C. (1968). *In* "Proceedings 2nd International Colloquium on Invertebrate Tissue Culture", Milan 1967 (C. Barigazzi, Ed.), pp. 254–263. Instituto Lombardo, Milan, Italy.
Vey, A., Quiot, J. M. and Vago, C. (1973). *C. r. hebd. Séanc. Acad. Sci. Paris. Sér. D.* **276**, 2489–2492.
Vinson, S. B. (1971). *J. Invertebr. Pathol.* **18**, 94–100.
Vinson, S. B. (1972). *J. Insect Physiol.* **18**, 1501–1516.
Vinson, S. B. (1977). *Expl. Parasit.* **41**, 112–117.
Werner, R. A. and Jones, J. C. (1969). *J. Insect Physiol.* **15**, 425–437.
Whitten, J. M. (1964). *J. Insect Physiol.* **10**, 447–469.
Wigglesworth, V. B. (1937). *J. exp. Biol.* **14**, 364–381.
Wigglesworth, V. B. (1943). *Proc. R. Soc. B.* **131**, 313–339.
Wigglesworth, V. B. (1955). *J. exp. Biol.* **32**, 649–663.
Wigglesworth, V. B. (1956). *Quart. Jl. microsc. Sci.* **97**, 89–98.
Wigglesworth, V. B. (1959). *A. Rev. Ent.* **4**, 1–16.

Wigglesworth, V. B. (1965). "The Principles of Insect Physiology", 6th edn. Methuen, London.
Wigglesworth, V. B. (1970). *J. Reticuolendothel. Soc.* **7**, 208–216.
Wigglesworth, V. B. (1973). *J. Insect Physiol.* **19**, 831–844.
Wigglesworth, V. B. (1979). *Tissue and Cell* **11**, 69–78.
Wilkinson, P. C. (1976). *Clin. exp. Immunol.* **25**, 355–366.
Wittig, G. (1965a). *Proc. Intern. Congr. Entomol. 12th. Lond.*, 1964, 743.
Wittig, G. (1965b). *J. Invertebr. Pathol.* **7**, 474–488.
Wittig, G. (1966). *J. Invertebr. Pathol.* **8**, 461–477.
Yeager, J. F. (1945). *J. agric. Res.* **71**, 1–40.
Yeager, J. F. and Munson, S. C. (1941). *J. agric. Res.* **63**, 257–294.
Zachary, D. and Hoffmann, J. A. (1973). *Z. Zellforsch. mikrosk. Anat.* **141**, 55–73.
Zachary, D., Brehélin, N. and Hoffmann, J. A. (1975). *Cell Tiss. Res.* **162**, 343–348.

Section VI

Lophophorates

14. Lophophorates

P. J. HAYWARD

Department of Zoology, University College of Swansea, Singleton Park, Swansea, SA2 8PP, U.K.

CONTENTS

I. Introduction

The lophophorates comprise three phyla of uncertain origin and phylogenetic relationships: Bryozoa, Phoronida and Brachiopoda. Habit and morphology of each phylum vary widely, from the shelled, sessile brachiopods to the tubicolous, worm-like phoronids and the colonial bryozoans. The common grouping, however, is based on a number of morphological similarities. For example, all three possess, primitively, a tripartite coelom; the mouth is surrounded by a feeding lophophore, a tentaculated extension of the body wall enclosing coelomic spaces, and the gut is U-shaped, with the anus opening at the base of the lophophore but outside the ring of tentacles. A common origin may be envisaged for the phoronids and bryozoans (Farmer, 1977), but relationships of both phyla with the brachiopods seem rather more obscure.

There has been little recent research on the circulatory systems or "blood" cells of the lophophorates. Most interest has focused on the phoronids which display a complex structure and are potentially more interesting. Accordingly, in this account prominence will also be given to the Phoronida; comparative information on the Brachiopoda and Bryozoa is given where available. In the present chapter, additional unpublished information is provided by the examination of thick plastic sections of *Phoronis hippocrepia*, collected from the Gower peninsula, South Wales.

II. Structure of the circulatory systems

The phoronids, alone among the lophophorates, have a closed vascular system consisting of two longitudinal trunk vessels: a dorsal or afferent vessel, and a ventral or efferent vessel. In the posterior half of the animal the two vessels are linked by an extensive haemal plexus in the peritoneum of the stomach wall (Figs 1, 2). Blood flows anteriorly in the dorsal vessel, which forks close to the oesophagus to produce an afferent ring vessel extending through the coelom of the lophophore. A single vessel extends from the afferent ring into each tentacle, linked at its base by a branch to an efferent ring. Blood flows to and fro in the tentacular vessels, passing back into the efferent ring from which it is drained by two branches; these run posteriorly, fusing at the posterior end of the oesophagus to form the ventral vessel (Hyman, 1959). The anterior half of the ventral vessel gives rise to a number of capillary caeca. The main blood vessels have a layer of circular muscle between the lining epithelium and the peritoneum which maintains a regular, rhythmic contraction; circulation in the tentacular vessels and the caeca is achieved by autonomic contraction independent of the main vessels.

The vascular system of brachiopods is little studied, but in all species it is reduced and open. A single main vessel lies along the dorsal surface of the oesophagus and stomach. Anteriorly the vessel divides, sending a branch into each of the arms of the lophophore; the vessel is enclosed within the peritoneum of one of the coelomic channels of the lophophore, and gives rise to small tentacular capillaries (Hyman, 1959). The main dorsal vessel forks again posterior to the stomach, each limb then bifurcating to send a branch to the dorsal and ventral mantle lobes on each side of the animal. These mantle vessels divide repeatedly, following the course of the coelomic channels. Above the stomach some sections of the dorsal vessel are

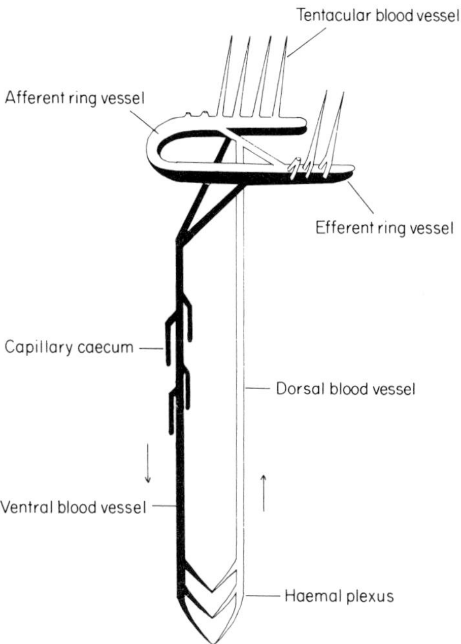

Fig. 1. Diagrammatic representation of the vascular system in *Phoronis*.

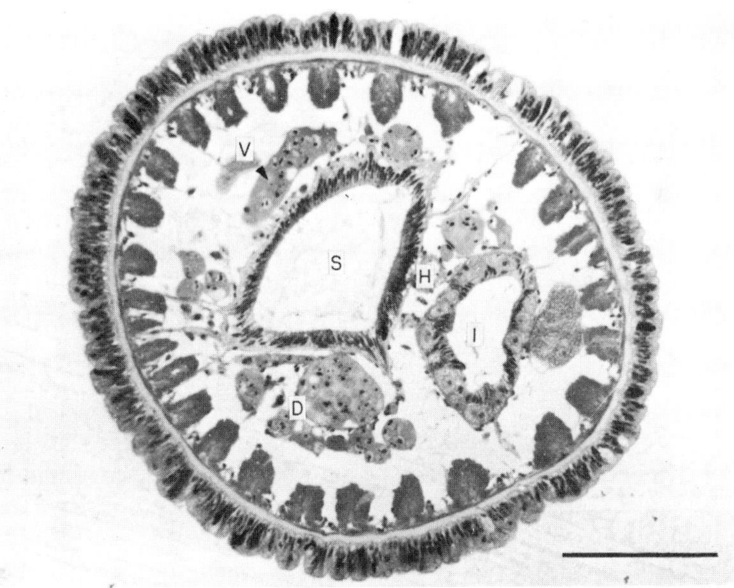

Fig. 2. Transverse section through posterior trunk region of *P. hippocrepia* showing dorsal (D) and ventral (V) blood vessels and the beginning of the haemal plexus (H). Stomach (S) and intestine (I) are also indicated. Scale = 100 μm.

thickened by layers of circular muscle to form small contractile vesicles; however, all authors have stated that contraction appears to be irregular and slow. Conversely, there is a steady circulation of the coelomic fluid, maintained by ciliary tracts of the lumen of the lophophore, mantle and pedicel, and by contraction of the gut and visceral muscles in the main coelom (Chuang, 1964).

In the Bryozoa, a vascular system is lacking altogether, its functions being performed wholly by coelomic fluids. Cilial circulation has been demonstrated in the freshwater genera, *Paludicella*, *Pectinatella* (Hyman, 1959) and *Lophopodella* (Mano, 1964) and is probably also present in many specialized Gymnolaemata and Phylactolaemata which possess large, common, colonial coelomic spaces (Cook, 1975).

III. Structure and classification of "blood" cells

The only comprehensive account of "blood" cell types in the Phoronida is that of Ohuye (1942), who studied *Phoronis australis* and *P. ijimae*. The cell types recognized by Ohuye are listed in Table I; leucocytes and erythrocytes were present. The erythrocytes were up to 12 μm in diameter with a small, round or oval, eccentric nucleus. Characteristically, the cytoplasm contained one to three refractile granules and the nucleus was often partly obscured by haemoglobin granules. The leucocytes included hyaline amoebocytes, of three different types, and both eosinophilic and basophilic granulocytes. The hyaline amoebocytes were almost as abundant as the erythrocytes, but the two granulocyte types were both generally rare. Ohuye's (1942) terminology is not always clear to the modern reader and several of the cell types he described were not recognized in *P. hippocrepia*. Further, he did not distinguish between coelomocytes and haemocytes; the erythrocytes, by virtue of their origin and distribution in the worm, may be regarded as haemocytes but it is clear that several of Ohuye's leucocyte types are more properly considered as coelomocytes.

Erythrocytes of *P. hippocrepia* are similar to those described in the Japanese species and formed the preponderance of cells present (Fig. 3). They are round or irregular in shape, up to 11 μm in diameter, and have a finely granular cytoplasm. The nucleus is distinctly eccentric in position and its outline is frequently obscured, presumably by granular deposits of haemoglobin. Most contain one or two large granules in the cytoplasm. A developmental sequence was illustrated by Ohuye (1942) showing differentiation of detached endothelial cells, in the tentacular blood vessels, and peritoneal cells in the lumen of the tentacles, to form proerythroblasts, with

TABLE I. The blood cells of *Choronis*. (After Ohuye 1942.)

Type		Size (μm)	Structure
Erythrocyte		8–12 × 2–4	spherical or slightly biconvex, smooth edges. Nucleus small, oval or round, eccentric, often partly obscured by haemoglobin. Cytoplasm homogeneous, with 1–3 refractile granules
Hyaline amoebocyte	A	4–8	large, round or oval nucleus; little cytoplasm.
	B	10–12	nucleus irregular–oval, lobed or u-shaped; little cytoplasm, sometimes a few large granules
	C	15–20	nucleus small, round, oval or rod-shaped, eccentric in position.
Eosinophilic granulocytes		10–16	(a) finely granular—granules 1–2 μm in diameter (b) coarsely granular—granules 2–6 μm in diameter } actively amoeboid, phagocytic
Basophilic granulocytes		not given	similar in structure to eosinophils, but less active
Russell body cells		variable	round or oval. Nucleus small, round or oval, eccentric, displaying signs of degeneration. Cytoplasm basophilic. Russell bodies spherical or angular, strongly eosinophilic
Spindle bodies		variable	elongate, fusiform, striated.

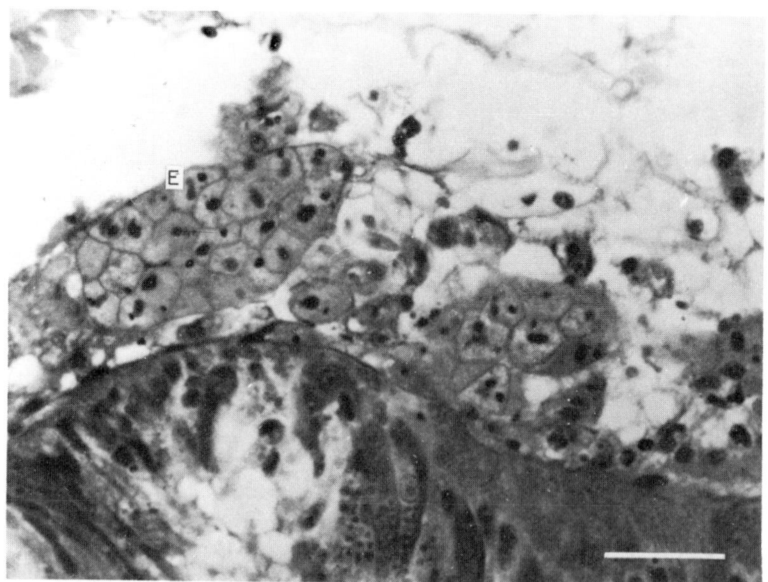

Fig. 3. Part of the haemal plexus in *P. hippocrepia*, showing numerous erythrocytes (E). Scale = 20 μm.

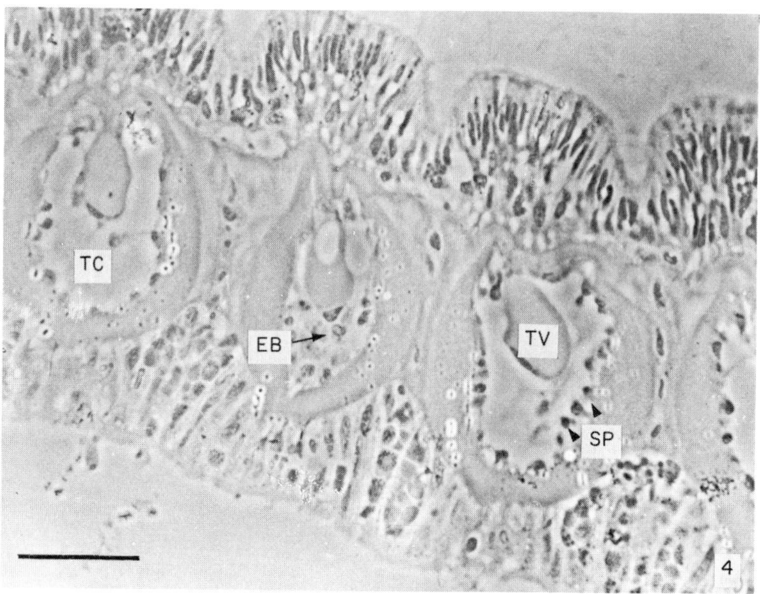

Fig. 4. Stained transverse section through tentacle bases of *P. hippocrepia*, viewed by phase contrast optics, showing peritoneal cells (SP) and liberated erythroblasts (EB) in the tentacular coelom (TC). Tentacular blood vessels (TV) may be clearly seen. Scale = 20 μm.

dense reticulate nuclei. Following haemoglobin deposition and rearrangement of the chromatin, these cells matured as polychromatophilic erythroblasts. After mitosis the erythroblasts were seen as small cells with relatively large nuclei which then increased their volume of cytoplasm to form erythrocytes. Sections of the tentacle bases of *P. hippocrepia* (Figs 4, 5) show proliferating peritoneum with swollen and stalked cells (=proerythroblasts) evident in the wall of the tentacle. Small round cells with large dense nuclei, visible in the tentacle lumen, appear to be liberated erythroblasts.

The leucocytes described by Ohuye (1942) present certain difficulties of interpretation. Three types of hyaline amoebocyte were distinguished (Table I), each characterized largely by size and by features of the nucleus. A particular type which occurs infrequently in *P. hippocrepia* may correspond to the Type B hyaline amoebocyte described by Ohuye; these are as large as erythrocytes (Fig. 6) but have a relatively homogeneous cytoplasm, with one or two large granules, and a central, lobed, U-shaped nucleus. The largest amoebocytes in the japanese phoronids (up to 20 μm diameter) were interpreted as tissue macrophages, and were distinguished by small, irregular, eccentric nuclei. Such cells were not found in *P. hippocrepia*, although

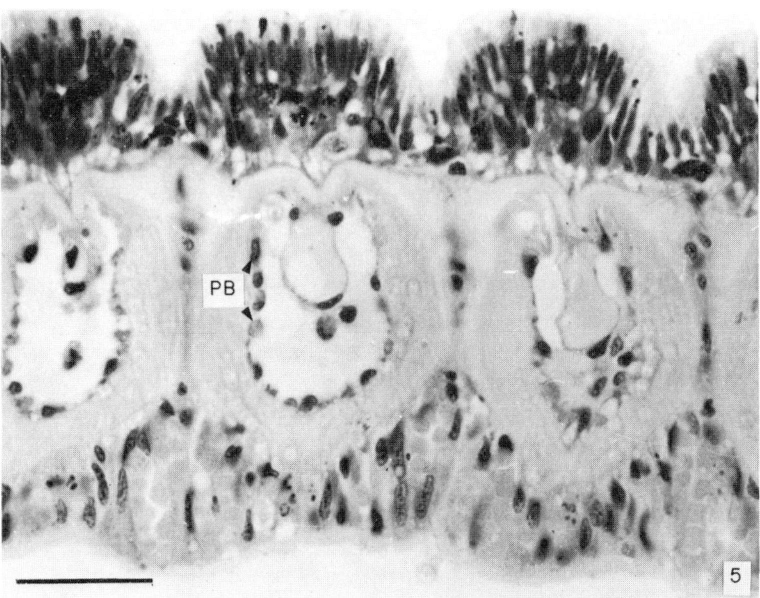

Fig. 5. A similar section showing proerythroblasts (PB) in the peritoneum of the tentacular coelom. Scale = 20 μm.

rare examples of what appears to be an amoeboid coelomocyte (Fig. 6) were present. Both the large amoebocytes and the granulocytes were shown by Ohuye (1942) to originate from the vasoperitoneal tissue and from the peritoneum in numerous parts of the worm. The peritoneum surrounding the blood sinus illustrated in Fig. 6 shows areas of active proliferation which may indicate differentiation of leucocytes.

Two further structures described by Ohuye (1942) remain enigmatic. Russell body cells were so called by the author after their resemblance to a particular cell type known in mammalian tissues. They were characterized as "free lymphoid cells", present in the coelom and vasoperitoneal tissue, with a basophilic cytoplasm and small, apparently degenerating, nuclei. The Russell bodies were round or irregular eosinophilic inclusions, often numerous, of unknown composition, although possibly at least partly composed of haemoglobin. These cells were also observed with spindle bodies enclosed within the cytoplasm; in some cases, the cell was ruptured

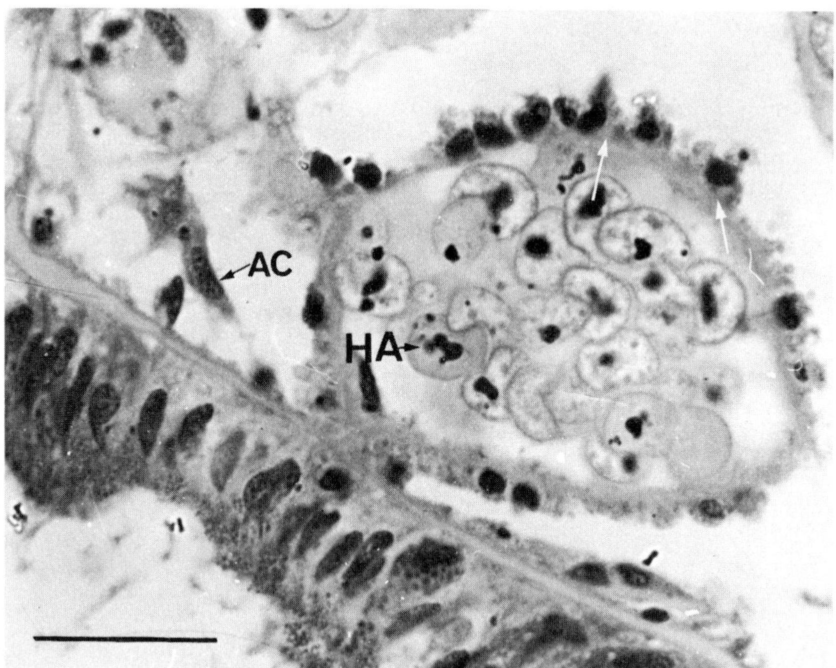

Fig. 6. Part of the haemal plexus of *P. hippocrepia*, showing a Type B hyaline amoebocyte (HA) and a presumed amoeboid coelomocyte (AC). The peritoneum enveloping the blood sinus shows signs of proliferation (arrows). Scale = 20 μm.

and its contents were free in the coelom. It seems most likely that Russell body cells represent phagocytic granulocytes in advanced stages of degeneration. None were found by the present author in *P. hippocrepia*. Spindle bodies have been reported in the coelomic cavity and the vasoperitoneal tissue of phoronids by several authors (e.g. Cori, 1891), and were found by Ohuye in both *P. australis* and *P. ijimae*. They were not described, but his drawings show elongate fusiform structures with a striated appearance, lacking both nuclei and discernible cytoplasmic features (Fig. 7). They varied in size from slightly larger than to less than half the size of an erythrocyte; perhaps significantly, they were most frequent in the vasoperitoneal tissue and increased in frequency as the animals' environmental conditions deteriorated. Despite careful searching, spindle bodies have not been seen in sections of *P. hippocrepia*.

Recently, Storch and Herrmann (1978) have described a cell type from the fine trunk sinuses of *P. muelleri*. These formed the lining of the blood vessels and could be recognized as podocytes; large stellate cells, the elongated processes of which radiated widely and were linked to those of neighbouring cells by filaments referred to as pedicels. Gaps between pedicels were crossed by a thin membrane, the slit membrane. In other invertebrates, and in vertebrates, such cell layers are known to function as sites of ultrafiltration (Storch and Herrmann, 1978).

The blood cells of brachiopods and bryozoans are less well-studied than those of phoronids. Mano (1964) has pointed out that much of the terminology of haematology is inappropriate to the Bryozoa, in which the only free cells found are more properly referred to as coelomocytes. This stricture should perhaps apply also to the Brachiopoda, in which the open blood system, and the fact the the majority of the free cells described are to be found in the coelom, makes it quite impossible at present to differentiate between blood cells, as strictly defined, and coelomocytes.

An early account by Yatsu (1902) of the free cell types of the brachiopod, *Lingula anatina* (= *L. unguis*) recognized three different cell types (Table II): (1) erythrocytes, which were simple transparent spheres, up to 20 μm in diameter, with clear cytoplasm and dense nuclei; (2) leucocytes, which were of a similar size to the erythrocytes, irregular in outline and tending to amoeboid movement, with a granular cytoplasm; (3) spindle bodies, similar to those of the phoronids but apparently much larger, up to 140 μm long (Fig. 7). Ohuye (1936, 1937) made more detailed observations on brachiopod blood cells, in two articulate species as well as *L. unguis*. For the latter he gave more comprehensive descriptions of the erythrocytes, discussed the structure and possible significance of the spindle bodies, and demonstrated that Yatsu's (1902) leucocytes could be divided into hyaline amoebocytes, and eosinophilic and basophilic granulocytes. The erythrocytes

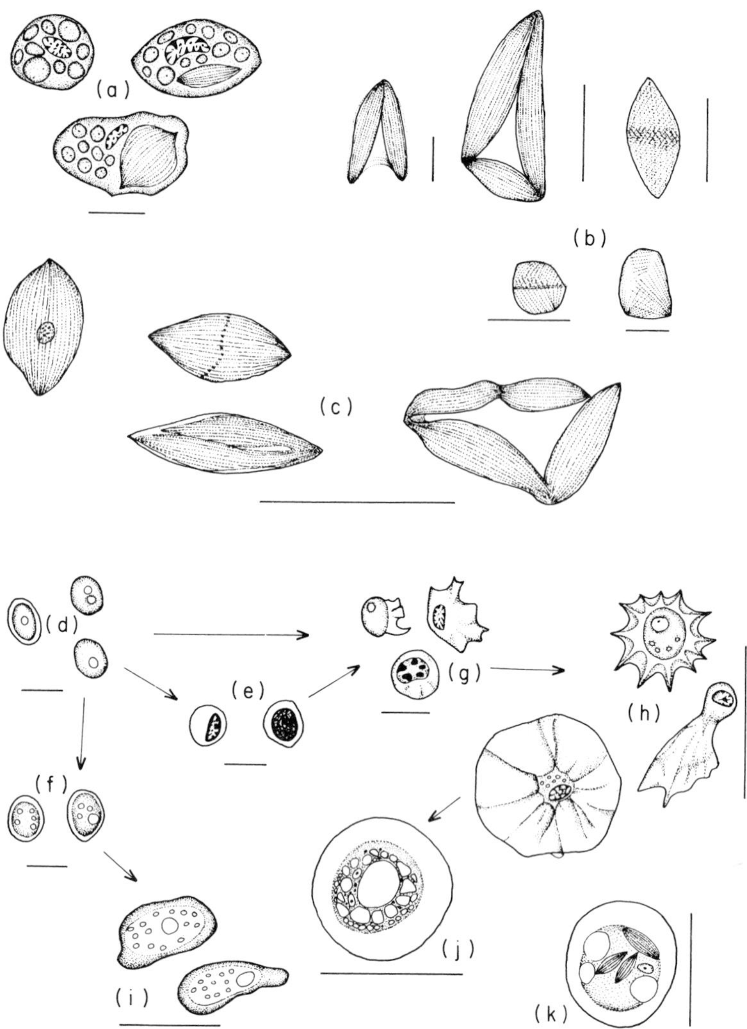

Fig. 7. (a), Russell body cells of *Phoronis*, two with ingested spindle bodies. (After Ohuye, 1942.) Scale = 15 μm; (b), Spindle bodies of *Lingula unguis*. (After Yatsu, 1902.) Scale = 20 μm; (c), Spindle bodies of *L. unguis*. (After Ohuye, 1937.) Scale = 30 μm; (d–k), Coelomocytes of *Lophopodella carteri*. (After Mano, 1964.) Arrows indicate the developmental sequences postulated by Mano; all scales are approximate; (d), Type A lymphocytes, scale = 10 μm; (e), Type B lymphocytes, scale = 10 μm; (f), Type C lymphocytes, scale = 10 μm; (g), small leucocytes, scale = 15 μm; (h), Hyaline amoebocytes, scale = 100 μm; (i), Granulocytes, scale = 40 μm; (j), Vacuolated cell, scale = 90 μm; (k), Spindle body cell, scale = 100 μm.

of *L. unguis* were spherical, often depressed in one or more places to form convex or biconvex discs; the cytoplasm contained a few large granules, and deposition of a blood pigment could be observed *in vitro*. The nucleus was typically small, oval and eccentric in position, and often U or Y-shaped.

The free coelomic cells of the two articulate brachiopods included hyaline amoebocytes and a range of granular amoebocytes in *Terebratalia coreanica* (Ohuye, 1936), and a granular amoebocyte series in *Coptothyris grayi* (Ohuye, 1937). Spindle bodies were present in both species. In the first of these two papers it was suggested that the hyaline amoebocytes were equivalent to the erythrocytes described by Yatsu (1902) in *L. unguis*. Comparison with *L. unguis* in the second paper showed this to be an error, and it is clear that erythrocytes do not occur in the two articulate species. The leucocytes described by Ohuye (Table II) for the three species of Brachiopoda are individually characterized by the number and type of granules in the cytoplasm. It is uncertain how they are related to each other, or whether they differ in both function and origin, although certain types seemed to be most frequent in the peritoneum of the lophophore. Both Yatsu (1902) and Ohuye (1937) gave detailed accounts of the curious spindle bodies and reviewed earlier theories and misconceptions of their structure, function and origin. However, neither author was able to account satisfactorily for them; Yatsu maintained that the spindle body was anucleate, whereas Ohuye claimed to have observed nuclei in some examples. In *L. unguis*, spindle bodies constituted the major element in the coelomic fluid of the pedicel, and Ohuye (1937) reported that their incidence increased in animals maintained in deteriorating environmental conditions. Yatsu (1902) observed stages in the formation of spindle bodies in the peritoneum of the brachial canals, and demonstrated convincingly that they were derived from erythrocytes. However, neither he nor Ohuye (1937) was prepared to infer a functional significance from this sequence, although it seems probable that spindle bodies represent the remnants of senescent blood cells.

Free cells have been described in the coelomic fluid of many species of bryozoans (e.g. Calvet, 1900; Borg, 1926) where they appear to fulfil a variety of functions; however, the nature of these cells is little understood. Borg (1926) considered some to be wandering mesenchymatous cells and others to be genuine coelomocytes. Vesicular amoebocytes and free phagocytes have been observed in active movement during budding, growth and tissue organization (Lutaud, 1961) and in the cyclic process of polypide degeneration (Gordon, 1977). Most types characterized appear to originate from the peritoneum of the main zooid coelom. Freshwater bryozoans which develop a large, colonial coelom, and those highly integrated marine species in which a common, coelomic space is an important functional adaptation, are potentially the most interesting as it might be expected that

TABLE II. Blood cells described in brachiopods and bryozoans.

Species	Cell type	Size (μm)	Description	Author
Lingula unguis (Brachiopoda)	blood corpuscle	10–20	colourless; spherical, biconcave or crescent-shaped. Nucleus compact. Cytoplasm homogeneous, with a small refractile spherule.	Yatsu, 1902
	erythrocyte		yellow or pink; spherical or biconcave. Nucleus round or irregular, compact. Cytoplasm homogeneous, with up to 3 granules	Ohuye, 1937
	leucocyte	13–20	spherical. Amoeboid, phagocytic. Frequently with enclosed spindle bodies	Yatsu, 1902
	eosinophilic granulocyte		amoeboid, phagocytic. Chtoplasm with uniform granules (0·6–2·0 μm diameter), often obscuring nucleus	Ohuye, 1937
	hyaline amoebocyte	5–12	colourless; amoeboid, phagocytic. Cytoplasm with several small vacuoles	Ohuye, 1937
	basophilic granulocyte	not given	similar to eosinophils, but with more granular cytoplasm	Ohuye, 1937
	spindle body	up to 100 × 30	elongate, fusiform. Thin cell membrane enclosing fibrillar contents orientated along long axis of spindle. Girdle of granules around middle of spindle. Form very variable. Enuclèate	Yatsu, 1902
			spherical, fusiform or moniliform. Nucleus sometimes visible, 4–6 μm diameter, oval, densely granular	Ohuye, 1937
Terebratalia coreanica (Brachiopoda)	hyaline amoebocyte	8–12	spherical, colourless. Nucleus small, compact. Phagocytic	Ohuye, 1936
	coarsely granular amoebocyte	12–20	cytoplasm with many granules, 2–4 μm diameter. Nucleus spherical, small, often obscured by granules	Ohuye, 1936
	finely granular amoebocyte	10–18	similar to above but with smaller granules (1–3 μm). More actively amoeboid	Ohuye, 1936
	amoebocyte with red granules	6–18	cytoplasm with 1–6 vermilion granules, 2–6 μm diameter. Rare in coelom but abundant in blood vessels	Ohuye, 1936
	amoebocyte with orange granules	10–18	distinguished by spherical orange granules. Distribution as for above	Ohuye, 1936
	amoebocyte with brown granules	8–16	with spherical brown granules. Rare in coelomic fluid, abundant in peritoneum	Ohuye, 1936
	spindle body		uncommon. Apparently identical to those of *Lingula unguis*	Ohuye, 1937

Coptothyris grayi (Brachiopoda)	hyaline amoebocyte coarsely granular amoebocyte finely granular amoebocyte amoebocyte with orange granules amoebocyte with brown granules		reported to be identical to those of *T. coreanica*	Ohuye, 1937
	amoebocyte with red granules		similar to those of *T. coreanica* but with up to 100 granules	Ohuye, 1937
	vesicular cell	6–15	with little cytoplasm; largely consisting of a single large vacuole, filled with a pale fluid	Ohuye, 1937
	spindle body		uncommon. Apparently identical to those of *Lingula unguis*	Ohuye, 1937
Lophopodella carteri (Bryozoa)	hyaline amoebocyte	50–110	round or irregular. Cytoplasm clear, forming inner endoplasm and outer ectoplasm, with several granules. Nucleus oval, lobed or u-shaped; strongly basophilic	Mano, 1964
	small leucocyte	15–20	spherical. Nucleus 5–7 μm diameter, large with little chromatin, or small, eccentric with compact chromatin	Mano, 1964
	lymphocyte (A)		nucleus occupying most of cell; fine diffuse chromatin, large nucleolus	
	(B)	7–15	nucleus large, eccentric, hemispherical; chromatin in compact granules	Mano, 1964
	(C)		characterized by refractile granules	
	granulocyte	7 × 7 – 15 × 40	irregular shape. Cytoplasm granular. Nucleus spherical, 3·5–4·5 μm	Mano, 1964
	phagocyte	50–100	irregular shape, displaying amoeboid movement. Cytoplasm containing vacuoles surrounding degenerating tissues etc. Nucleus eccentric; often polynuclear	Mano, 1964
	vacuolated cell	80–100	not amoeboid or phagocytic. Cytoplasm transparent, with numerous fluid-filled vacuoles. 1 or 2 oval nuclei, with diffuse chromatin	Mano, 1964
	spindle body	10–30	observed in phagocytes and vacuolated cells. Eosinophilic	Mano, 1964
	vibrating corpuscle	30–60	with filaments up to 20 μm long: moves actively by vibration of filaments	Mano, 1964
	neutral red body cell		not characterized. Corpuscles with large bodies staining with neutral red	Mano, 1964

in such species transport within the coelom is an important feature of physiological functions. Mano (1964) studied the coelomic corpuscles of the freshwater species, *Lophopodella carteri* and recognized nine distinct types (Table II) (Fig. 7), including examples of the curious spindle bodies described in brachiopods and phoronids by Yatsu (1902) and Ohuye (1937, 1942).

IV. Origin and formation of "blood" cells

Blood corpuscles are visible in the early phoronid larva as one or more red spots in the anterior end of the animal, situated close to the stomach (Hyman, 1959). These differentiate from masses of mesenchyme cells in the remnant of the blastocoel, which in the actinotroch larva constitutes the pre-septal cavity. At the same stage, the longitudinal blood vessels develop between the epithelium and peritoneum of the stomach, elongating anteriorly to communicate with the pre-septal space, and posteriorly developing to form the haemal plexus. At metamorphosis, part of the pre-septal space forms the ring vessels and tentacular capillaries; the enclosing blood cell masses break up and pass anteriorly into the longitudinal vessels (Hyman, 1959).

In the phoronids, blood cell formation occurs in the endothelial lining of blood vessels and in peritoneal tissue in many parts of the animal (Ohuye, 1942). No specific haemopoietic centre is known, although there is usually a high concentration of developing cells in the region of the haemal plexus, where the peritoneum is developed as a conspicuous mass enveloping the capillaries, and is referred to as vasoperitoneal tissue (Fig. 8). Ohuye (1942) described the formation of erythrocytes in the fine vessels of the tentacles. Flat endothelial cells were seen to swell, and project into the lumen of the blood vessel. The cells enlarged and rounded off, as the nuclei increased in size; the points of attachment narrowed to slender stalks, and eventually the cells broke free and continued development in the lumen of the blood vessel. These cells differentiated as either erythrocytes or granulocytes, although according to Ohuye (1942) the former predominated.

The cell layer lining the lumen of the tentacles is also regarded as a site of haemopoiesis. Ohuye (1942) observed cells in active proliferation; some appeared to differentiate as erythroblasts but the majority seemed to develop as "free histiocytes" and were assumed to migrate into the main coelom upon their release. The peritoneum lining the tentacles of *P. hippocrepia* shows active proliferation, with swollen and stalked cells protruding into the tentacle lumen (Figs 4, 5). Numerous liberated cells were also seen, but these appear to be identifiable as proerythroblasts, and granulocytes were not apparent.

The peritoneum is an important site of haemopoiesis in phoronids, particularly where it envelops the blood vessels of the trunk. This tissue seems to be the most important site for the production of granulocytes, although Ohuye (1942) reported the presence of erythroblasts as well. Peritoneal haemopoiesis is marked by a hypertrophy of the tissue; proliferating cells with enlarged, round nuclei may be seen bulging from the surface (Fig. 6). Subsequent differentiation may produce granulocytes, which migrate into the lumen of the blood vessel, or "free histiocytes" which are liberated into the coelom. Within the haemal plexus, the vasoperitoneal tissue may be greatly hypertrophied, forming diffuse masses around the capillaries (Fig. 8). This tissue is the source of sex cells and regresses seasonally as the gonads develop (Hyman, 1959). All types of blood cells were reported by Ohuye (1942) to occur in the vasoperitoneal tissue; erythroblasts and developing eosinophilic granulocytes were observed, but basophilic granulocytes were present only as mature cells. The vasoperi-

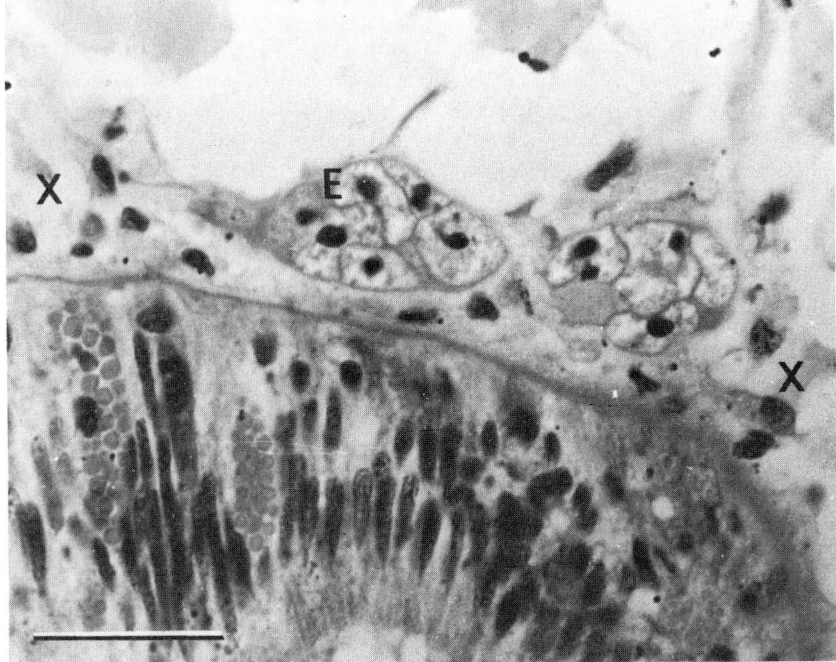

Fig 8. Vasoperitoneal tissue of *P. hippocrepia*; small blood sinuses packed with erythrocytes (E), surrounded by cells (X) which may represent the developing granulocytes of earlier authors. Scale = 20 μm.

toneal tissue is also a site of cell breakdown and many granulocytes were observed containing ingested and degenerated erythrocytes (Ohye, 1942).

In both brachiopods and bryozoans, haemopoiesis occurs in regions of the peritoneum, although there have been no precise studies in either case. Yatsu (1902), discussing the distribution of blood cells in the inarticulate brachiopod *L. unguis*, indicated that cell differentiation was concentrated in two special areas: a prominent ridge of peritoneum in the branches of the pallial sinus, and restricted regions of the peritoneum of the dorsal and ventral body walls. Mano (1964), studying the coelomocytes of the fresh-water bryozoan, *Lophopodella carteri*, cultured tissues from different parts of the zooid and was able to demonstrate that the stem cells of the different coelomocytes originated in the peritoneum of the zooid wall and the lophophore. By careful experimentation she was able to demonstrate that two different developmental series of leucocytes could be recognized. The inferred stem cell, of all types, was a "lymphoblast", derived from peritoneal cells of the body wall. These gave rise to three types of juvenile cells, "lymphocytes", each with an average diameter of 10 μm. Type A lymphocytes had very little cytoplasm and a very large nucleus, with a large nucleolus and fine granular chromatin. They differed only in the distribution of chromatin from cells in the zooid epithelium. Type B lymphocytes had slightly smaller, eccentric nuclei, with large chromatin granules, and Type C contained active refractile granules (Fig. 7). Mano (1964) suggested that Type B and Type C lymphocytes both matured from Type A; either Type A or Type B might then develop as small leucocytes (Fig. 7), but the Type C lymphocytes had a different fate. The small leucocytes, their diverse origins apparent from their nuclear morphology, were up to 20 μm in diameter and eventually matured as the hyaline amoebocytes which constituted up to 90% of the coelomocytes in each of the specimens studied. Type C lymphocytes appeared to mature as irregularly-shaped granulocytes, up to 40 μm long; these were rarely seen free in the coelom, occurring instead on the surfaces of tissues, and their origin may be distinct from those of the rest of the leucocyte series. Hyaline amoebocytes of the largest size, up to 80 μm diameter, became actively phagocytic, and both these and the granulocytes seemed eventually to form gerontic vacuolated cells, which constituted about 5% of the coelomic corpuscles.

V. Functions of "blood" cells

The functions of the various kinds of free cells described from different lophophorates have been largely a matter for speculation by the authors quoted above. Published research is limited to descriptive accounts of the morphology and origin of blood cells and there is an absence of both observational and experimental data on cell functions. An exception is the work of Ohuye (1942) who conducted a few simple experiments, injecting *Phoronis* spp. with suspensions of coloured dyes and observing phagocytosis of the particles by most of the cell types of the leucocyte series. Repeated injection appeared to stimulate the development of the larger granulocytes.

The erythrocytes of phoronids are perhaps the most obvious of the blood cell types in these worms, yet their respiratory physiology is completely unknown. Ohuye (1937) considered the blood pigment of the brachiopod, *Lingula unguis*, to be a type of haemoglobin, but Kawaguti (1941) later showed it to be a haemerythrin. Subsequently two haemerythrins were isolated in *L. unguis*, each distinguished by particular chemical and physical properties (Joshi and Sullivan, 1973). Distinct vascular and coelomic haemerythrins are known in certain other invertebrates (Joshi and Sullivan, 1973) but the significance and distribution of the two types in *L. unguis* are still not understood. Red pigment granules present in the cytoplasm of certain amoebocytes of the articulate brachiopod *Terebratalia* were tentatively identified by Ohuye (1936) as an echinochrome, and were considered to be similar to pigments thought to act as respiratory agents in echinoids (see Chapter 15). Finally, Mano (1964), observing mitochondria in the small leucocytes and hyaline amoebocytes of the bryozoan. *Lophopodella carteri*, suggested that these cells might contain oxidative enzymes of importance in respiration.

Among phoronids, potentially the most interesting aspect of blood cell functions is their role in regeneration. All species of *Phoronis* regularly autotomize the lophophore in response to deteriorating environmental conditions, or may lose them through regular grazing by predators (Emig, 1979). The worms are able to replace the lophophore swiftly, and detached lophophores of at least one species, *P. ovalis*, may themselves regenerate as complete worms (Silén, 1955). Following autotomy the wound is sealed by rapidly proliferating peritoneum, part of which differentiates to form the new body wall; the rest then forms a dense mass in the coelomic cavity, similar in appearance to the vasoperitoneal tissue, which constitutes a source of new blood cells (Ohuye, 1942). Silén (1955) observed that after autotomy and wound healing, the number of erythrocytes in the coelom of a regenerating lophophore increases rapidly.

Bryozoans have been shown to possess equally well-developed reparative powers (e.g. Lutaud, 1961) but the role of their coelomic corpuscles in regeneration is unclear. Cyclic regression and regeneration of the lophophore, gut and associated musculature (collectively the polypide) is a feature of most bryozoan life cycles and involves the breakdown and compaction of large areas of tissue to form dense residual "brown bodies". Brown body formation includes extensive phagocytosis of regressing tissues, and several authors (Matricon, 1960; Bobin and Prenant, 1972) have described free coelomic cells which they suggest might play a part in the process. However, Gordon (1977), in a comprehensive review of polypide regression, has shown that in several species large phagocytic cells form from the epidermis of the lophophore, and although coelomic cells might well act as phagocytes during polypide regression, it would be difficult to distinguish them from other cell types present in the degenerating tissues simply because they have yet to be adequately characterized. Gordon (1977) rejects the notion that polypide regression may be intimately associated with excretion, and thereby implies that phagocytosis observed during the process itself has no direct excretory function. Mano (1964) noted a regular loss of coelomic fluid through the coelomopore of *L. carteri*, occurring when coelomic pressure was increased by simultaneous contraction of all the polypides of a colony. Concentrations of coelomocytes appeared close to the coelomopore prior to the loss of fluid and she speculated that this might be a means of eliminating excretory products, and that gerontic vacuolated cells might be disposed of in this way. However, no evidence was offered in favour of this supposition.

VI. Concluding remarks

Lophophorates are, in general, poorly studied, and unsurprisingly there is a dearth of information on the ultrastructure and physiology of their blood cells. Both phoronids and bryozoans display remarkable regenerative powers; the importance of coelomic cells in the processes of repair and regeneration is known, but the functions of the different cell types are not understood and require further investigation. Among the Bryozoa, evolutionary trends towards highly integrated colonies involve increasing development of large, colonial coelomic spaces which must require common systems for nutrition, excretion and defence, processes in which coelomic corpuscles probably play vital, but as yet undetermined, roles. In all three Phyla the cell types present in vascular and coelomic fluids are still scarcely characterized (many enigmatic features described by earlier authors remain to be elucidated) and there is a need for additional research before the range of types, and their developmental relationships, can be fully and satisfactorily defined.

Acknowledgements

I am grateful to Dr N. A. Ratcliffe and Dr A. F. Rowley, Department of Zoology, University College of Swansea, for their advice and encouragement, and much practical assistance, during the preparation of this account.

References

Bobin, G. and Prenant, M. (1972). *Cah. Biol. mar.* **13**, 479–510.
Borg, F. (1926). *Zool. Bidr. Upps.* **10**, 181–507.
Calvet, L. (1900). *Trav. Inst. Zool. Univ. Montpellier* **8**, 1–488.
Chuang, S. H. (1964). *Proc. Zool. Soc. Lond.* **143**, 221–237.
Cook, P. L. (1975). *Docum. Lab. Géol. Fac. Sci. Lyon.* H.S.**3**, 161–168.
Cori, G. J. (1891). *Z. wiss. Zool.* **51**, 480–568.
Emig, C. C. (1979). "British and other Phoronids". Academic Press, London and New York.
Farmer, J. D. (1977). *In* "Biology of Bryozoans" (R. M. Woollacott and R. L. Zimmer, Eds), pp. 487–517. Academic Press, New York and London.
Gordon, D. P. (1977). *In* "Biology of Bryozoans" (R. M. Woollacott and R. L. Zimmer, Eds), pp. 335–376. Academic Press, New York and London.
Hyman, L. H. (1959). "The Invertebrates", Vol. 5. McGraw-Hill, New York.
Joshi, J. G. and Sullivan, B. (1973). *Comp. Biochem. Physiol.* **44B**, 857–867.
Kawaguti, S. (1941). *Mem. Fac. Sci. Taihoku imp. Univ.* **23** (Zool., 12), 95–98.
Lutaud, G. (1961). *Ann. Soc. roy. zool. Belg.* **91**, 157–300.
Mano, R. (1964). *Sci. Rep. Tokyo Kyoiku Daig. 11B*, **172**, 211–235.
Matricon, I. (1963). *Archs Zool. exp. gén.* 102, notes et rev. **2**, 79–93.
Ohuye, T. (1936). *Sci. Rep. Tôhoku Univ. ser. 4, Biol.* **11**, 231–238.
Ohuye, T. (1937). *Sci. Rep. Tôhoku Univ. ser. 4, Biol.* **12**, 241–253.
Ohuye, T. (1942). *Sci. Rep. Tôhoku Univ. ser. 4, Biol.* **17**, 167–185.
Silen, L. (1955). *Acta Zool.* **36**, 159–165.
Storch, V. and Herrmann, K. (1978). *Cell. Tiss. Res.* **190**, 553–556.
Yatsu, N. (1902). *J. Coll. Sci. imp. Univ. Tokyo* **17**, 1–29.

Section VII

The Echinoderms

15. The echinoderms

V. J. SMITH

University Marine Biological Station, Millport, Isle of Cumbrae, Scotland

---

CONTENTS

I. Introduction

The echinoderms are deuterostome invertebrates that are exclusively marine and amongst the most abundant of all benthic animals. They have a number of characteristic features including, possession of a spiny skin, pedicellariae, a complex tubular hydrocoel, and the secondary adoption of pentamerous symmetry. The existing phylum is usually divided into five main classes, namely, the crinoids (feather stars); asteroids (star fishes); ophiuroids (brittle stars); echinoids (sea urchins) and holothurians (sea cucumbers). The crinoids are usually regarded as the most primitive and the echinoids and holothurians as the most advanced.

The echinoderms have been the subject of considerable scientific interest, and their fascination may be partly attributed to two factors. First, they exhibit many unique and highly specialized features, such as the water vascular system and tube feet, and secondly, they occupy a phylogenetically strategic position in the animal kingdom, near the chordates. This supposed evolutionary link with the chordates has tempted many workers to look to the echinoderms for the origin of vertebrate characteristics (Jefferies, 1967; Carton, 1974; Bang, 1975). The validity of such generalizations, however, is questionable since the Echinodermata is an ancient phylum which probably evolved in the early Paleozoic, so that present day representatives are not closely related to any other group.

Although many studies of echinoderm biology have been concerned with understanding the structure and functions of the coelomic systems, many aspects are still poorly understood and there is some confusion regarding the structure and functions of the cellular components of the coelomic fluids. Previous reviews of the coelomic systems and coelomocytes have been made by Geddes (1880), Cuénot (1887), Kindred (1921, 1924, 1926), Hyman (1955), Boolootian and Giese (1958, 1959), Boolootian (1962), Burton (1964, 1966), Hetzel (1963, 1965), Andrew (1962, 1965), Endean (1958, 1966), Stang-Voss (1971, 1974) and Ratcliffe and Rowley (1979). The present review attempts to integrate the early descriptions of the coelomocytes, with the more recent ultrastructural analyses, to unify the classification and nomenclature of the cell types and to clarify their various roles and functions.

II. Structure of the circulatory systems

Echinoderms lack a distinct directional circulation of "blood". The coelom, however, is well-developed and has become structurally and physiologically specialized to carry out some of the functions of a vascular and haemocoelic system (Fig. 1, Table I). Embryologically, the coelom arises as enterocoelic

TABLE I. Summary of circulatory systems of echinoderms.

	Crinoidea	Asteroidea	Ophiuroidea	Echinoidea	Holothuroidea
Perivisceral coelom	reduced to a series of intercommunicating spaces in the body and to five coeliac canals in the arms and stalk	reduced, but occurs as a single cavity which extends into the arms	reduced to a single cavity in disc and to aboral side of arms	large, well-developed, divided by mesenteries into five distinct cavities	large, well-developed, divided by mesenteries into four distinct cavities
Water vascular system	composed of oral water ring and five radial canals which connect to tube feet. Ampullae absent. Madreporite absent and oral ring connects with perivisceral cavity through numerous ciliated pores. Polian vesicles absent. Spongy bodies similar to Tiedemann's bodies may be present	composed of oral ring with stone canal leading through madreporite to exterior. Five radial canals connect tube feet and ampullae. Polian vesicles and Tiedemann's bodies present	composed of oral ring with stone canal leading through madreporite (which has a single pore). Five radial canals connect with tube feet. Ampullae absent. Four Polian vesicles present and Tiedemann's bodies absent	composed of oral ring with stone canal leading through madreporite to exterior. Five radial canals which connect with tube feet and ampullae, pass upward aborally. Polian vesicles and Tiedemann's bodies absent but replaced by spongy bodies	composed of circum-pharyngeal ring with short stone canal and internal madreporite. Five radial canals, which connect tube feet and ampullae pass backwards inside body. Variable number of Polian vesicles, and Tiedemann's bodies absent
Haemal system	reduced, lacunar, composed of oral rings with five radial strands to arms. Axial organ and spongy body present, connected to alimentary canal	reduced, lacunar, composed of oral and aboral rings joined together by axial organ, connected to alimentary canal. Five radial strands to each arm	reduced, lacunar, composed of oral and aboral rings joined together by axial organ, connected to the alimentary canal. Five radial strands extend to each arm	reduced, composed of oral and aboral rings joined by axial organ, branches to alimentary canal and gonad. Five radial strands extend upwards aborally	well-developed, composed of gut plexus, oral ring and five radial canals
Perihaemal system	composed of oral ring and axial sinus. Radial canals extend to arms	surrounds haemal system. The axial sinus encircles axial organ and stone canal and opens into it below madreporite	surrounds haemal system. Axial sinus divided by axial organ and stone canal into axial sinus proper and dorsal sac	composed of oral and aboral rings. Axial sinus absent. Radial canals do not connect with oral ring	perihaemal system absent

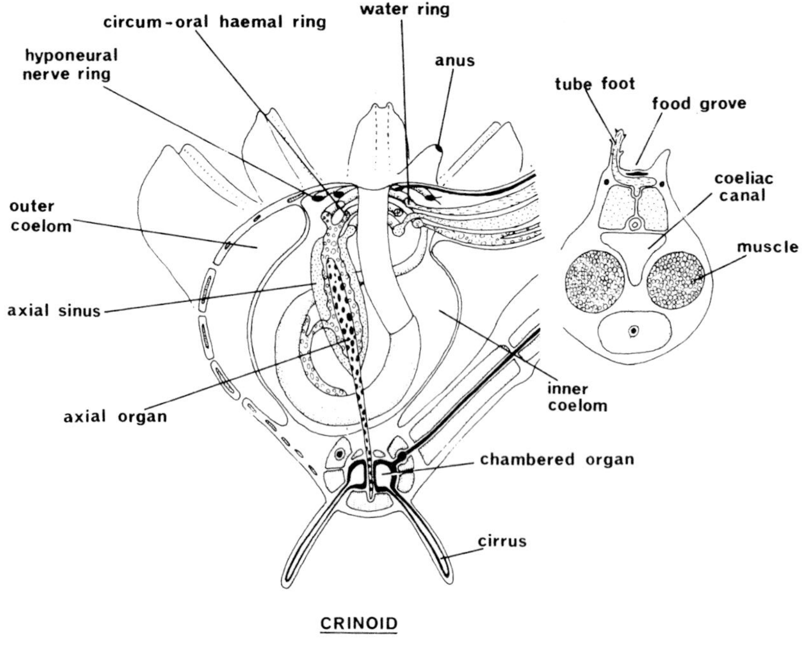

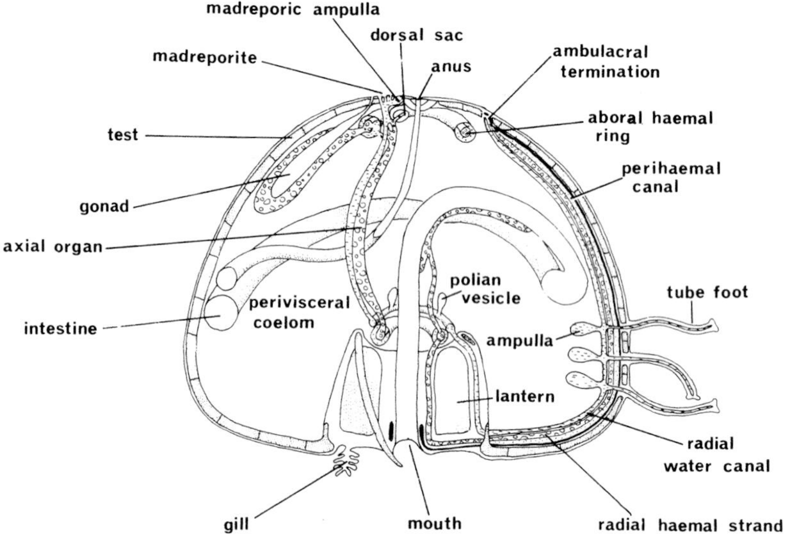

ECHINOID

KEY to systems

- water vascular
- haemal
- perihaemal
- skeletal
- nervous

Fig. 1. The "circulatory" systems and body plans of the five echinoderm classes. Redrawn from Nichols (1969).

peribuccal coelom
perivisceral coelom
'oral' perihaemal ring
water ring
stomach
bursa
gonad
madreporite
mouth
'aboral' haemal ring
radial nerve
tube-foot

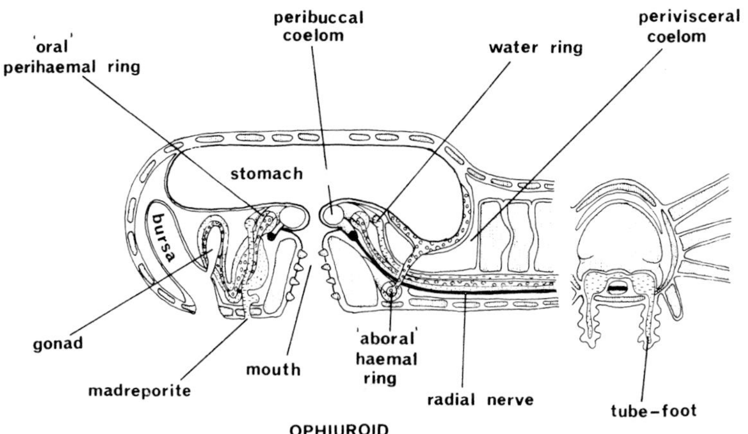

OPHIUROID

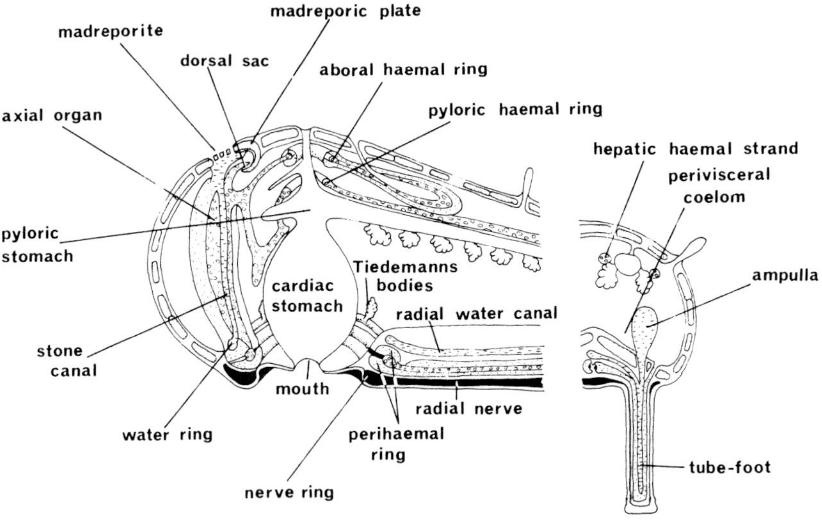

madreporic plate
madreporite
dorsal sac
aboral haemal ring
axial organ
pyloric haemal ring
hepatic haemal strand
perivisceral coelom
pyloric stomach
Tiedemanns bodies
cardiac stomach
ampulla
radial water canal
stone canal
mouth
radial nerve
water ring
perihaemal ring
tube-foot
nerve ring

ASTEROID

madreporic body
gonad
buccal tube-foot
perivisceral coelom
haemal plexus
anus
tube foot
respiratory tree
polian vesicle
buccal ampulla

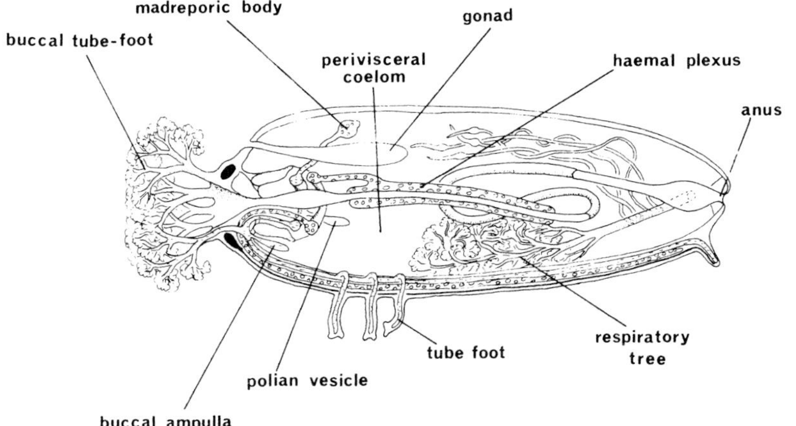

HOLOTHURIAN

pouches from the gut, a form of development that distinguishes the echinoderms from those animals in which the coelom forms by a split in the mesoderm to produce a schizocoel, and as such gives them greater affinity with the sipunculids, phoronids, brachiopods and hemichordates, etc. than with the annelids, molluscs and arthropods (see Chapter 1).

In the adult, the coelom is unusual in being divided into two distinct portions:

(i) the perivisceral coelom, which is the cavity surrounding the gut and other organs;
(ii) a tubular component, which includes the water vascular system, the haemal system and the perihaemal system.

The latter, because of its close proximity to the major nerves of the body is sometimes referred to as the hyponeural sinus. There is, in addition, a gonadial coelom, but for the purposes of this review this will not be considered within the concept of the circulatory systems.

The three tubular systems (ii, above) of echinoderms are isolated, highly complex, specialized sub-divisions of the coelom and their arrangement varies between the different classes. Their structure has been described by many authors, including Nichols (1969) and Millott (1967), so that the present review is limited to a brief general description with the main differences between each class summarized in Table I.

A. Perivisceral coelom

The perivisceral coelom takes the form of fluid-filled spaces around the main body organs. It is usually lined with ciliated endothelium which covers the gut and maintains circulation of the coelomic fluid. There is little doubt that the perivisceral coelom is involved in internal transport of dissolved nutrients, gases and waste materials, and serves to convey the coelomocytes to various parts of the body.

B. Tubular coelomic systems

1. Water vascular system

The water vascular system supplies sufficient hydrostatic pressure to the hydraulic organs, the tube feet, for their effective participation in locomotion, feeding and burrowing. The system generally opens to the exterior via a calcified pore, the madreporite, which serves as a pressure compensator. Extending from the madreporite, along the axis of the body to the circum-oral ring (Fig. 1), is a calcified vessel, the stone canal, which may be associated with the axial organ. Five radial canals arise at intervals from the circum-oral ring and pass, one into each arm (Fig. 1). These canals, in turn, branch alternately and form numerous lateral canals which feed each tube foot and its accompanying ampulla (Fig. 1). Also associated with the circum-oral ring may be a variable number of bulbous protrusions, the Polian vesicles, and, in asteroids, spongy structures known as Tiedemann's bodies whose function is not fully understood.

2. *Haemal system*

The haemal system is composed of interconnecting lacunae in the spongy connective tissues, which send elements to all parts of the body. It comprises a number of ring elements, the oral, aboral, gastric and pyloric rings, joined together by a vessel running parallel to the stone canal (Fig. 1). This vessel is often in close association with a structure known as the axial organ and may communicate directly with the madreporite via the dorsal sac. Vessels, termed radial haemal strands, also extend from the oral haemal ring into each arm alongside the radial canals of the water vascular system (Fig. 1). The haemal system appears to function for the long term slow translocation of elaborated molecules (Farmanfarmaian, 1968) and not simply for the transportation of dissolved gasses.

3. *Perihaemal system*

The perihaemal system generally surrounds and mimicks the vessels (or lacunae) of the haemal system (Fig. 1). An axial sinus encircles the axial organ and stone canal, and often connects with them below the madreporite (Fig. 1). In holothurians, a perihaemal system is almost totally absent, but, in these animals, the haemal system is more highly developed. The precise function of the perihaemal system is unknown but it probably assists with internal transport.

Table I summarizes the main features of the circulatory systems of the five echinoderm classes.

III. Coelomic fluid and "circulation"

The perivisceral cavity and the tubular systems of the coelom are filled with a watery fluid, the coelomic fluid. By virtue of its embryological origin, the coelomic fluid cannot strictly be regarded as equivalent to the blood of vertebrates or even to the haemolymph of arthropods. However, in the absence of any other circulatory system the coelomic fluid of echinoderms has taken over many vascular activities.

It is generally accepted that the coelomic fluid can move freely between all the coelomic systems either directly through interconnecting junctions at the axial organ (Boolootian and Campbell, 1964), madreporite etc., or, indirectly, through the tissues and across the coelomic epithelium. A few authors, notably Cuénot (1901), believe that the perivisceral coelom, water vascular system, haemal and perihaemal systems are quite separate. Vanden Bossche and Jangoux (1976) have recently provided some experimental evidence, in support of this hypothesis.

There has been some controversy over the existence of a heart in the echinoderms and the axial organ has frequently been ascribed this role (Tiedemann, 1816; Boolootian and Campbell, 1964). More recent studies, however, have refuted this notion (Millott and Vevers, 1964; Farmanfarmaian, 1968), and the "circulation" (or more accurately, oscillating movements) of the coelomic fluid is now believed to be achieved by movements of the body together with contractions of some of the internal structures and beating of the endothelial cilia (Farmanfarmaian, 1966, 1968).

The composition of the coelomic fluid resembles that of seawater except that it has a higher concentration of potassium ions and contains small amounts of dissolved lipid, protein, non-protein nitrogen and reducing sugars (Endean, 1966). More importantly, it also possesses large populations of circulating cells, the coelomocytes.

IV. Structure and classification of coelomocytes

Of all aspects of echinoderm biology, perhaps the one most in need of clarification and reappraisal is that of the structure and classification of the coelomocytes. Although numerous studies have been made, an understanding of the cell types for the phylum as a whole is complicated by the unwieldy number of names used by some workers often to describe the same or similar cells in different species or classes. For example, Boolootian and Giese (1958) identified thirteen distinct cell types in fifteen species of echinoderms while Endean (1966) lists eighteen well characterized cell populations in five classes. There is also considerable disagreement between authors over the diagnostic features of each cell type, frequently because insufficient attention has been paid to variations induced through the experimental conditions or the method of observation. Furthermore, most attention has been paid to the echinoids and holothurians, while the crinoids, ophiuroids and asteroids are relatively neglected. In addition, apart from the recent investigations of Fabre *et al.* (1969), Johnson *et al.* (1970), Chien *et al.* (1970), Stang-Voss (1971), Vethamany and Fung (1972), Fontaine and Lambert (1973, 1977) and Edds (1980), very few ultra-structural analyses have been carried out, so that general trends for the phylum as a whole are difficult to assess. However, for the present review, some new light and electron microscopy observations have been made on the coelomocytes of the crinoid, *Antedon bifida*, the asteroid, *Asterias rubens*, the ophiuroid, *Ophicomina nigra*, the echinoid, *Echinus esculentus* and the holothurian, *Cucumaria normani* (*Aslia lefevrei*).

From these and previous studies, the coelomocytes appear to fall into six main categories (Tables II, III), the phagocytic amoebocytes, the spherule cells, the vibratile cells, the haemocytes, the crystal cells and the progenitor cells. Some authors have subdivided the spherule cells on the basis of their inclusions into coloured or colourless forms (Tables II, III) but these probably represent different developmental states of the same cell line and, in the present review, are described together.

Regarding the relative proportions of each cell types, few values have been quoted by the various investigators. Preliminary observations of the coelomic fluids of the five species examined for the present review, however, reveal that the coelomocyte profiles can vary dramatically not only between species but also between individuals of the same species according to their size, and physiological condition. Similar variations in proportions of the different coelomocyte types have also been noted by Bang and Lemma (1962) in animals collected from different geographical locations. Wherever possible, however, some indication of the abundance of the various coelomocyte types has been given.

A. Phagocytic amoebocytes

The phagocytic amoebocytes (Figs 2–8) are the most common of all the echinoderm coelomocytes and have been found in every species studied. They have been given a variety of names by different authors (Table II).

The cells are large (*ca.* 14·0–30·0 μm in diameter), variable in shape with a round, ovoid or central nucleus (Fig. 2) (Bookhout and Greenburg, 1940; Hetzel, 1963; Vethamany and Fung, 1972; Fontaine and Lambert, 1977; Bertheussen and Seljelid, 1978) (Table III). The cytoplasm contains some yellow or brown granules (Figs 3, 4) and under the electron microscope, a number of membrane-bound electron-dense bodies, mitochondria, multi-vesicular bodies (possibly lysosomes), vacuoles, vesicles, a well-developed Golgi and some rough and smooth endoplasmic reticulum may also be observed (Figs 5, 6) (Chien *et al.*, 1970; Vethamany and Fung, 1972; Fontaine and Lambert, 1977) (Table III).

TABLE II. Summary of cell types and their synonyms in various echinoderm classes.

Reference/species studied	Phagocytic amoebocytes	Spherule cells Colourless	Spherule cells Coloured	Vibratile cells	Haemocytes	Crystal cells	Progenitor cells	Other
Kindred (1924) review	leucocytes	spherule cells	spherule cells	vibratile cells				
Boolootian and Giese (1958) review								
Crinoids	small spherical corpuscles		red corpuscles					fusiform cells large spherical corpuscles
Asteroids	bladder/filiform amoebocytes	morula cells					small spherical corpuscles	
Ophiuroids	amoebocytes	morula cells					small spherical corpuscles	fusiform cells
Echinoids	bladder/filiform amoebocytes	colourless amoebocytes	eleocytes	vibratile cells			hyaline haemocytes	
Holothurians	bladder/filiform amoebocytes	colourless spherical amoebocytes		vibratile cells	haemocytes	crystal cells		
Endean (1966) review								
Crinoids	amoeboid cells	morula cells	morula cells					fusiform cells cells with rods and granules
Asteroids	phagocytes						small pigment cells	reniform cells, leucocytes, osmiphil cells, hyaline cells
Ophiuroids	phagocytes	morula cells		vibratile cells	haemoglobin-containing cells			
Echinoids	amoebocytes	spherule cells	eleocytes				small spherical cells	red cells, ex-plosive cells
Holothurians	phagocytes	morula cells	morula cells	vibratile cells	haemocytes	crystal cells	lymphocytes	fusiform cells

Andrew (1962) review Ophiuroids	leucocytes	spherule cells			haemocytes	crystal cells		revolving cysts
Holothurians	petaloid leucocytes	spherule cells			haemocytes	crystal cells		
Fabre et al. (1969) Echinoid and Holothurian review	grandes coelomocytes	granulocytes and amoebocytes du réserve			hyaline coelomocytes		coelomocytes miniscules	fusiform cells, reniform cells (echinoids)
Ratcliffe and Rowley (1979) review	phagocytic amoebocytes	spherule cells	spherule cells	vibratile cells	haemocytes	crystal cells	progenitor cells	
Johnson and Beeson (1966) *Patiria miniata*	phagocytic/ filiform amoebocytes			flagellated/ golden cells		crystal cells		revolving cysts
Bookhout and Greenburg (1940) *Mellita quinquiperforatus*	amoebocytes/ leucocytes	spherule amoebocytes	spherule amoebocytes					
Liebman (1950) *Arbacia puntulata*	phagocytes	trephocytes	nephrocytes					
Holland et al. (1965) *Strongylocentrotus purpuratus*	bladder/ filiform amoebocytes	spherule amoebocytes	eleocytes	vibratile cells				
Johnson (1969a) *Strongylocentrotus purpuratus* and *Chien et al. (1970)* *S. franciscanus*	phagocytic leucocytes	colourless spherule cells	red spherule cells	vibratile cells				
Stang-Voss (1974) *Psammechinus miliaris*	amoeboid phagocytes	colourless spherule amoebocytes	eleocytes				coelomic endothelial cells	

TABLE II—*cont.*

Reference/species studied	Phagocytic amoebocytes	Spherule cells Colourless	Spherule cells Coloured	Vibratile cells	Haemocytes	Crystal cells	Progenitor cells	Other
Vethamany and Fung (1972)								
Strongylocentrotus droebachiensis	phagocytic leucocytes	spherule cells	red spherule cells	vibratile cells			small spherical cells	granulocytes
Bertheussen and Seljelid (1978)								
Strongylocentrotus droebachiensis	phagocytes	white morula cells	red morula cells	vibratile cells				
Hetzel (1963)								
Holothurian review	bladder/filiform amoebocytes	colourless morula cells		vibratile cells	haemocytes	crystal cells	lymphocytes, small spherical cells	minute corpuscles
Hetzel (1965)								
Holothuria leucospilota	phagocytes	morula cells	morula cells		haemocytes	crystal cells	homogeneous amoebocytes	spindle cells
Fontaine and Lambert (1973, 1977)								
Cucumaria miniata	bladder/filiform/ transitional amoebocytes	morula cells	morula cells	vibratile cells	haemocytes	crystal cells	lymphocytes	

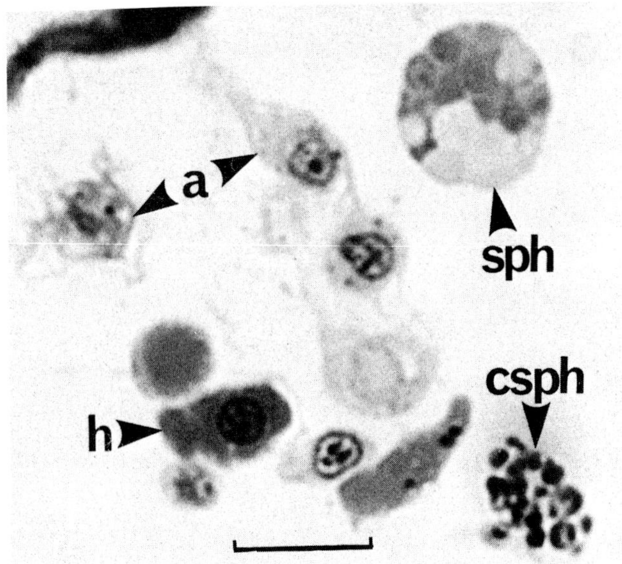

Fig. 2. Thick plastic section of coelomocytes from *Cucumaria normani* showing phagocytic amoebocytes (a), a haemocyte (h), colourless spherule cell (sph) and coloured spherule cell (csph). Scale bar = 10 μm.

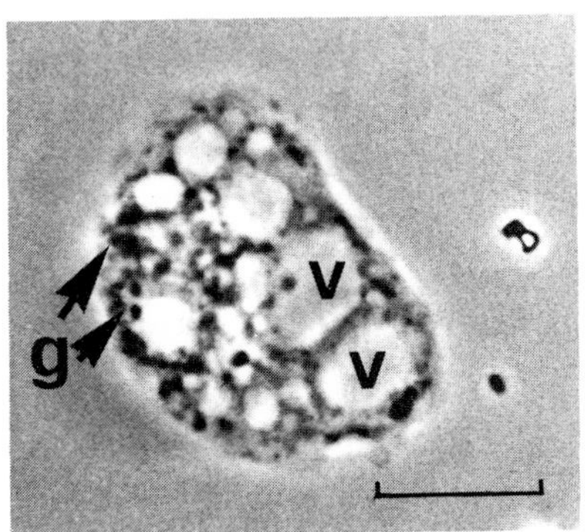

Fig. 3. Phase contrast micrograph of a petaloid-type amoebocyte of *Asterias rubens*, with prominent bladder like vacuoles (v) and phase-dark granules (g). Scale bar = 10 μm.

TABLE III. Summary of main features of echinoderm coelomocytes.

Cell type	Size	Shape	Nucleus	Cytoplasmic inclusions
Phagocytic amoebocytes	large *ca*. 20 μm in diameter	variable, either petaloid, filopodial or transitional	small, round or ovoid, central, encloses some condensed chromatin	yellow or brown inclusions. Some electron-dense bodies, mitochondria, lysosomes (?). Golgi complex, RER and SER
Spherule cells	variable *ca*. 15 μm in diameter	usually round, sometimes ovoid	small, irregular, eccentric, with a variable amount of condensed chromatin	numerous large mucopolysaccharide-containing spherules, either red, green, yellow or colourless. Some mitochondria, RER and a Golgi
Vibratile cells	small *ca*. 7 μm in diameter	usually spherical	large, spherical, central, with some condensed chromatin	variable, some small coloured granules. Mitochondria, Golgi, RER, flagellar basal body, some microfilaments
Haemocytes	variable *ca*. 15 μm in diameter	variable, often spherical or biconvex	small, round or ovoid, variable in position, with some condensed hetero-chromatin	infrequent, Golgi complex, mitochondria, ribosomes, lysosomes (?), microtubules, SER, vacuoles
Crystal cells	variable, usually small *ca*. 5 μm in diameter	rhomboidal or round	small, sometimes absent	1–3 rhomboidal or star-shaped crystals, other organelles infrequent
Progenitor cells	small, *ca*. 7 μm in diameter	spherical	large, spherical, central, with some peripheral chromatin	infrequent, some RER, mitochondria, a Golgi and a few granules

Behaviour *in vitro*	Total coelomocyte count (%)	Special features	Origin	Key references
stable, usually spread and attach to glass surfaces, actively motile by amoeboid movement	*ca.* 50% in asteroids and echinoids. *ca.* 10% in holothurians	can rapidly transform from one morphological phase to another, each phase exhibits functional characteristics	from progenitor cells	Kindred (1924), Bookhout and Greenburg (1940), Endean (1958), Hetzel (1963), Johnson (1969a), Chien *et al.* (1970), Stang-Voss (1971), Vethamany and Fung (1972), Fontaine and Lambert (1977), Edds (1980).
fairly stable, exhibit some motility by amoeboid movement. Sometimes despherulate	abundant 50–70% in echinoids and holothurians	napthaquinone pigments (= echinochrome) present in red spherule cells	possibly from phagocytic amoebocytes or progenitor cells	as above and Kindred (1926), Cowden (1968).
semi-stable, actively motile by flagellar movement. May release mucoid substances in blood clots. Non-adherent	variable, often very abundant in echinoids	possess one or two long flagella	not known	Kindred (1924), Hetzel (1963), Johnson and Beeson (1966), Johnson (1969a), Chien *et al.* (1970), Vethamany and Fung (1972), Stang-Voss (1974), Fontaine and Lambert (1977).
stable, non-motile and non-adherent	abundant	contain haemoblogin-like pigments homogeneously distributed in cytoplasm	probably from progenitor cells or amoebocytes	Foettinger (1880), Kindred (1924), Kawamoto (1927), Endean (1958), Hetzel (1963), Stang-Voss (1974), Fontaine and Lambert (1973).
unstable, crystal dissolves, cytoplasm breaksdown. Non-adherent	infrequent, *ca.* 5% in most species	nature and function of crystals unknown	not known	Théel (1921), Kawamoto (1927), Hetzel (1963), Johnson and Beeson (1966), Fontaine and Lambert (1977).
stable, non-motile, and non-adherent	variable, may be very frequent		from leucopoietic stem cells in various tissues or organs	Kindred (1924), Kawamoto (1927), Endean (1958), Hetzel (1963), Doyle and McNeil (1964), Fabre *et al.* (1969), Fontaine and Lambert (1977).

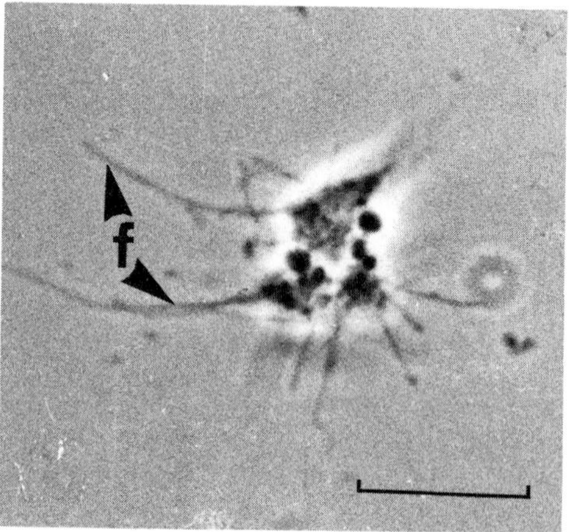

Fig. 4. Phase contrast micrograph of a filopodial-form amoebocyte of *Ophicomina nigra* showing the numerous filopodial extensions (f). Scale bar = 10 μm.

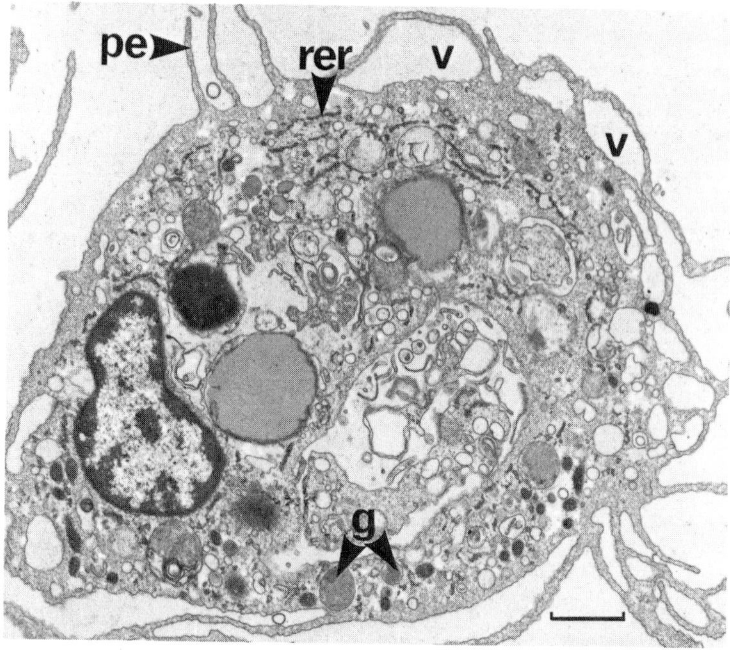

Fig. 5. Electron micrograph of a petaloid phagocytic amoebocyte from *Cucumaria normani*. Note the cytoplasmic granules (g), rough endoplasmic reticulum (rer) and fine pseudopodia (pe) surrounding bladder-like vacuoles (v). Scale bar = 1 μm.

Characteristically, the cells exhibit two morphologically distinct phases, the petaloid form, in which the cytoplasm is extruded into a number of bladder-like flaps (Figs 3, 5, 7) and the filopodial stage, where the cytoplasm is extended into long fine filiform pseudopodia (Figs 4, 8). Transformation, from the petaloid to the filopodial state occurs rapidly *in vitro*, after wounding or osmotic shock (Chien *et al.*, 1970; Fontaine and Lambert, 1977; Edds, 1977a,b; Otto *et al.*, 1979) and is preceded by collapse of the cytoplasmic bladders. During this change microtubular filamentous rods of actin are formed at the cell periphery (Edds, 1977a,b, 1979, 1980; Otto *et al.*, 1979), and Otto *et al.* (1979) and DeRosier and Edds (unpublished) have recently shown that the formation of these rods is controlled by fascin, an actin cross-linking protein.

In vivo, the majority of the cells adopt either the petaloid or an intermediate (transitional) form, but the exact proportion varies from species to species. For example, in the urchin, *Strongylocentrotus droebachiensis*, *ca.* 20% of the amoebocytes are petaloid, and the rest are intermediate (Bertheussen and Seljelid, 1978), while in the sea cucumber, *Cucumaria miniata*, *ca.* 35% are petaloid, *ca.* 7% filopodial and the rest are transitional (Fontaine and Lambert, 1977). The transitional cells probably

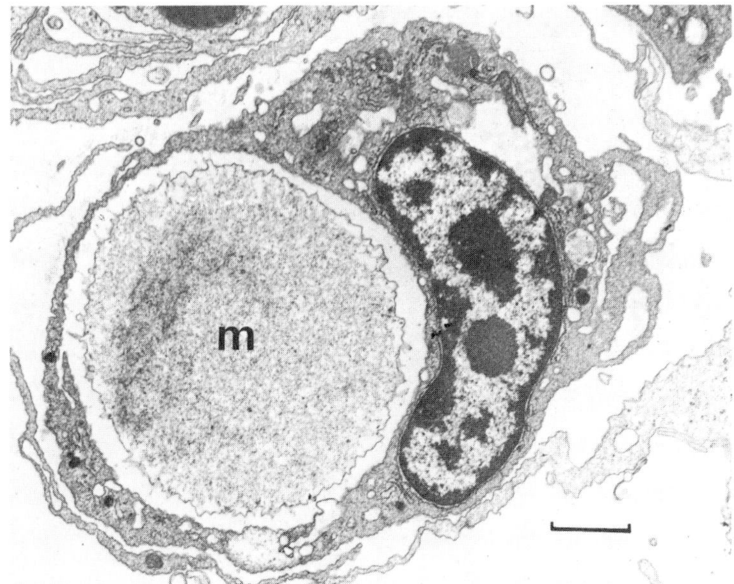

Fig. 6. Electron micrograph of a petaloid phagocytic amoebocyte of *Cucumaria normani* containing ingested material (m) of unknown origin. Scale bar = 1 μm.

represent a reservoir of undifferentiated cells capable of rapid conversion after appropriate stimulation (Fontaine and Lambert, 1977; Edds, 1977a,b).

The two phases of the amoebocytes exhibit different functional properties (Table IV). The petaloid form, which is capable of strong amoeboid movement, being actively phagocytic (see section on phagocytosis) (Fig. 6), while the filopodial stage appears to be important in cell clotting (Fig. 8) (see section on clotting). The biphasic nature of the amoebocytes is shown by all groups except the crinoids, the coelomocytes of which rarely produce extensive pseudopodia (Cuénot, 1891; Andrew, 1962; Endean, 1966). Crinoid amoebocytes, however, are capable of limited locomotion and are clearly phagocytic (Cuénot, 1891; Endean, 1966).

In *in vitro*, hanging drop cultures, the phagocytic amoebocytes are very stable with the majority being either petaloid or transitional (Johnson,

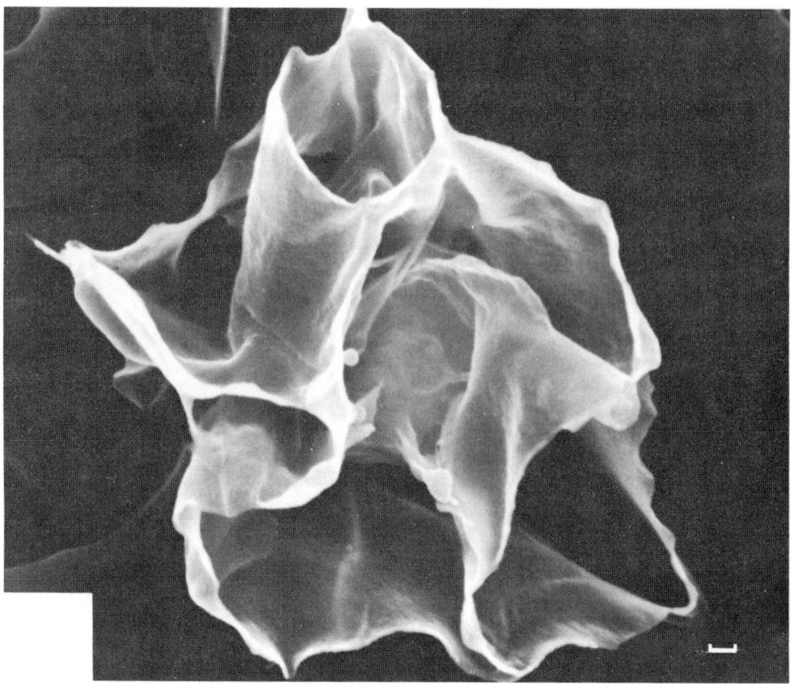

Fig. 7. Scanning electron micrograph of a petaloid-form amoebocyte from *Strongylocentrotus droebachiensis*. [From Edds (1980).] Scale bar = 1 μm.

1969a). On contact with glass coverslips, however, many of the cells rapidly settle and spread out, often up to 60 μm in diameter, to form confluent monolayers (Bertheussen and Seljelid, 1978). This spreading behaviour is inhibited by anticoagulants, particularly caffeine, and is probably an encapsulation-type response (Bertheussen and Seljelid, 1978).

In asteroids and echinoids, the phagocytic amoebocytes are the most numerous of all the coelomic cells (Endean, 1966; Johnson, 1969a; Vethamany and Fung, 1972), and in *Arbacia puntulata* comprise *ca*. 50% of the total coelomocyte population (Liebman, 1950). They are less abundant in holothurians, where they are usually outnumbered by the haemocytes (Fontaine and Lambert, 1977). In *Holothuria leucospilota*, only 10% of the circulating cells are phagocytic amoebocytes with a further 10% represented by fusiform cells (Endean, 1958) (see section on progenitor cells).

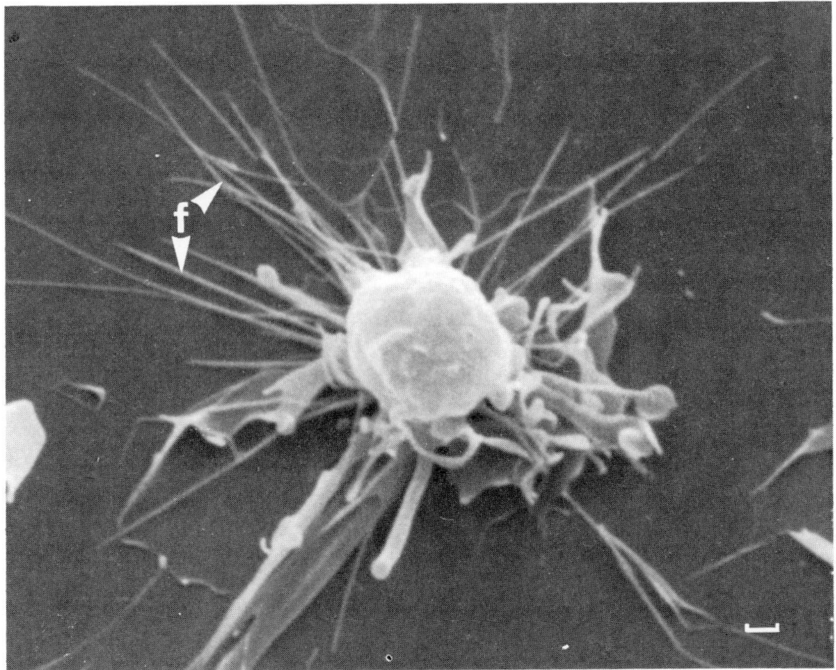

Fig. 8. Scanning electron micrograph of a filopodial-form of the petaloid amoebocyte from *S. droebachiensis* which arises from a morphological transformation of the latter under the influence of hypotonic shock or just settling onto a glass slide. Note the numerous filopodia (f). [From Edds (1980).] Scale bar = 1 μm.

TABLE IV. Summary of functions of echinoderm coelomocytes.

Cell type	Function	Key references	Comments
Phagocytic amoebocytes	phagocytosis	Durham (1887), Cuénot (1891), Kindred (1921), Ohuye (1934), Bookhout and Greenburg (1940), Hetzel (1965), Johnson and Beeson (1966), Hilgard *et al.* (1967), Hilgard and Phillips (1968), Johnson (1969c)	chiefly by petaloid form. Few *in vitro* studies
	cell clumping/ encapsulation	Davidson (1953), Bang and Lemma (1962), Ghiradella (1965), Johnson and Beeson (1966), Johnson (1969c), Reinisch and Bang (1971)	possibly also brown body formation
	clotting/coagulation	Kindred (1921), Donnellon (1938), Bookhout and Greenburg (1940), Boolootian and Giese (1959), Noble (1970), Vethamany and Fung (1972)	chiefly by filopodial form. Three distinct types of clot observed
	wound repair	Rollefsen (1965), Menton and Eisen (1973), Heatfield and Travis (1975a)	probably acts in phagocytic capacity
	graft rejection	Hildemann and Dix (1972), Coffano and Hinegardner (1977), Bertheussen (1979)	phagocytic or cytotoxic
	transport	Cuénot (1891), Kindred (1921)	variety of materials in phagocytic vacuoles—probably unlikely

Spherule cells	cell clumping/ encapsulation	Ghiradella (1965), Johnson and Beeson (1966), Johnson (1969c), Reinisch and Bang (1971)	function not known but, probably acts in bactericidal capacity
	wound repair	Rollefsen (1965), Menton and Eisen (1973), Heatfield and Travis (1975b)	
	graft rejection	Coffano and Hinegardner (1977)	
	bactericidal activity	Vevers (1963), Johnson and Chapman (1970), Wardlaw and Unkles (1978), Messer and Wardlaw (1980)	possibly due to presence of echinochrome in red spherule cells
	storage/transport	MacMunn (1885), Cuénot (1891), Liebman (1950), Boolootian and Lasker (1964)	probably transport of elaborated materials and not oxygen
	synthesis-pigment	MacMunn (1885), Millott (1950, 1953), Jacobson and Millott (1953)	chiefly red spherule cells
	collagen	Endean (1958, 1966), Hetzel (1963), Menton and Eisen (1973)	chiefly colourless cells
Vibratile cells	clotting	Johnson (1969a,b,c), Chien *et al.* (1970), Vethamany and Fung (1972), Bertheussen and Seljelid (1978)	probably by release of acid mucopolysaccharides
	immobilization of invading microbes	Johnson (1969a,b,c)	
Haemocytes	transport of dissolved oxygen	Van der Heyde (1927), Hiestand (1940), Crescitelli (1945), Manwell (1959), Hetzel (1963, 1965), Fontaine and Lambert (1973)	contains haemoglobin-like pigment
Crystal cells	ossicle formation	Hetzel (1963)	inconclusive evidence
Progenitor cells	leucopoiesis/stem cells	Kollmann (1908), Kindred (1926), Ohuye (1934), Endean (1958), Hetzel (1965), Brillouet *et al.* (1981)	

B. Spherule cells

The spherule cells (Figs 2, 9–12) occur in crinoids (Cuénot, 1891; Boolootian and Giese, 1958), ophiuroids (Kindred, 1924; Boolootian and Giese, 1958; Andrew, 1962), echinoids (Kindred, 1924; Behre, 1932; Bookhout and Greenburg, 1940; Boolootian and Giese, 1958; Andrew, 1962; Holland *et al.*, 1965; Johnson, 1969a; Chien *et al.*, 1970; Vethamany and Fung, 1972) and holothurians (Kindred, 1924; Kawamoto, 1927; Ohuye, 1934; Boolootian and Giese, 1958; Endean, 1958, 1966; Andrew, 1962; Hetzel, 1963; Doyle and McNeil, 1964; Cowden, 1968; Fontaine and Lambert, 1977) (Table II).

The cells are round or ovoid and range from 8·0 to 20·0 μm in diameter (Figs 2, 9–11). The nucleus is small, irregular and eccentrically placed, with a variable amount of condensed chromatin (Fig. 10) (Table III). Typically, the cytoplasm is filled with numerous, large (*ca.* 2·0–5·0 μm diameter) spherical inclusions which at the ultrastructural level are seen to range in

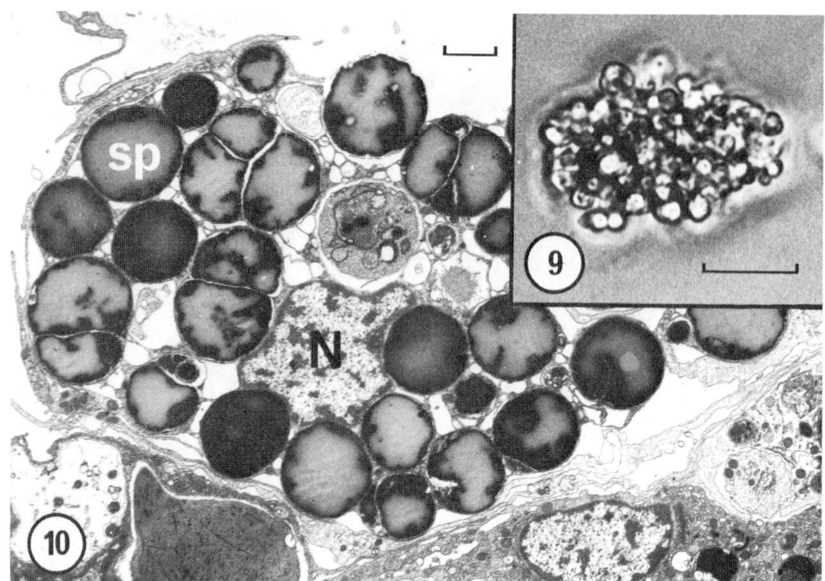

Fig. 9. Phase contrast micrograph of a spherule cell from *Cucumaria normani*. Scale bar = 10 μm.

Fig. 10. Electron micrograph of a coloured spherule cell from *Cucumaria normani*. Note the numerous membrane-bound spherules (sp) and nucleus (N). Scale bar = 1 μm.

form from membrane-bound and amorphous to heterogeneous microtubule-containing structures (Figs 10–12) (Table III). Also present in the cytoplasm may be microtubules, a Golgi complex, and some rough endoplasmic reticulum, which probably synthesizes the spherules by accretion. Histochemically, the spherules are composed of mucopolysaccharides and protein (Hetzel, 1963; Cowden, 1968; Fontaine and Lambert, 1977), but they may show considerable variation in staining properties (Kindred, 1924; Kawamoto, 1927; Ohuye, 1934; Endean, 1958; Hetzel, 1963; Doyle and McNeil, 1964; Holland *et al.*, 1965; Rollefsen, 1965; Burton, 1966). It has been suggested (Kindred, 1926; Johnson, 1969b) that the cells undergo a cycle during which the spherules pass from a basophilic to an eosinophilic state.

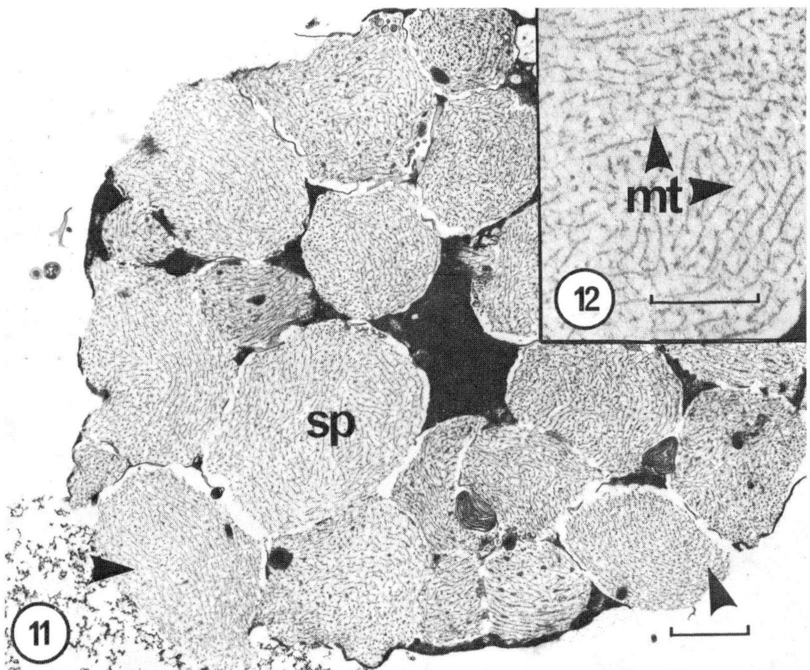

Fig. 11. Electron micrograph of a colourless spherule cell from *Echinus esculentus* with microtubule-containing spherules (sp). Some spherules are in the process of being discharged (unlabelled arrows) which is probably caused by poor fixation. Scale bar = 1 μm.

Fig. 12. High power electron micrograph of part of a spherule from a colourless spherule cell of *Echinus esculentus* showing in detail the microtubular (mt) substructure. Scale bar = 0·5 μm.

The spherule cells may be either colourless or enclose red, green or yellow pigments. Colourless forms are present in most species, but, in addition, yellow or green forms may occur in crinoids and some holothurians (Fig. 2), with red spherule cells (sometimes considered a separate coelomocyte type) described in all echinoids (Endean, 1966).

In echinoids this red pigmentation is due to the presence of napthaquinone compounds, termed echinochromes (MacMunn, 1885; Kuhn and Wallenfels, 1940). Several subclasses of echinochrome have now been identified (Goodwin and Srisukh, 1950; Fox and Hopkins, 1966) and related compounds (spinochromes) occur in the test and spines of sea urchins (Millott, 1950). The chief echinochrome located in the spherule cells is echinochrome A, a 6-ethyl-2-3, 7-trihydroxynaphthazarin compound, bound to PAS-positive proteins (Goodwin and Srisukh, 1950; Holland *et al.*, 1967; Anderson *et al.*, 1969; Johnson, 1970). The nature of the green and yellow pigments of crinoids and holothurian spherule cells is uncertain, but is probably also echinochrome, since this is known to be yellow at high and green at low hydrogen ion concentrations (Johnson, 1969c).

In vitro, the spherule cells are fairly stable and may exhibit amoeboid movement by the formation of short blunt pseudopodia (Johnson, 1969a; Johnson and Chapman, 1971). Upon fixation, however, some of the cells despherulate (Fig. 11) and under the electron microscope it is not always possible to distinguish pigment-bearing cells from colourless forms. When present, however, echinochrome is seen as amorphous flocculent material (Fig. 10).

The spherule cells are frequently quite numerous and in *Holothuria leucospilota* may comprise *ca.* 70% of the total coelomocyte count (Endean, 1958). Similarly in echinoids, Liebman (1950) records a value of *ca.* 50% in *Arbacia punctulata*, of which *ca.* 48% are red, 41% are white and 10% are green or yellow (Table III).

C. *Vibratile cells*

The vibratile cells (Fig. 13) are unusual coelomocytes occurring chiefly in echinoids (Cuénot, 1891; Behre, 1932; Boolootian and Giese, 1958; Andrew, 1962; Boolootian, 1962; Endean, 1966; Johnson, 1969a; Chien *et al.*, 1970; Vethamany and Fung, 1972; Bertheussen and Seljelid, 1978) and holothurians (Kindred, 1924; Kawamoto, 1927; Boolootian and Giese, 1958; Endean, 1958; Boolootian, 1962; Stang-Voss, 1971; Fontaine and Lambert, 1977) (Table II). They have also been found in the ophiuroid, *Ophiopholis aculeata* (Kindred, 1924; Boolootian and Giese, 1958; Boolootian, 1962) and flagellated structures (sometimes termed golden cells) resembling vibratile cells have been observed in the asteroid, *Patiria miniata* (Johnson and Beeson, 1966) (Table II). Because of their inconsistent distribution the vibratile cells have been the subject of some controversy, some workers regarding them as protozoan parasites, detached peritoneal cells, gametes or artefacts (see reviews by Hetzel, 1963; Endean, 1966). However, the close similarity of the vibratile cells to sipunculid urn cells (Bang, 1967; Johnson, 1969c) has encouraged their acceptance as a distinct coelomocyte category.

Surprisingly, vibratile cells were not seen in any of the species studied for the present review, possibly because they may rapidly loose structural integrity upon fixation (Hetzel, 1963; Endean, 1966; Johnson, 1969b; Vethamany and Fung, 1972). In fresh preparations, however, they have been observed to be small (5·0–10·0 μm diameter), spherical structures usually with a single long 20–50 μm flagellum (Hetzel, 1963; Endean, 1966; Bertheussen and Seljelid, 1978), though in some holothurians, two flagella may be present (Hetzel, 1963; Endean, 1958). The nucleus is large, irregular

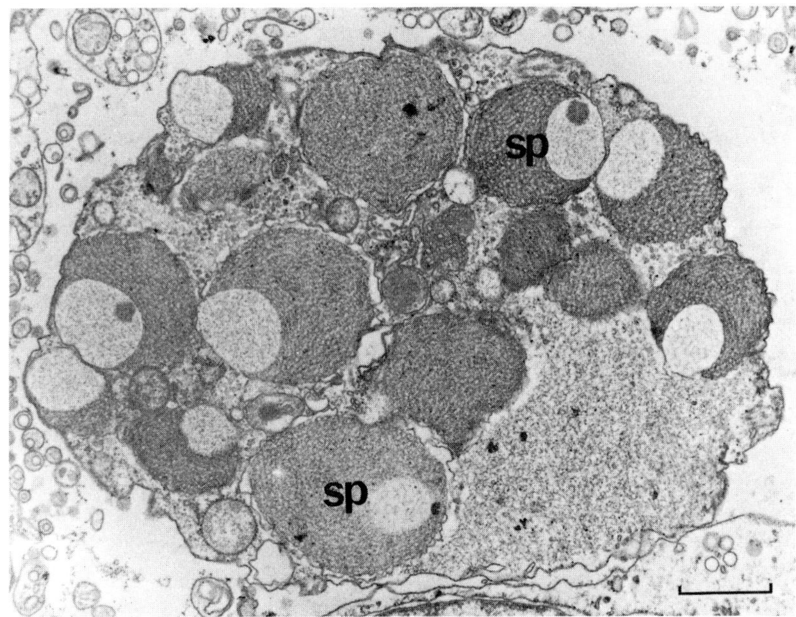

Fig. 13. Electron micrograph of part of a vibratile cell from the sea urchin, *Strongylocentrotus franciscanus*. Spherule-like inclusions (sp). The flagellum characteristic of these cells is absent in this particular section. [From Chien *et al.* (1970).] Scale bar = 1 μm.

and has some central condensed chromatin (Chien *et al.*, 1970; Vethamany and Fung, 1972). The cytoplasm which is sometimes yellow or brown in colour, contains a number of membrane-bound, microtubule-containing granules (Fig. 13), a few mitochondria, a well-developed Golgi complex, some rough ER and the basal body of the flagellum together with its associated microfibrils (Johnson, 1969a; Chien *et al.*, 1970; Vethamany and Fung, 1972) (Table III). The nature of the granule contents has not been fully elucidated but the cells are rich in substances which have a similar fine structural appearance to complex polysaccharides (Vethamany and Fung, 1972) and stain strongly with PAS and Alcian blue (Johnson, 1969b).

The cells are actively motile but do not appear to respond chemotactically to foreign or other materials (Johnson, 1969a,c). Cuénot (1901) believed that the rapid movement of these cells assists in the "circulation" of the coelomic fluid through the various body cavities.

In vitro, the cells are often quite stable, but some may release mucoid substances which appear as semi-transparent veils in freshly drawn coelomic fluid (Johnson, 1969a; Chien *et al.*, 1970) (Table III).

As with other echinoderm "blood cells", the size of the vibratile cell population is very variable, but in the sea urchins, *Strongylocentrotus purpuratus* and *S. franciscanus* is the second most abundant after the phagocytic amoebocytes (Johnson, 1969a).

D. Haemocytes

The haemocytes (Figs 2, 14, 15) have been found only in holothurians where they are restricted to the orders Dendrochirota and Molpadonia (Théel, 1921; Van der Heyde, 1922; Kindred, 1924; Kawamoto, 1927; Boolootian and Giese, 1958; Endean, 1958; Andrew, 1962; Boolootian, 1962; Hetzel, 1963; Fontaine and Lambert, 1973) (Table II).

A haemoglobin-containing cell has also been detected in the ophiuroid, *Ophiactis viriens* (Foettinger, 1880), but, to date, there are no other reports of such cells outside the Holothuroidea.

The cells are large (10·0–23·0 μm diameter), variable in shape but usually biconvex or spherical (Fig. 14), and, typically, enclose haemoglobin (Van der Heyde, 1922), homogeneously distributed throughout the cytoplasm, which imparts a yellow or red colour to the cells (Table III). The nucleus is round or ovoid, variable in position and has some peripheral condensed heterochromatin (Fig. 15). Also present in the largely homogeneous haemocyte cytoplasm (Fig. 15), may be a Golgi complex, a few mitochondria, some ribosomes, lysosome-like structures, containing electron-dense material, some marginal microtubules and vacuoles, and a small amount of ER.

The haemoglobins from different holothurian species display wide variation in their absorption banding spectra (Hogben and Van der Lingen, 1928; Kobayashi, 1932; Crescitelli, 1945) so that several classes of haemoglobin probably exist in different animals. Structurally, these pigments resemble the haemoglobins of vertebrates, but usually have lower molecular weights (*ca.* 23 600) (Farmanfarmaian, 1966) and slightly different absorption spectra (Crescitelli, 1945). Thus, despite the similarity of the haemocytes to the nucleated erythrocytes of lower vertebrates and the early erythroblasts of mammals, they are probably analogous rather than homologous structures (Fontaine and Lambert, 1973).

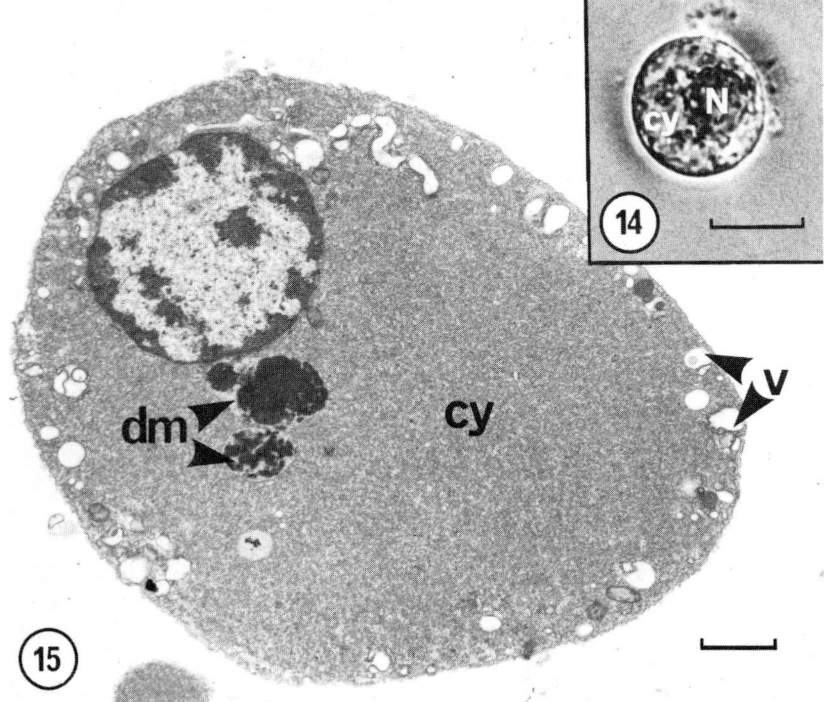

Fig. 14. Phase contrast micrograph of a haemocyte from *Cucumaria normani*. Note the eccentric nucleus (N) and relatively homogeneous cytoplasm (cy). Scale bar = 10 μm.

Fig. 15. Electron micrograph of a haemocyte from *Cucumaria normani* with homogeneous cytoplasm (cy) presumably containing haemoglobin, peripheral vacuoles (v) and vacuoles containing electron-dense material (dm). Scale bar = 1 μm.

In vitro, the haemocytes are fairly stable but sometimes produce bleb-like cytoplasmic protuberances after *ca.* 1 h (Hetzel, 1963). The cells are rarely motile, but a few may extend short filiform pseudopodia (Hetzel, 1963) and occasionally have been observed to ingest a small number of injected carbon particles (Hetzel, 1965).

When present, these cells may be very abundant (Fontaine and Lambert, 1973) and in *Paracaudina* sp. may number *ca.* 15.0×10^4 per ml of coelomic fluid (Andrew, 1962) (Table III).

E. Crystal cells

The crystal cells are unusual coelomocytes present in holothurians (Théel, 1921; Kawamoto, 1927; Ohuye, 1934; Endean, 1958; Boolootian and Giese, 1958; Andrew, 1962; Hetzel, 1963; Fontaine and Lambert, 1977). They have also been reported in *Patiria miniata* (Johnson and Beeson, 1966) but rarely in other groups (Table II).

The cells are generally rhomboidal and vary from 2·0 to 24·0 μm in length with the majority being 6–10 μm (Hetzel, 1963; Endean, 1966) (Table III). Characteristically, the cells enclose one to three rhomboidal or star-shaped crystals of unknown material, and which are surrounded by a thin rim of cytoplasm (Hetzel, 1963). The nucleus is often difficult to detect and few cytoplasmic organelles or inclusions are present (Hetzel, 1963; Endean, 1966) (Table III).

The crystals within the coelomocyte cytoplasm are extremely fragile and rapidly dissolve under slight osmotic stress, so that the cells are very difficult to fix and stain for light and electron microscopy, which may account for the failure to find crystal cells in *Cucumaria normani* in the present investigation.

These coelomocytes are relatively infrequent in most species and in *Holothuria leucospilota* comprise only *ca.* 5% of the total cell count (Burton, 1958; Endean, 1958) (Table III).

F. Progenitor cells

Although progenitor cells (Figs 16, 17) are probably present in most echinoderm species, detailed reports exist only for the asteroids (Boolootian and Giese, 1958) and holothurians, where they have sometimes been termed lymphocytes (Kawamoto, 1927; Ohuye, 1934; Endean, 1958; Hetzel, 1963; Doyle and McNeil, 1964; Fabre *et al.*, 1969; Fontaine and Lambert, 1977) (Table II). They were observed in *Echinus esculentus* in the present study and it is likely that the small spherical cells found in other echinoids by Boolootian and Giese (1958), Stang-Voss (1971) and Bertheussen and Seljelid (1978) also correspond to the progenitor cells (Table II).

Structurally, the cells are small (6·0–8·0 μm diameter) and usually round or ovoid (Figs 16, 17). The nucleus is large and round, with prominent nucleoli, some peripheral condensed chromatin, and is surrounded by a thin rim of hyaline cytoplasm (Figs 16, 17) (Table III). There are relatively few organelles within the cytoplasm but abundant RER, free ribosomes and some vesicles are usually present and, occasionally, a Golgi body and a few granules (Fig. 17) may also occur in more mature cells (Table III).

The progenitor cells are undoubtedly the stem cells from which other coelomocytes are derived (Kindred, 1924; Ohuye, 1934; Endean, 1958;

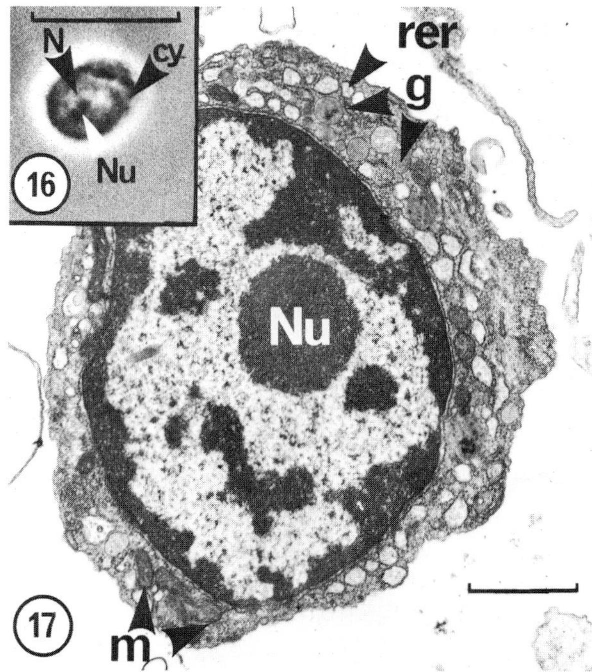

Fig. 16. Phase contrast micrograph of a progenitor cell from *Echinus esculentus*. Note the prominent nucleoli (Nu) and large nuclear (N): cytoplasmic (cy) ratio. Scale bar = 10 μm.

Fig. 17. Electron micrograph of a progenitor cell from *Cucumaria normani*. Note the characteristic large nuclear: cytoplasmic ratio, prominent nucleolus (Nu) and cytoplasm containing rough endoplasmic reticulum (rer) a few granules (g) and mitochondria (m). Scale bar = 1 μm.

Hetzel, 1965; Ratcliffe and Rowley, 1979) and intermediate, differentiating cells were frequently observed in all species examined for the present review. Furthermore, the long spindle-shaped, fusiform cells (Fig. 18) described in the crinoid, *Antedon rosacea* (Endean, 1966), the ophiuroid, *Gorgonocephalus euneumis* (Boolootian and Giese, 1958) and the holothurians, *Caudina chilensis* (Ohuye, 1934) and *Cucumaria plankii* (Fabre *et al.*, 1969) probably also represent progenitor cells, possibly undergoing maturation into amoebocyte types cells (Table III).

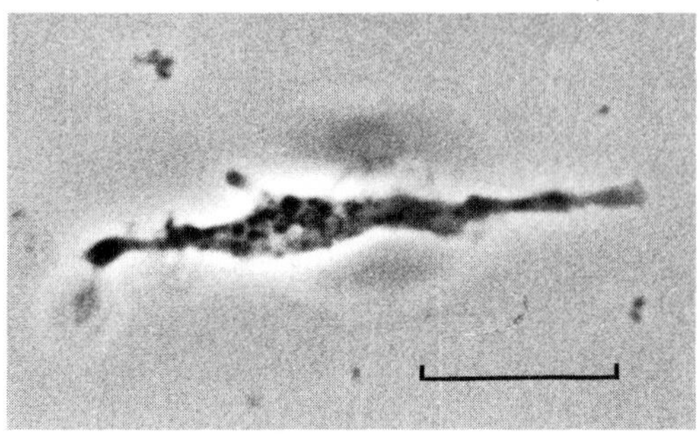

Fig. 18. Phase contrast micrograph of a fusiform cell from *Ophicomina nigra*. Scale bar = 10 μm.

Since progenitor cells represent a transitional stage, their numbers will vary not only from species to species but also depending upon the physiological status of the host. Fabre *et al.* (1969) has estimated that in *Cucumaria plankii* they comprise *ca.* 69% of the total population, with a further 7·5% being fusiform cells. However, in other species they are likely to represent a much smaller percentage. Equivalent cells in *Cucumaria miniata* are the third most abundant coelomocytes, after the haemocytes and phagocytic amoebocytes, and Fontaine and Lambert (1977) found that they averaged $1{\cdot}6 \times 10^6$ cells/ml (Table III).

G. Other coelomocytes

Occasionally, other atypical coelomocyte types have been reported for some species which do not fit readily into any of the above categories (Table II). Whilst some of these forms may be intermediate or transitional cells, others are probably artefacts.

1. Cells with rods and granules

These cells described by Cuénot (1891), Reichensparger (1912) and Endean (1966) are round or elongate with a small spherical nucleus and a large number of rod-like cytoplasmic inclusions which stain strongly with safranin. They have been found only in crinoids, and although their origin and function are unknown they may represent vibratile and/or spherule cell type precursors (Table II).

2. Minute corpuscles

In a review of holothurian coelomocytes, Hetzel (1963) described a number of anucleate cytoplasmic structures which he termed either minute or fusiform cells, according to their size. The number of these cells was usually small (values not given) but apparently increased with handling or stress of bleeding. Similar cells have not been found in other species, and they are probably cytoplasmic fragments derived from either degraded crystal cells, vibratile cells or coelomic epithelial cells (Table II).

3. Explosive cells

The explosive cells, sometimes termed Hardy's corpuscles because of their similarity to the fragile, refractile type cells of crustaceans (see Chapter 12) have been described for some echinoids and holothurians by Boolootian and Giese (1958, 1959) and Endean (1966). According to these authors, the cells are yellow, amoeboid structures (9·0–14·0 μm diameter) with a vacuolar hyaline cytoplasm. They are reputed to be extremely fragile and to lyse rapidly upon injury. Equivalent cells have not been reported by other workers and, although they may be atypical vibratile cells, their existence as a separate coelomocyte category is doubtful (Table II).

4. Brown bodies

Brown bodies, or revolving cysts, have been found in the coelomic cavities of asteroids (Johnson and Beeson, 1966), echinoids (Johnson, 1969a) and holothurians (Hetzel, 1965). They are spherical, yellow or brown aggregates of cells or cell fragments measuring 25·0–50·0 μm in diameter (Table II). Typically, these structures exhibit a rapid rotating motion and in hanging drop culture have been observed to continue revolving for up to 40 days. They often contain ingested carbon particles (Hetzel, 1965), gregarine parasites (Johnson and Beeson, 1966) or other cell debris (Fontaine and Lambert, 1973), and Hetzel (1965) has suggested that they may be important in the elimination of foreign or waste materials. Clearly, these structures are not discrete coelomic cells, but it has yet to be established whether they are equivalent to arthropod nodules or similarly named bodies in bivalves (see Chapters 12, 13).

Finally, regarding the miscellaneous cells such as the osmiphil cells, reniform cells, pigment cells, hyaline cells, red cells, spherical cells and granulocytes described for various species by Boolootian and Giese (1958), Boolootian (1962), Endean (1966) and Fabre *et al.* (1969) (Table II), there is insufficient information about their structure, behaviour and occurrence to conclude in the present review, to which of the six major coelomocyte categories these cells belong.

V. Origin and formation of coelomocytes

Despite a dearth of convincing experimental evidence, many suggestions have been made for the origin and formation of echinoderm coelomocytes. The various theories fall generally into two broad categories, namely those that advocate self replication of the circulating cells in the coelomic fluid, and those that propose the existence of a specific leucopoietic organ or tissue.

Among those ascribing to the former hypothesis are Kollmann (1908) and Ferguson (1966), and recently, Holland *et al.* (1965) have demonstrated proliferation of coelomocytes in the circulation of *Strongylocentrotus purpuratus*, although these authors failed to ascertain the extent of mitosis.

Great interest has been generated in the search for coelomocyte-producing organs or tissues, and several possible sites have been implicated.

For asteroids, Tiedemann (1816), Cuénot (1887) and Bargman and Behrens (1964) suggested the Tiedemann's bodies, but recent evidence by Vanden Bossche and Jangoux (1976) using tritiated thymidine indicates that in *Asterias rubens* the sole origin of the coelomocytes is the coelomic epithelium. In contrast, Panijel *et al.* (1977) and Brillouet *et al.* (1981) have found, also in *A. rubens*, that the axial organ can be stimulated by mitogens to produce different populations of progenitor-type coelomocytes. In the light of these new discoveries, it is interesting to speculate whether similar events occur in the axial organ of the closely related ophiuroids and possibly also in the spongy bodies of crinoids, as suggested by Cuénot (1891). Certainly, in echinoids, the axial organ has received most favour as the likely site for coelomocyte proliferation. This claim was first made by Kollmann (1908), and Millott (1969) has subsequently observed discharge of cells and structural changes in the axial organ following injury. The situation, however is not fully resolved since leucopoiesis appears to take place in other echinoid tissues, such as the epithelial cells of the peritoneum (Geddes, 1880; Liebman, 1950; Millott, personal communication), and the dermal connective tissue of the body wall (Schinke, 1950). An autoradiographic investigation of the coelomocytes of *Strongylocentrotus purpuratus* (Holland *et al.*, 1965) also showed active cell division in the visceral peritoneum, parietal peritoneum, hydrocoel peritoneum, Polian vesicles, haemal strands and dermal connective tissue as well as in the axial organ.

Finally, in the Holothuroidea, the literature reveals no clear evidence of any individual leucopoietic organ or tissue. Cuénot (1891) proposed the Polian vesicles while Herouard (1889) and Endean (1958) believe the cells originate in the connective tissue of the respiratory trees, and, Prosser and Judson (1952) and Hetzel (1965) claim they are derived from the haemal connective tissue.

Thus, although current research indicates that the axial organ, or its equivalent, is the main source of coelomocytes in echinoderms, it is also possible that a number of different tissues may have independently acquired this ability during the evolution of the specialized cavities and tubular systems of the coelom. Clearly, further investigations are necessary particularly in the crinoids, ophiuroids and holothurians.

Whatever the tissue of origin, one consistent feature does emerge, however, and that is, that most coelomocytes appear to be derived from a single lymphoid-like progenitor cell (Kollmann, 1908; Kindred, 1926; Ohuye, 1934; Endean, 1958, 1966; Hetzel, 1965), although the exact sequence of events leading to the differentiation of the various cell types has not been fully elucidated. Kindred (1926) believed that the spherule cells are derived from the phagocytic amoebocytes by active accumulation of ingested material, but Hetzel (1965) considered that the amoebocytes, spherule cells and haemocytes develop independently from the precursor cells. The origin of the crystal cells and vibratile cells remains a mystery. Théel (1921) claimed that the crystal cells were derived from amoeboid cells, but the presence of pigmented inclusions in both the crystal and vibratile cells could indicate some relationship with the spherule cells, and they may represent terminal stages in this line of maturation.

VI. Functions of coelomocytes

The coelomocytes of echinoderms carry out a number of important physiological functions, such as host defence, clotting, transport, storage, synthesis and excretion (Endean, 1966). However, the precise role of each cell type in these processes has not always been clearly defined.

A. Host defence reactions

Although little is known about echinoderm pathology, the enormous success of these large, active animals in the microbe-rich marine environment must be attributed, at least in part, to their ability to defend themselves against parasitism and microbial invasion. No doubt, the possession by many species of a tough, external, calcareous test affords some measure of protection, but certain areas of the body, e.g. tube feet and skin are extremely vulnerable to injury and could serve as a route of entry for potential pathogens.

As with most invertebrates, threats to the homeostatic integrity of the host are dealt with in echinoderms by the phagocytic, clumping and immobilizing activities of the "circulating blood cells". In addition, the coelomocytes are important in wound repair, liberation of toxic or lytic substances and graft rejection (Table IV).

1. Phagocytosis

Phagocytosis by echinoderm coelomocytes was first observed in the perivisceral coelom of *Asterias rubens* by Durham (1887) after injection of India ink or aniline blue. Phagocytosing cells were also found in the tube feet, intestinal wall and all other organs of the body by Cuénot (1891), and, to date, numerous workers have reported the uptake of various materials, including bacteria, inert particles, foreign cells, spherule cells and cell debris, in many echinoderm species (Chapeaux, 1893; Cuénot, 1901; Reichensparger, 1912; Kindred, 1921; Lison, 1930; Ohuye, 1934; Bertolini, 1937; Millott, 1950; Boolootian and Giese, 1958; Boolootian, 1962; Bang and Lemma, 1962; Ghiradella, 1965; Johnson and Beeson, 1966; Johnson, 1969c; Johnson *et al.*, 1970; Johnson and Chapman, 1971; Reinisch and Bang, 1971; Heatfield and Travis, 1975a; Kaplan and Bertheussen, 1977). (Table IV).

Ingestion of particles appears to be carried out chiefly by the petaloid form of the phagocytic amoebocytes (Kindred, 1921; Ohuye, 1934; Boolootian and Giese, 1958; Johnson, 1969c) (Fig. 6) although Ohuye (1934) also found uptake in the minute corpuscles (=progenitor cells), and Boolootian and Giese (1958) claim that both the filopodial and petaloid phases are phagocytic.

Surprisingly, few *in vitro* studies of phagocytosis have been carried out and little information is available on the rates and efficiencies of uptake by different species, or of the influence of temperature, incubation time, presence/absence of opsonins and the nature of the test particle on the process. Some degree of specificity is shown by the phagocytes, however, since Johnson (1969c) has found that in hanging drop cultures, the coelomocytes of *Strongylocentrotus purpuratus* and *S. franciscanus*, ingest Gram-positive bacteria more readily than Gram-negative forms. Also in *S. purpuratus*, Hilgard *et al.* (1967) and Hilgard and Phillips (1968) report that the coelomocytes are capable of discriminating between self and non self proteins, and that *in vivo* pretreatment with bovine serum albumin (BSA) markedly reduces the uptake of secondary doses of BSA but not of bovine gamma globulin by the coelomocytes, thus indicating that receptor molecules of different combining specificities are present on the cells and are actively involved in ingestion (Hilgard, 1970). Kaplan and Bertheussen (1977), also found in *Strongylocentrotus droebachiensis*, receptors for C3 on the phagocytic amoebocytes whose distribution was similar to those of rat Kupffer cells and mouse peritoneal cells.

Following ingestion, the phagocytes appear to migrate to the gills, respiratory trees and/or axial organ, from where they may be discharged to the exterior (Durham, 1891; Bertolini, 1937; Millott, 1950; Bang and Lemma, 1962). The extent of intracellular breakdown of phagocytosed material is not clear. Johnson *et al.* (1970) failed to observe the formation of primary lysosomes in the amoebocytes of *Strongylocentrotus* sp. even after 48 h incubation with bacteria. However, at present, there is insufficient data to draw any definite conclusions regarding the fate of ingested material.

2. *Cell clumping and encapsulation*

Alternative cellular reactions to the presence of foreign particles in the coelom are cell clumping/nodule formation and encapsulation (Table IV). These responses have been reported to occur in asteroids and echinoids to a variety of substances including bacteria, inert materials and foreign tissue implants (Davidson, 1953; Bang and Lemma, 1962; Ghiradella, 1965; Johnson, 1969c; Reinisch and Bang, 1971; Bertheussen and Seljelid, 1978). Some degree of specificity is also demonstrated in these reactions, with Gram-negative bacteria or allogeneic cells more effectively contained than Gram-positive bacteria or autogeneic cells (Johnson, 1969c; Reinisch and Bang, 1971).

Both phagocytic amoebocytes and spherule cells appear to be involved in clump and capsule formation (Johnson, 1969c) (Table IV), but further detailed ultrastructural studies are necessary to elucidate the exact roles of these two cell types. The vibratile cells do not appear to play any significant part in these responses, and Johnson (1969c) found that they frequently retreated from the area of the inoculum.

The development of the clumps or capsules is always preceded by the initial attachment of amoebocytes to the foreign material, and, as with other invertebrates (Chapters 12, 13), this first stage of recognition is followed by the adherence of large numbers of other amoebocytes to the cell: foreign particle complexes (Johnson, 1969c). Phagocytosis has not been observed within the clumps (Johnson, 1969c; Reinisch and Bang, 1971), but insufficient studies have been made to conclude that ingestion is not involved in this phenomenon. Inside the clumps, the spherule cells are invariably found adjacent to the foreign material (Johnson, 1969c; Reinisch and Bang, 1971) and it is possible that they release acid mucopolysaccharides and/or echinochrome (Johnson, 1969c) which may influence later cell adhesion and/or effect extracellular killing.

The fate of secluded material and the enclosing cells is, at present, unknown, and this, together with most other aspects of cell clumping and encapsulation responses are areas in need of further research.

3. Wound repair

Although some echinoderms possess a rigid calcite skeleton, this is often covered by a thin ectoderm, through which protrude the hydrostatic organs or tube feet. The ectoderm and tube feet are delicate structures easily damaged by abrasion, rough handling or violent dislodgement of the body through strong currents or predation. Since all echinoderms depend entirely on hydrostatic changes in the water vascular system for locomotion, feeding and other activities (Nichols, 1969), damage to the tube feet, and consequent loss of coelomic fluid, can seriously affect many behavioural and physiological functions. Thus, efficient plugging and repair of injured tissues is essential, not only to prevent infection but also for the maintenance of normal homeostasis.

Most studies of wound repair processes have been conducted on holothurians, and in these animals the normal response to injury is the initial aggregation of the coelomocytes to prevent "blood" loss, followed by migration of fibroblast epidermal cells to the wound site (Cowden, 1968; Menton and Eisen, 1973). In the holothurian *Thyone briareus*, healing of incisional wounds is usually complete within fourteen days, but is more prolonged after excision of part of the test (Menton and Eisen, 1973). Mitotic activity by adjacent epidermal cells does not appear to be important, at least in the early stages of incisional tissue recovery (Menton and Eisen, 1973), but coelomocyte accumulation at the site is usually rapid and pronounced (Rollefsen, 1965; Menton and Eisen, 1973). Cowden (1968), however, failed to observe marked leucocyte infiltration and exudation in damaged cutaneous tissues of the sea cucumber, *Strichopus bodionotus*, and concluded that the coelomocytes do not serve any special purpose in the repair response. The coelomocyte accumulations noted at wound sites by Rollefsen (1965) and Menton and Eisen (1973) consisted of significant numbers of spherule cells which rapidly broke down and despherulated (Table IV). Menton and Eisen (1973) suggested that the function of these cells is to produce the collagen for the fibrous matrix of the cuticle, but it is also possible that substances released from the spherules may act as chemotactic agents for the migratory epidermal cells and/or help to disinfect the area against microbial invasion (Table IV).

Red spherule cells and phagocytic amoebocytes have also been observed in the dermis and other tissues of regenerating spines of the sea urchins, *Echinus esculentus* (Pilkington, 1969) and *Strongylocentrotus purpuratus* (Heatfield and Travis, 1975a,b) (Table IV). The amoebocytes have a structural similarity to the skeletogenic cells (sclerocytes) present in echinoid spines (Johnson and Chapman, 1970), and Pilkington (1969) postulated that these sclerocytes may represent a skeletal phase of the migratory coelomocytes. Heatfield and Travis (1975a), however, could find no ultrastructural evidence for the transformation of the amoebocytes to sclerocytes (termed calcoblasts by Heatfield and Travis), and it appears that the phagocytic amoebocytes serve chiefly to remove cell debris and/or invading microorganisms. In addition, other factors may contribute to the injury response and Millott (1969) has reported the release of acid mucopolysaccharides from the axial organ following incisional injury to the body which may influence the cellular reactions. The precise role of these mucopolysaccharides is at present unknown.

4. *Clotting*

Clotting of echinoderm coelomic fluid occurs rapidly in response to injury, trauma or contact with foreign materials (Schäfer, 1882; Geddes, 1880; Théel, 1896; Kindred, 1921; Donnellon, 1938; Bookhout and Greenburg, 1940; Davidson, 1953; Boolootian and Giese, 1959; Bang and Lemma, 1962; Abraham, 1964; Endean, 1966; Bang, 1970; Noble, 1970) (Table IV). The response is mediated only by the coelomocytes and gelation of the plasma, similar to that of arthropods, has not been observed in any echinoderm species. The main coelomocyte types involved in the clotting process are the phagocytic amoebocytes (Donnellon, 1938; Johnson, 1969a), but some workers (Vethamany and Fung, 1972; Bertheussen and Seljelid, 1978), believe the vibratile cells also participate, as these are often seen in association with coelomocyte clots (Johnson, 1969a) and appear to release mucoid substances in freshly drawn coelomic fluid (Johnson, 1969a; Chien *et al.*, 1970) (Table IV).

Boolootian and Giese (1959), carried out a detailed survey of clotting in several echinoderm species and they recognized three distinct types of clot formation:

(a) *Type I*. Temporary cellular agglutination, characteristic of crinoids and some ophiuroids, in which the coelomocytes retain their structural integrity, and from which they may later dissociate.
(b) *Type II*. More permanent cellular agglutination, seen commonly in asteroids and some holothurians, in which the cells break down and fuse together to form "plasmodia".
(c) *Type III*. Cellular agglutination, usually exhibited by echinoids and holothurians, which is initiated by lysis of explosive or hyaline cells, and involves the formation of fibre-networks which entrap other cells and cell debris.

The major criticism of this scheme is the questionable existence of the explosive cells, described by Boolootian and Giese (1958), which are essential for Type III clotting. However, this type of clotting occurs chiefly in echinoids and holothurians and it is possible that the fibre-like networks, reported by Boolootian and Giese (1959) are strands of mucoid substances released by the vibratile cells, in a manner similar to that observed by Bertheussen and Seljelid (1978).

The formation of cytoplasmic plasmodia, distinctive of Type II clots is also a matter of controversy (Geddes, 1880; Kindred, 1921, 1926; Johnson and Beeson, 1966; Bertheussen and Seljelid, 1978), and confirmatory ultrastructural studies are necessary to resolve this problem.

Nevertheless, the work of Boolootian and Giese (1959) does show a clear correlation between the level of complexity of the clotting response and the diversity of the coelomocyte populations present in the various echinoderm groups, and could shed some light on the evolution of certain coelomocyte types. Certainly, in those animals, such as the crinoids, in which the amoebocytes do not produce filopodial extensions, a modified form of clotting would be expected. Furthermore, with the development of larger coelomic cavities in the echinoids and holothurians, a more efficient clotting sytem would be necessary, a requirement perhaps fulfilled by the evolution of the vibratile cells.

Regarding the clotting mechanism itself, a number of factors are known to enhance the rate of cell agglutination (e.g. calcium chloride, potassium chloride, barium chloride and fat solvents) (Donnellon, 1938), while others retard or completely inhibit clot formation (e.g. sodium citrate, potassium oxalate, cysteine, sodium bisulphite, *n*-ethyl maleimide, EDTA, EGTA, mercaptoethanol and caffeine) (Donnellon, 1938; Bertheussen and Seljelid, 1978). In most species, clotting is preceded by transformation of the phagocytic amoebocytes from the petaloid or transitional states into the filopodial stage (Kindred, 1921; Davidson, 1953; Boolootian and Giese, 1959; Endean, 1966; Noble, 1970), and this change is independent of the presence of calcium, but is inhibited by reducing, chelating or SH binding reagents (Boolootian and Giese, 1959; Noble, 1970). The second stage of clotting is the agglutination of the cells by interlacing of their long filopods (Kindred, 1921; Boolootian and Giese, 1959; Johnson, 1969a; Noble, 1970), and this process is strongly dependent upon calcium ions (Donnellon, 1938; Bookhout and Greenburg, 1940; Davidson, 1953; Noble, 1970). In their scheme, Boolootian and Giese (1959), consider that only Type I clots are calcium dependent, with Type II clots achieved by the formation of disulphide linkages between adjacent cells. A few workers also believe a tissue factor, released from damaged cells or tissues is also essential for the induction of clotting (Donnellon, 1938; Davidson, 1953).

5. *Antibacterial factors*

In addition to phagocytosis and cell clumping, many invertebrates are capable of protecting themselves against microbial exploitation by the production of antibacterial factors such as agglutinins, bacteriolysins and bactericidins, all of which may be found free in the body fluids. However, in a comprehensive survey of the responses of bacteria to invertebrate body fluids, Johnson and Chapman (1971) found that the coelomic fluid of the sea cucumber, *Strichopus tremulens* had bacteriostatic properties, and that the factor responsible appeared to reside in the coelomocytes. The cell types involved in the phenomenon were not defined, so the possibility of phagocytic intervention cannot be ruled out. Johnson (1969a,b,c) also considers that acid mucopolysaccharides released from the vibratile cells act as immobilizing agents on bacteria, both *in vitro* and *in vivo* (Table IV).

Recently, Wardlaw and Unkles (1978) have found strong bactericidal activity in the coelomocytes of *Echinus esculentus*. This was not due to phagocytosis or cell clumping since the effect was still obtained in cell free extracts after ultrasonic disruption of the cells. Subsequent fractionization of *E. esculentus* coelomocytes on density gradients, has revealed that the cells responsible for this phenomenon are the red spherule cells (Messer and Wardlaw, 1980) (Table IV).

Further evidence for the participation of the spherule cells in bacterial killing is provided by the observations of Johnson (1969c) who reports that in *S. purpuratus* and *S. franciscanus*, the spherule cells *in vitro* are strongly attracted to some strains of bacteria, and in conjunction with the phagocytic amoebocytes effectively contain and kill them. Moreover, red spherule cells have also been detected in the internal organs and regenerating spine tips of *S. franciscanus*, infected with epibiotic diatoms, and other microorganisms (Johnson and Chapman, 1970) (Table IV). The red spherule cells are known to contain naphthaquinone compounds (echinochrome) which have algistatic properties (Vevers, 1963), and Vevers (1966) has suggested that these substances may also function as general disinfecting agents (Table IV).

It is not known whether other pigments, commonly found in echinoderms, have similar antibacterial properties. In many invertebrates, melanin deposition has been found to accompany host cellular defence responses (Unestam and Nylund, 1972; Schmit *et al.*, 1977; Smith and Ratcliffe, 1980) and intermediary compounds in melanin synthesis are believed to have antibacterial properties (Taylor, 1969). Since melanin and melanin precursors have been detected in the amoebocytes of *Thyone briareus* (Millott, 1950) and the colourless and red spherule cells and axial organ of *Diadema antillarum* (Millott and Jacobson, 1952; Jacobson and Millott, 1953; Vevers, 1966) it would be interesting to discover the role of these substances in echinoderm host defence.

6. *Graft rejection*

Because of the close ancestral relationship of the echinoderms to the vertebrates, many studies have been directed towards the search in this phylum for the precursors of vertebrate immunocompetent cells and molecules (Hilgard and Phillips, 1968; Burnet, 1968; Prendergast and Suzuki, 1970; Prendergast and Unanue, 1970, Hilgard, 1970; Reinisch and Bang, 1971; Prendergast, 1971; Carton, 1974; Prendergast *et al.*, 1974; Bang, 1975). Experiments with allogeneic and xenogeneic transplants, in particular, provide useful models for the study of specificity and anamnestic responses, and several such investigations have been carried out in asteroids, echinoids and holothurians (Ghiradella, 1965; Truslé, 1967; Hildemann and Dix, 1972; Karp and Hildemann, 1975, 1976; Coffano and Hinegardner, 1977; Hildemann *et al.*, 1977; Bertheussen, 1979). The results of the earlier transplantation experiments, however, are conflicting, with some species of asteroids accepting xenogeneic transplants (Truslé, 1967), while others exhibit rejection (Ghiradella, 1965). As pointed out by Hildemann and Reddy (1973), these studies are indecisive, chiefly because of the limitations of the experimental methods. More recently, Hildemann and Dix (1972) have demonstrated slow allogeneic rejection to first set integumentary grafts in the asteroid, *Protoreaster nodosus*, and the holothurian, *Cucumaria tricolor*. During the rejection processes, numerous coelomocytes, particularly phagocytic amoebocytes, granulocytes (=spherule cells?) and lymphocytes (=progenitor cells or transitional amoebocytes?) were seen to infiltrate the grafts (Hildemann and Dix, 1972), and were probably directly responsible for destruction of the foreign tissues (Table IV). Similar events were found to accompany rejection of second and third set allografts in the sea star, *Dermasterias imbricata* (Karp and

Hildemann, 1975; Karp, 1976), but the response (i.e. rejection) occurred much more rapidly and more intensely than in first set rejections, indicating that the coelomocytes can not only discriminate between self- and non-self, but are also capable of a specific, adaptive response. Similar rejection of first set allografts with accelerated rejection of second set allografts have also been reported in the echinoid, *Lytechinus pictus* (Coffano and Hinegardner, 1977), and in these animals, there was a direct correlation between the proportion of accepted allografts and the extent of inbreeding between host and donor.

The exact mechanism(s) by which graft rejection is achieved in echinoderms is still largely unknown but is unlikely to be mediated by production of immunoglobulins in a manner equivalent to vertebrate systems. However, Bertheussen (1979) has recently demonstrated strong cytotoxicity of echinoid phagocytes to allogeneic and xenogeneic coelomocyte mixtures *in vitro*. This lytic response was found to be contact dependent and not influenced by the presence of other, non-phagocytic cells, such as the vibratile or spherule cells. Bertheussen (1979) thus concludes, that in echinoderms, the phagocytic amoebocytes are the recognition and effector cells in transplant reactions. The participation of other cell types in graft destruction cannot be entirely ruled out, especially as Coffano and Hinegardner (1977) detected the accumulation of massive numbers of red spherule cells at the site of both first and second set allografts in *L. pictus*. No doubt, some of these cells were responding non-specifically to wounding since a few were also seen in the control autografts, which were not rejected. Nevertheless, it is possible that their presence in the autografts was stimulated by chemotactic factors released either from the damaged tissue cells or, alternatively, from the host effector (phagocytic) cells, and again they may be acting as general disinfecting agents.

B. Transport and storage

Echinoderms lack an extensive, directional vascular system, characteristic of most other animals, and so translocation of materials, particularly in the large echinoids and holothurians, may be carried out, to some extent, by populations of migratory coelomocytes (Table IV).

1. Oxygen transport

Many echinoderms are large active animals and possess a number of specialized respiratory structures, including the tentacles and respiratory trees in holothurians and the podia and gills in echinoids, asteroids and ophiuroids (Farmanfarmaian, 1966). Transport of dissolved oxygen from these organs to the various parts of the body takes place via the coelomic fluid and is probably aided, in some species, notably the holothurians, by the large populations of haemoglobin-containing coelomocytes (haemocytes) (Foettinger, 1880; Théel, 1921; Van der Heyde, 1922; Hogben and Van der Lingen, 1928; Kobayashi, 1932; Crescitelli, 1945; Endean, 1958; Manwell, 1959; Andrew, 1962; Hetzel, 1963; Fontaine and Lambert, 1973) (Table IV).

However, the efficiency of the haemocytes in oxygen uptake is a matter of some controversy. Nomura (1926) found no marked affinity for oxygen in *Paracaudina chilensis*, while Hiestand (1940) showed that the oxygen consumption of *Thyone briareus* is independent of the oxygen concentration of the surrounding seawater, and that the animal is capable of compensating for low oxygen partial pressures. It is possible that such differences are due to variations in the amount of haemoglobin present in the cells, or to the size of the haemocyte populations at the time of the experiments (Manwell, cited by Farmanfarmaian, 1966). An alternative suggestion is that the haemocytes do not serve primarily to enhance uptake of oxygen, but merely act as storage vehicles during transportation within the body (Farmanfarmaian, 1966).

Finally, haemoglobin-containing cells are absent from echinoids and other groups and MacMunn (1885) and Freidheim (1932) considered that the echinochrome-bearing spherule cells have an equivalent function. Other studies, however, failed to confirm this hypothesis (Tyler, 1939; Farmanfarmaian, 1966) and it appears that in these animals, oxygen is dissolved directly in the coelomic fluid.

2. *Nutrient transport*

The role of the coelomocytes in digestion, transport and storage of nutrients (Table IV) has also been the subject of much controversy. The cells have frequently been observed closely associated with the digestive tract of several species (Anderson, 1966; Endean, 1966) and some workers regard this to be indicative of enzyme secretion (Cuénot, 1887; Frenzel, 1892; Chapeaux, 1893; Stott, 1955). However, the mere presence of the cells in the gut is not, in itself, sufficient evidence for their participation in digestion and in crinoids and asteroids, breakdown of food appears to take place entirely within the pyloric caeca (Anderson, 1953, 1966). Other workers believe that the coelomocytes are important in the translocation and/or storage of food materials (Cuénot, 1891; Kindred, 1926; Liebman, 1950; Hyman, 1955; Tanako, 1958; Boolootian and Lasker, 1964), and both the phagocytic amoebocytes (Cuénot, 1891; Kindred, 1926) and the spherule cells (Cuénot, 1891; Liebman, 1950; Boolootian and Lasker, 1964) have been implicated in these processes (Table IV). In an autoradiographic study, however, Ferguson (1964, 1970) has shown that in the starfish, *Asterias forbesi*, the amoebocytes play only a minor, secondary role in the dispersion of food substances, and concludes that the coelomic fluid is the chief medium for nutrient transport, with continual exchange of materials taking place between this fluid and the various body organs.

In contrast to the asteroids and echinoids, digestive enzymes associated with the yellow or green spherule cells are found in holothurians (Anderson, 1966) and these cells often lie in close proximity to the digestive tract, possibly suggesting an involvement in nutrient digestion and/or transport (Endean, 1966). Thus it is only in holothurians that the coelomocytes seem to participate in the nutritive processes, and Endean (1966) speculates that this ability may have arisen with the development of respiratory trees in this group, so that food materials, which enter these structures, via the respiratory currents, may be utilized.

C. Synthesis

The synthetic activities of the coelomocytes appear to be concerned primarily with the production of pigments, collagen and/or, polysaccharide-type materials (Table IV). In addition, suggestions have been made that some cells, chiefly the crystal cells, may be involved in ossicle formation (Hetzel, 1963) (Table IV) although the function(s) of these cells is still poorly understood.

1. Pigments

Pigments, particularly melanin and echinochrome are widely distributed throughout members of the phylum and are deposited in the ectoderm and other regions of the body (Vevers, 1966). Melanin and its precursors have also been found in the red and colourless spherule cells of the sea urchin, *Diadema antillarum* (Jacobson and Millott, 1953) and the spherule cells of the holothurians, *Thyone briareus* (Millott, 1950) and *Holothuria forskali* (Millott, 1953). The pigment is always found associated with the spherular inclusions and does not appear to be present in the enclosing cytoplasm or free in the coelomic fluid (Jacobson and Millott, 1953; Millott, 1953). The biochemical pathway for melanin synthesis is the serial enzymic oxidation of phenol precursors, often with dopa quinone and/or dopa-chrome formed as intermediary compounds (Mason, 1959). An enzyme system, with mono- and poly-phenolase activity, capable of synthesizing melanin has been found in the spherule cells of *Diadema antillarum*, together with the substrate tyrosine (Jacobson and Millott, 1953). An inhibitory factor present in the coelomic fluid appears to prevent melanogenesis until the cells have migrated to the skin, and/or other tissues, where deposition takes place. A similar synthetic pathway has been demonstrated in the spherule cells of *Thyone briareus* and *Holothuria forskali*, but in these animals, a coelomic fluid inhibitory factor is wanting and so melanin granules are often present on the outside of the cytoplasmic spherules (Millott, 1953).

Naphthaquinones (or echinochromes) are also commonly found in echinoderms and they are particularly abundant in the red spherule cells (Vevers, 1966) (Table IV) in which they are probably synthesized. Related compounds, spinochromes, also occur in the test and spines of many echinoids (Millott, 1950) and may be deposited by the spherule cells. The precise function of the echinochromes is not clear. Suggested roles include oxygen transport (MacMunn, 1885) (see section on oxygen transport), photoreception (Yoshida, 1966), excretion (Fox, 1953) and algistasis (Vevers, 1963) (see section on antibacterial factors). More recently, there has been some indication that they have a bactericidal effect (Service, unpublished) and they may be important in keeping the test free from microbial colonization (Vevers, 1966).

2. *Other materials*

In addition to pigment synthesis, the coelomocytes may elaborate other materials, including collagen and mucopolysaccharides (Table IV).

Collagen is a major component of the connective tissue and Cuvierian tubules of echinoderms (Giese, 1966), and coelomocytes, principally the colourless spherule cells, have often been found closely associated with these structures (Endean, 1958; Burton, 1966). The spherular inclusions of these cells are known to contain polysaccharide and protein (Endean, 1958; Hetzel, 1963; Johnson, 1969b) which upon release may form fibres (Endean, 1958, 1966). Since despherulation has frequently been observed in regions of connective tissue growth or repair (Endean, 1958; Rollefsen, 1965; Menton and Eisen, 1973; Heatfield and Travis, 1975b) (see section on wound repair), it is most likely that they are responsible for the synthesis and deposition of collagen materials (Burton, 1966; Doyle and McNeil, 1964; Endean, 1966; Cowden, 1968).

D. Excretion

Echinoderms lack distinct excretory organs and, presumably, the chief nitrogenous waste products, ammonia and urea, pass directly to the exterior through the respiratory surfaces, such as the dermal papillae, buccal branchiae and respiratory trees (Delaunay, 1931). It is not known whether the coelomocytes participate in this elimination, although injected dyes are rapidly taken up and transported to the outside by the phagocytic amoebocytes (Durham, 1891; Cuénot, 1901; Bertolini, 1937) (Table IV).

Fox (1953) suggested that the polyhydroxy-naphthaquines present in the red spherule cells of echinoids are excretory products which are stored in the skin and other tissues before incorporation into the skeleton as calcium salts. However, there is little evidence to support this hypothesis, and recent research indicates a different function for these compounds (see sections on antibacterial factors and pigments).

VII. Summary and concluding remarks

In contrast to many of the previous accounts of echinoderm coelomocytes, only six morphologically and functionally distinct cell types have been identified in the present review, and these include the phagocytic amoebocytes, the coloured and colourless spherule cells, the vibratile cells, the haemocytes, the crystal cells and the progenitor cells.

A variety of important physiological functions, such as host defence, oxygen transport and pigment synthesis are carried out by these cells, most of which are highly specialized for their task(s).

Not all six cell types are present in every species, however, and in general the highest coelomocyte diversity occurs in the more advanced echinoids and holothurians, probably as a consequence of the greater development of their coelomic cavities. Certainly in echinoids, the vibratile cells may have evolved in order to prevent the rapid loss of coelomic fluid which occurs after wounding due to the exceptionally large body cavities of these animals and their inability to contract the body wall. Furthermore, this clotting process may be even more efficient than its analogue in the arthropods (which possess true plasma gelation) since the possession of flagella by the vibratile cells enables them to be more readily mobilized to the site of injury.

Likewise, the acquisition of specialized haemoglobin-containing cells in some holothurians may be correlated with the relatively high oxygen requirement of these benthic, muscular animals, although the reason for the absence of these cells from the Apoda and Aspidochirotida is not clear.

To date the crystal cells remain enigmatic, and until their chemical and structural characteristics have been elucidated, their origins and functions will remain a matter of speculation.

The phagocytic amoebocytes, on the other hand, are abundant stable structures, found throughout the phylum. They probably represent an ancestral type of coelomocyte, with equivalent cells present in nearly all invertebrate species. Echinoderm amoebocytes, however, are unusual and display a relatively sophisticated recognition system, capable of discriminating between closely related proteins or cells. Whether this ability has any significance in terms of the phylogeny of immunocompetent cells is debatable. However, these recent findings do emphasize that in invertebrates specific "immune" responses can be achieved without the intervention of immunoglobulins.

Without doubt, the state of knowledge regarding echinoderm coelomic cells has increased dramatically over the last fifteen years, but there are many areas where further research is urgently required. For example, much is still unknown about the structure and function of crinoid and ophiuroid coelomocytes, despite the fact that these animals represent ancient and unique taxonomic groups, perhaps of greater phylogenetic significance than the more abundant and predominant echinoids and holothurians. Additional studies are also necessary on many aspects of the host cellular defences, particularly with respect to phagocytosis. It would be interesting to determine whether sub-populations of amoebocytes capable of responding differentially to various types of foreign substances exist in echinoderms, and the extent to which the cells co-operate and interact in cell clumping and wound repair. Finally, the mode of origin and formation of the coelomocytes needs clarification, as do the biochemical events responsible for the initiation of cell activity, chemotaxis and/or microbial killing and cytotoxicity.

Acknowledgements

I would like to express my gratitude to the editors for their assistance with the electron microscopy and manuscript preparation, and to the Royal Society and Science Research Council (Grant No. GR/B/1014.4) for the provision of equipment used in this study. I would also like to thank Prof. N. Millott and Mr M. Service for much helpful advice and discussion; Mr A. Osborn and Mr B. Bullimore for collection of specimens; Mr P. Llewellyn for drawing Fig. 1; Dr K. Edds for supplying Figs 7, 8; Dr P. Chien for allowing me to use Fig. 13; and to Professors J. A. Allen and E. W. Knight-Jones in whose departments this work was carried out.

References

Abraham, M. (1964). *Pubbl. Stanz. Zool. Napoli* **34**, 43–52.

Anderson, H. A., Mathieson, J. W. and Thomson, R. H. (1969). *Comp. Biochem. Physiol.* **28**, 333–345.

Anderson, J. M. (1953). *Biol. Bull., Woods Hole* **105**, 47–61.

Anderson, J. M. (1966). *In* "Physiology of Echinodermata" (R. A. Boolootian, Ed.), pp. 329–358. J. Wiley (Interscience), London and New York.

Andrew, W. (1962). *Amer. Zool.* **2**, 285–297.

Andrew, W. (1965). "Comparative Hematology". Grune and Stratton, New York and London.

Bang, F. B. (1967). *Fed. Proc.* **26**, 1680–1684.

Bang, F. B. (1970). *J. Reticuloendoth. Soc.* **7**, 161–172.

Bang, F. B. (1975). *Annls N.Y. Acad. Sci.* **266**, 344.

Bang, F. B. and Lemma, A. (1962). *J. Insect. Pathol.* **4**, 401–414.

Bargman, W. and Behrens, B. (1964). *Z. Zellforsch. mikrosk. Anat..* **63**, 120–128.

Behre, E. (1932). *Anat. Rec.* **54** (Suppl.), 92.

Bertheussen, K. (1979). *Exp. Cell Res.* **120**, 373–381.

Bertheussen, K. and Seljelid, R. (1978). *Exp. Cell Res.* **111**, 401–412.

Bertolini, F. (1937). *Proc. 12th Int. Congr. Zool.* **2**, 759–760.

Bookhout, C. G. and Greenburg, N. P. (1940). *Biol. Bull., Woods Hole* **79**, 309–320.

Boolootian, R. A. (1962). *Amer. Zool.* **2**, 275–284.

Boolootian, R. A. and Campbell, J. L. (1964). *Science* **145**, 173–175.

Boolootian, R. A. and Giese, A. C. (1958). *Biol. Bull., Woods Hole* **115**, 53–63.

Boolootian, R. A. and Giese, A. C. (1959). *J. exp. Zool.* **140**, 207–229.

Boolootian, R. A. and Lasker, R. (1964). *Comp. Biochem. Physiol.* **11**, 273–289.

Brillouet, C., Luquet, C. and Leclerc, M. (1981). Proc. 1st Congr. Dev. Comp. Immunol. Pergamon Press, Aberdeen (in press).

Buslé, J. (1967). *Cah. Biol. mar.* **8**, 417.

Burnet, F. M. (1968). *Nature* **218**, 426–430.

Burton, M. P. M. (1964). *Nature* **204**, 1218–1219.

Burton, M. P. M. (1966). *Nature* **211**, 1095–1096.

Carton, Y. (1974). *Ann. Immunol. (Inst. Pasteur)* **125c**, 731–745.

Chapeaux, M. (1893). *Bull. Acad. r. Belg. Cl. Sci, ser 3* **26**, 227–232.

Chien, P. K., Johnson, P. T., Holland, N. D. and Chapman, F. A. (1970). *Protoplasma* **71**, 419–442.

Coffano, K. A. and Hinegardner, R. T. (1977). *Science* **197**, 1389–1390.

Cowden, R. R. (1968). *J. Invertebr. Pathol.* **10**, 151–159.

Crescitelli, F. (1945). *Biol. Bull., Woods Hole* **88**, 30–36.

Cuénot, L. (1887). *Archs Zool. exp. gén. ser. 2* **5**, 1–44.

Cuénot, L. (1891). *Archs Zool. exp. gén. ser. 2* **9**, 593–670.

Cuénot, L. (1901). *Archs Zool. exp. gén. ser. 3* **9**, 233–259.

Davidson, E. (1953). *Biol. Bull., Woods Hole* **105**, 372.

Delaunay, H. (1931). *Biol. Rev.* **6**, 265–301.

Donnellon, J. A. (1938). *Physiol. Zoöl.* **11**, 389–397.

Doyle, W. L. and McNeil, G. F. (1964). *Quart. Jl. Microsc. Sci.* **105**, 7–12.

Durham, H. E. (1887). *Proc. R. Soc., B* **43**, 327–330.

Durham, H. E. (1891). *Quart. Jl. Microsc. Sci.* **33**, 81–121.

Edds, K. T. (1977a). *Exp. Cell Res.* **108**, 452–456.

Edds, K. T. (1977b). *J. Cell Biol.* **73**, 479–491.

Edds, K. T. (1979). *J. Cell Biol.* **83**, 109–115.

Edds, K. T. (1980). *Cell Motility* (in press).

Endean, R. (1958). *Quart. Jl. Microsc. Sci.* **99**, 47–60.

Endean, R. (1966). *In* "Physiology of Echinodermata" (R. A. Boolootian, Ed.), pp. 301–328. J. Wiley (Interscience), London and New York.

Fabre, T., Fayollas, G., Richoilleu, G. and Lecal, J. (1969). *Bull. Soc. Hist. nat. Toulouse* **105**, 234–262.
Farmanfarmaian, A. (1966). *In* "Physiology of Echinodermata" (R. A. Boolootian, Ed.), pp. 245–265. J. Wiley (Interscience), London and New York.
Farmanfarmaian, A. (1968). *Comp. Biochem. Physiol.* **24**, 855–863.
Ferguson, J. C. (1964). *Biol. Bull., Woods Hole* **126**, 33–53.
Ferguson, J. C. (1966). *Trans. Amer. Microsc. Soc.* **85**, 200.
Ferguson, J. C. (1970). *Biol. Bull., Woods Hole* **138**, 14–25.
Foettinger, A. (1880). *Archs Biol., Paris* **1**, 405–415.
Fontaine, A. R. and Lambert, P. (1973). *Can. J. Zool.* **51**, 323–332.
Fontaine, A. R. and Lambert, P. (1977). *Can. J. Zool.* **55**, 1530–1544.
Fox, D. L. (1953). "Animal Biochromes and Structural Colours." Cambridge University Press.
Fox, D. L. and Hopkins, T. S. (1966). *In* "Physiology of Echinodermata" (R. A. Boolootian, Ed), pp. 277–300. J. Wiley (Interscience), London and New York.
Frenzel, J. (1892). *Archs Anat. Physiol.* (*Physiol. Abt.*), pp. 81–114.
Friedheim, E. A. H. (1932). *C. r. Seanc. Soc. Biol.* **111**, 505–507.
Geddes, P. (1880). *Archs Zool. exp. gén.* **8**, 483–496.
Ghiradella, H. T. (1965). *Biol. Bull., Woods Hole* **128**, 77–89.
Giese, A. C. (1966). *In* "Physiology of Echinodermata" (R. A. Boolootian, Ed.), pp. 757–797. J. Wiley (Interscience), London and New York.
Goodwin, T. W. and Srisukh, S. (1950). *Biochem. J.* **47**, 69–76.
Heatfield, B. M. and Travis, D. F. (1975a). *J. Morphol.* **145**, 13–50.
Heatfield, B. M. and Travis, D. F. (1975b). *J. Morphol.* **145**, 51–72.
Hérouard, E. (1889). *Archs Zool. exp. gén. ser 2.* **7**, 535–704.
Hetzel, H. R. (1963). *Biol. Bull., Woods Hole* **125**, 289–301.
Hetzel, H. R. (1965). *Biol. Bull., Woods Hole* **128**, 102–111.
Hiestand, W. A. (1940). *Trans. Wis. Acad. Sci. Arts Lett.* **32**, 167–174.
Hildemann, W. H. and Dix, T. G. (1972). *Transplantation* **15**, 624–633.
Hildemann, W. H. and Reddy, A. L. (1973). *Fed. Proc.* **32**, 2188–2194.
Hildemann, W. H., Raison, R. L., Cheung, G., Hull, C. J., Akaka, L. and Okamoto, J. (1977). *Nature* **270**, 219–223.
Hilgard, H. R. (1970). *Transpl. Proc.* **11**, 240–242.
Hilgard, H. R. and Phillips, J. R. (1968). *Science* **161**, 1243–1245.
Hilgard, H. R., Hinds, W. E. and Phillips, J. H. (1967). *Comp. Biochem. Physiol.* **23**, 814–824.
Hogben, L. and Van der Lingen, J. (1928). *J. exp. Biol.* **5**, 292–294.
Holland, L. Z., Giese, A. C. and Hopkins, J. H. (1967). *Comp. Biochem. Physiol.* **21**, 361–371.
Holland, N. D., Phillips, J. H. and Giese, A. C. (1965). *Biol. Bull., Woods Hole* **128**, 259–270.
Hyman, L. H. (1955). "The Invertebrates. Vol. IV, Echinodermata: the Coelomate Bilateria." McGraw Hill, New York.
Jacobson, F. W. and Millott, N. (1953). *Proc. R. Soc.* **141**, 231–247.
Jefferies, R. P. S. (1967). *In* "Echinoderm Biology" (N. Millott, Ed.). Symp. Zool. Soc. Lond., 20, 163–208.
Johnson, P. T. (1969a). *J. Invertebr. Pathol.* **13**, 25–41.
Johnson, P. T. (1969b). *Histochemie* **17**, 213–231.
Johnson, P. T. (1969c). *J. Invertebr. Pathol.* **13**, 42–62.
Johnson, P. T. (1970). *Comp. Biochem. Physiol.* **37**, 289–300.

Johnson, P. T. and Beeson, R. J. (1966). *Life Sci.* **5**, 1641–1666.
Johnson, P. T. and Chapman, F. A. (1970). *J. Invertebr. Pathol.* **16**, 268–276.
Johnson, P. T. and Chapman, F. A. (1971). *J. Invertebr. Pathol.* **17**, 95–106.
Johnson, P. T., Chien, P. K. and Chapman, F. A. (1970). *J. Invertebr. Pathol.* **16**, 466–469.
Kaplan, G. and Bertheussen, K. (1977). *Scand. J. Immunol.* **6**, 1289–1296.
Karp, R. D. (1976). *In* "Phylogeny of Thymus and Bone Marrow-Bursa Cells" (R. K. Wright and E. L. Cooper, Eds), pp. 37–44. Elsevier, Amsterdam.
Karp, R. D. and Hildemann, W. H. (1975). *In* "Immunologic Phylogeny" (W. H. Hildemann and A. A. Benedict, Eds), Vol. 54, pp. 137–150. Plenum Press, New York and London.
Karp, R. D. and Hildemann, W. H. (1976). *Transplantation* **22**, 434–439.
Kawamoto, N. (1927). *Sci. Rep. Tôhoku. Imp. Univ. Biol.* **2**, 239–264.
Kindred, J. E. (1921). *Biol. Bull., Woods Hole* **41**, 144–152.
Kindred, J. E. (1924). *Biol. Bull., Woods Hole* **46**, 228–251.
Kindred, J. E. (1926). *Biol. Bull., Woods Hole* **50**, 147–154.
Kobayashi, S. (1932). *Sci. Rep. Tôhoku. Imp. Univ. Biol.* **7**, 211–227.
Kollmann, M. (1908). *Annls. Sci. nat (b). ser. 9* **8**, 1–240.
Kuhn, K. and Wallenfels, K. (1940). *Ber. at. chem. Ges.* **73**, 458–464.
Liebman, E. (1950). *Biol. Bull., Woods Hole* **98**, 46–59.
Lison, L. (1930). *Archs Biol., Paris* **40**, 175–203.
MacMunn, C. A. (1885). *Quart. Jl. Microsc. Sci.* **25**, 469–490.
Manwell, C. (1959). *J. Cell. Comp. Physiol.* **53**, 75–83.
Mason, H. S. (1959). *In* "Pigment Cell Biology" (M. Gordon, Ed.), pp. 563–582. Academic Press, London and New York.
Menton, D. N. and Eisen, A. Z. (1973). *J. Morphol.* **141**, 185–204.
Messer, L. I. and Wardlaw, A. C. (1980). *Proc. Europ. Coll. on Echinoderms, Brussels* (M. Jangoux, Ed.), pp. 319–323. A. A. Balkema, Rotterdam.
Millott, N. (1950). *Biol. Bull., Woods Hole* **99**, 343–344.
Millott, N. (1953). *J. mar. biol. Ass. U.K.* **31**, 529–539.
Millott, N. (1966). *Nature* **209**, 594–596.
Millott, N. (1967). "Echinoderm Biology". Symp. Zool. Soc., London, Vol. 20. Academic Press, London and New York.
Millott, N. (1969). *Experientia* **25**, 756–757.
Millott, N. and Jacobson, F. (1951). *Nature* **168**, 878–879.
Millott, N. and Jacobson, F. (1952). *J. Invest. Derm.* **18**, 91–95.
Millott, N. and Vevers, H. G. (1964). *Nature* **204**, 1216–1217.
Nichols, D. (1969). "Echinoderms", 4th edn. Hutchinson University Library, London.
Noble, P. B. (1970). *Biol. Bull., Woods Hole* **139**, 549–556.
Nomura, S. (1926). *Sci. Rep. Tôhoku, Imp. Univ. ser. 4. Biol.* **2**, 133–138.
Ohuye, T. (1934). *Sci. Rep. Tôhoku, Imp. Univ. ser. 4, Biol.* **9**, 47–52.
Otto, J. J., Kane, R. E. and Bryan, J. (1979). *Cell* **17**, 285–293.
Panijel, J., Leclerc, M., Redziniack, G. and Labidu, M. E. (1977). *In* "Developmental Immunobiology" (J. B. Solomon and J. D. Horton, Eds), pp. 91–97, Elsevier, Amsterdam.
Pilkington, J. B. (1969). *J. mar. Biol. Ass. U.K.* **49**, 857–877.
Prendergast, R. A. (1971). *Fed. Proc.* **30**, 647–655.
Prendergast, R. A. and Suzuki, M. (1970). *Nature* **227**, 277–279.
Prendergast, R. A. and Unanue, E. R. (1970). *Fed. Proc.* **29**, 771–782.

Prendergast, R. A., Cole, G. A. and Henney, C. S. (1974). *N.Y. Acad. Sci* **234**, 7–17.
Prosser, C. L. and Judson, C. L. (1952). *Biol. Bull., Woods Hole* **102**, 249–251.
Ratcliffe, N. A. and Rowley, A. F. (1979). *Devl. Comp. Immunol.* **3**, 189–221.
Reichensparger, A. (1912). *Z. wiss. Zool.* **101**, 1–69.
Reinisch, C. and Bang, F. B. (1971). *Cell. Immunol.* **2**, 496–503.
Rollefsen, I. (1965). *Arbok. Univ. Bergen. mar. Nat. Ser.* **8**, 3–12.
Schäfer, E. A. (1882). *Proc. R. soc.* **34**, 370–371.
Schinke, H. (1950). *Z. Zellforsch. mikrosk. Anat.* **35**, 311–331.
Schmit, A. R., Rowley, A. F. and Ratcliffe, N. A. (1977). *J. Invertebr. Pathol.* **29**, 232–234.
Smith, V. J. and Ratcliffe, N. A. (1980). *J. Invertebr. Pathol.* **35**, 65–74.
Stang-Voss, C. (1971). *Z. Zellforsch. mikrosk. Anat.* **122**, 76–84.
Stang-Voss, C. (1974). *In* "Contemporary Topics in Immunobiology" (E. L. Cooper, Ed.), Vol. IV, pp. 65–75. Plenum Press, New York and London.
Stott, F. C. (1955). *Proc. R. Soc.* **125**, 63–72.
Tanaka, Y. (1958). *Bull. Fac. Fish. Hokkaido. Univ.* **9**, 14–28.
Taylor, R. L. (1969). *J. Invertebr. Pathol.* **14**, 427–428.
Théel, H. (1896). *Terstskrift für Lillyeborg, Uppsala*, pp. 47–58.
Théel, H. (1921). *Arch. für Zool.* **25**, 1–40.
Tiedemann, F. (1816). Preisschr. Parisen. Akad., Paris, Landshut.
Tyler, A. (1939). *Proc. Nat. Acad. Sci. Wash.* **25**, 523–528.
Unestam, T. and Nylund, J. E. (1972). *J. Invertebr. Pathol.* **19**, 94–106.
Vanden Bossche, J. P. and Jangoux, M. (1976). *Nature* **261**, 227–228.
Van der Heyde, H. C. (1922). *Biol. Bull., Woods Hole* **42**, 95–98.
Vethamany, V. G. and Fung, M. (1972). *Can. J. Zool.* **50**, 77–81.
Vevers, G. (1963). Proc. 16th Int. Congr. Zool. Washington D.C., pp. 120–122.
Vevers, G. (1966). *In* "Physiology of Echinodermata" (R. A. Boolootian, Ed.), pp. 267–275. J. Wiley (Interscience), New York.
Wardlaw, A. C. and Unkles, S. E. (1978). *J. Invertebr. Pathol.* **32**, 25–34.
Yoshida, M. (1966). *In* "Physiology of Echinodermata" (R. A. Boolootian, Ed.). J. Wiley (Interscience) London and New York.

Section VIII

Urochordates

16. Urochordates

R. K. WRIGHT

Department of Anatomy, School of Medicine, Center for the Health Sciences, University of California, Los Angeles, California 90024, U.S.A.

CONTENTS

I. Introduction

Lesser Deuterostomes include the subphyla Urochordata and Cephalochordata of the phylum Chordata. They possess all the chordate characteristics at least in some stage of their life. The Cephalochordata, often collectively called *Amphioxus* (*Branchiostoma*), are small, translucent, free-living marine animals. Their circulatory system has the characteristics of both an open and closed system (Moller and Philpott, 1973) and has been described by several investigators (Lankester, 1889; Benham, 1894; Franz, 1927; von Skramlik, 1938). They have no true heart or capillaries and blood vessels occur as lacunae within the connective tissue matrix or as contractile vessels consisting of a single layer of myoepithelial cells (Moller and Philpott, 1973). No circulating cellular elements have been observed within the blood (Franz, 1927; Moller and Philpott, 1973) and the presence of analogous counterparts within the coelom (coelomocytes) is uncertain. Thus, the main focus of this chapter will be on the Urochordata.

The Urochordata, commonly referred to as tunicates or ascidians, are marine animals with world-wide distribution. The larval stage is free living while adults are generally sessile. There are, however, some pelagic species. As a group, the tunicates are divided into three classes: Ascidiacea, Thaliacea and Larvacea (Table I). The Ascidiacea contain the majority of species and are the most common and typical tunicates. They may be colony-forming or solitary. The Thaliacea, colony-forming and solitary ascidians, and Larvacea, solitary tunicates, are pelagic and specialized for a planktonic existence.

Literature on the tunicate circulatory system, blood and blood cells is extensive, spanning 145 years. Historically, the circulatory system was first described by Lister (1834), Milne-Edwards (1842) and Van Beneden (1847). Recognition of the systematic position of tunicates (Kowalevsky, 1867, 1871) stimulated widespread interest in the group. Between 1866 and 1901, the embryological development of the heart was investigated (reviewed by Selys-Longchamps, 1901) and reviews on blood cell types were published (Cuénot, 1891; Kollmann, 1908). Comparative and systematic studies on

TABLE I. Tunicate classification.

Class	Order	Suborder	Families
Ascidiacea	Enterogona	Aplousobranchiata	Clavelinidae
			Polyclinidae
			Didemnidae
		Phlebobranchiata	Cionidae
			Diazonidae
			Perophoridae
			Corellidae
			Ascidiidae
	Pleurogona	Stolidobranchiata	Styelidae
			Pyuridae
			Molgulidae
Thaliacea	Pyrosomida		
	Doliolida		
	Salpida		
Larvacea	Copelata		

blood cells followed with the publications of Azéma (1937), George (1939) and Pérès (1943). High concentrations of vanadium were first reported by Henze (1911), followed by the demonstration that vanadium was concentrated by blood cells (Henze, 1913a). Numerous studies since then have been devoted to the subject of heavy metal accumulation, its chemistry and distribution within tunicates. In the past 20 years, functional studies on blood cells have appeared and recently the first comprehensive review was published on the circulatory system, blood and blood cells (Goodbody, 1974). Since its publication, additional investigations have provided new information on blood cell functions, interrelationships and origins.

II. Structure of the circulatory system

For complete descriptions on the circulatory system, the publications of Brien (1948), Berrill (1950), Millar (1953), Burighel and Brunetti (1971) and Mukai *et al.* (1978) should be consulted. The circulatory system consists of a tubular heart enclosed in a pericardium. Blood is pumped through the system by means of peristaltic contractions originating at one end of the heart. Due to the presence of two pacemakers, one at each end of the heart, the direction of peristalsis and blood flow reverses periodically. The heart contains no valves. A single blood vessel exits from each end of the heart, distributing blood throughout the animal.

A. Circulation

The principal features of the circulatory system have been reviewed (Goodbody, 1974). For ease of reference, the general disposition of principal blood vessels in an adult solitary tunicate is illustrated in Fig. 1. At the abvisceral end of the heart, a large vessel is given off, running under the endostyle and a second vessel crosses the mantle to supply the test. The subendostylar vessel supplies branches to the mantle and branchial sac. From the branchial sac, blood collects into a dorsal branchial sinus which also receives blood from the body and delivers it to the alimentary canal. A series of blood spaces and channels circulate the blood around the viscera

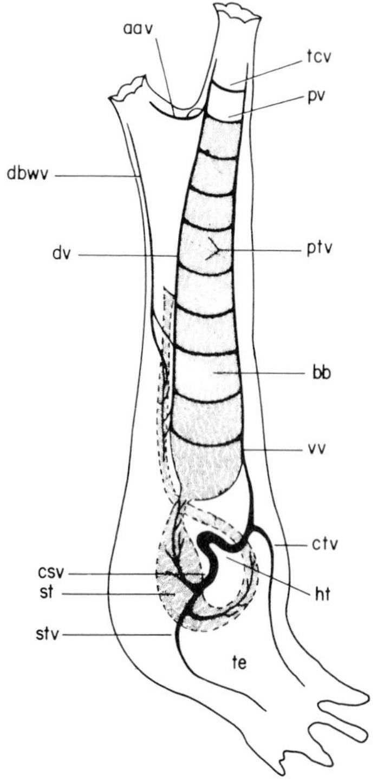

Fig. 1. Diagram showing the principal blood vessels in an adult solitary tunicate, *Ciona intestinalis*, as viewed from the right side. Redrawn from Millar (1953). Abbreviations: aav, anterior atrial vessel; bb, branchial basket (pharynx); csv, cardio-stomachic vessel; ctv, cardio-test vessel; dbwv, dorsal body wall vessel; dv, dorsal vessel; ht, heart; ptv, pharyngeal transverse vessels; pv, peripharyngeal band vessel; st, stomach; stv stomacho-test vessel; tcv, tentacle circular vessel; te, test; vv, ventral vessel.

before collecting into a visceral vessel that rejoins the heart along with a second test vessel at the visceral end.

The two test vessels form a network of vessels that ramify throughout the test in many tunicates. In some species, this network of vessels ends in terminal ampullae at the periphery of the test. In colonial tunicates, the ampullae and vessels are capable of autonomous, coordinated contractions which are unaffected by the reversal of heart beat. No evidence of nervous elements in the vascular system is known.

B. Heart

The embryogenesis of the heart has been studied in *Clavelina rissoana* (Van Beneden and Julin, 1885), *Ciona intestinalis* (Selys-Longchamps, 1901) and *Morchellium argus* (Brien and Blanjean, 1939). In all three, the heart arises as a mesodermal plate lying between the ventral endoderm and ectoderm. The plate thickens laterally and a groove appears along the centre to form a long tubular pericardium. One side of the pericardium invaginates, forming a longitudinal fold with the lips approximated. The tube thus formed constitutes the heart which remains attached to the pericardium along the length of the original suture (raphe). A band of undifferentiated cells runs the length of the heart opposite and parallel to the raphe and may be responsible for the increase in circumference of the heart during growth (Millar, 1953).

The heart consists of a single layer of fusiform shaped myoepithelial cells whose size varies from species to species. The basal or luminal part of each cell contains a bundle of cross striated myofibrils. At the raphe, the myoepithelial cells are fused together by a thin layer of connective tissue. There are conflicing reports on the question of cardiac innervation, but on the basis of numerous physiological studies, this appears to be wanting (see reviews of Krijgsman, 1956; Ebara, 1971; Goodbody, 1974). Heart ultrastructure has been studied in *C. intestinalis* (Kawaguti and Ikemoto, 1958; Schulze, 1964; Ichikawa, 1966; Kriebel, 1968). *Ascidia sidneyensis* (Kalk, 1970), *Corrella willmeriana* (Oliphant and Cloney, 1972), *Ascidiella* sp. (Lorber and Rayns, 1972), *Boltenia ovifera* (Weiss and Morad, 1974; Weiss *et al.*, 1976) and *Corella eumyota* (Lorber and Rayns, 1977).

C. Blood vessels

The blood channels through which the blood circulates are called vessels. True blood vessels however, are lacking and the vascular system is essentially a haemocoel (Berrill, 1950) with blood flowing into various sinuses or lacunae in the connective tissue. There are no muscular arteries, valvular veins or dilatable capillaries. The lacunae are not lined with an endothelium except at the end of the heart where there is a loose reticulum of cells lining the large vessels (Millar, 1953). These cells are irregular in outline and have several processes which make contact with those of neighbouring cells. Principal channels have a connective tissue lining, one cell thick. In the larger efferent vessels, smooth muscle fibres may be present (Fernandez, 1904; von Skramlik, 1929). Test vessels are lined with an epithelium consisting of a single layer of large columnar epidermal cells. Blood cells can be observed migrating across the walls of the vessels, penetrating the test substance. In many monoascidians and colonial tunicates, the test vessels terminate in knob-like bulbils (ampullae) near the periphery of the test. Fine structural features of these ampullae have been described in *Botryllus primigenus* (Katow and Watanabe, 1978).

III. Blood plasma

The plasma or fluid portion of the blood is colourless although in many species it may appear coloured due to the presence of various pigments within the blood cells. Analysis of plasma components have been determined in *Phallusia mamillata* (Henze, 1911, 1912; Bialaszewicz, 1933; Webb, 1939; Robertson, 1954), *Ascidia atra* (Hecht, 1918; Fulton, 1920), *C. intestinalis* (Bialaszewicz, 1933), *Pyura stolonifera* (Webb, 1939, 1956; Endean, 1955a), *Boltenia ovifera* (Weiss *et al.*, 1976) and *Salpa maxima* (Robertson, 1954). Ascidian plasma is iso-osmotic with sea water, slightly alkaline, acid or neutral in pH and contains a low concentration of sulphate ions and protein. It has a low carbon dioxide capacity and oxygen concentrations are similar to those of sea water. There is no loosely bound oxygen in the plasma. No specialized respiratory carriers for oxygen are present. Contrary to early suggestions that the vanadium chromogen present in some blood cells may function as a respiratory catalyst, subsequent studies have demonstrated that this is not concerned with oxygen transport (Webb, 1939, 1956; Macara *et al.*, 1979).

Plasma proteins probably do not function in controlling osmotic intake of water or loss of salts. Instead, they may be part of the ascidian internal defence system and analogous to vertebrate globulins. Ascidian plasma can agglutinate a variety of vertebrate erythrocytes (Fuke and Sugai, 1972; Wright, 1973, 1974; Bretting and Renwrantz, 1973; Renwrantz and Uhlenbruck, 1974; Parrinello and Patricolo, 1975; Anderson and Good, 1975). The chemical and biophysical characteristics of these agglutinins, called haemagglutinins (Table II), suggests they are high molecular weight

TABLE II. Chemical and biophysical characteristics of the haemagglutinin in tunicate blood plasma.

Characteristics	*Ciona intestinalis*	*Ascidia malaca*	*Phallusia mamillata*	*Halocynthia pyriformis*	*Styela plicata*
Agglutinating activity towards	human, rabbit, rat, sheep, guinea pig, mouse, duck and fish erythrocytes	human, dolphin, rat, rabbit, calf and swine erythrocytes	human, calf, horse, swine, sheep, rabbit, rat, dolphin, chicken, toad, frog and eel erythrocytes	human, rabbit, ox, sheep, goat, swine, calf, guinea pig, horse, pigeon, duck, goose, chicken and turkey erythrocytes	rabbit and mouse erythrocytes
Heat lability	70°C	75°C	75°C	50°C	>140°C
pH activity range		2–10	2–10	6–10	2–10
Dialyzable	no	no	no	no	no
Ca^{2+} or Mg^{2+} required for activity	yes	no	no	yes	no
Precipitated by $(NH_4)_2SO_4$ or distilled water		yes	yes	yes	yes
Trypsin sensitive				yes	no
Pepsin sensitive		yes	yes		
2-Mercaptoethanol sensitive		yes	yes		
Periodate sensitive		no	no		yes
Saccharide inhibitor				*N*-acetyl-neuraminic acid	
Molecular weight					>800 000
Chemical nature	protein	protein	protein	protein	polysaccharide or mucopolysaccharide
Reference	Wright (1973, 1974)	Parrinello and Patricolo (1975)	Parrinello and Patricolo (1975)	Anderson and Good (1975)	Fuke and Sugai (1972)

proteins except in *Styela plicata*. They appear to be part or all of the plasma proteins since haemagglutinin levels (titres) are proportional to protein concentrations (Wright, 1973; Wright and Cooper, 1975) and titres can be reduced or abolished by removal of plasma proteins (Parrinello and Patricolo, 1975; Anderson and Good, 1975). The erythrocyte binding proteins of *Pyura stolonifera* are a heterogeneous population of molecules (800 000 daltons) consisting of a single 65 000–70 000 dalton subunit (Marchalonis and Warr, 1978; Form *et al*., 1979). These molecules resemble vertebrate immunoglobulin in charge heterogeneity and polyacrylamide gel analysis shows that the subunit resembles the μ heavy immunoglobulin chain (Marchalonis and Warr, 1978). The source of these haemagglutinins is unknown, but they may be synthesized and released by the blood cells. Their physiological significance is as yet undefined and it has been suggested that they function as opsonins, enhancing phagocytosis (Wright, 1974), as humoral recognition factors (Anderson and Good, 1975), are necessary for cell to cell adherence (Fuke and Sugai, 1972), or represent a primitive μ-like chain that is ancestral to vertebrate immunoglobulin polypeptide chains (Marchalonis and Warr, 1978).

IV. Origin and formation of blood cells

A. Blood cell ontogeny

Embryological origins of ascidian blood cells have been investigated only in the colonial tunicate *Clavelina picta* (Cowden, 1968). Within developing embryos, prospective blood forming mesodermal cells arise from a cell mass formed by cells of the archenteron. Morphologically, these cells resemble the haemoblasts found in adult haematogenic tissue (Ermak, 1976). In early tail bud stages, the haemoblasts extend around the coelom, lying adjacent to the ectoderm.

Continued development of the embryo leads to an elongated "tadpole" larvae. Upon hatching, the free swimming larvae have a functional blood vascular system and circulating blood cells (Andrew, 1961). Haemoblasts have migrated to the tissues of the gill slits (pharynx), localizing in the transverse bars of the stigmata epithelium (Ermak, 1976) and have also migrated to the sides of the intestine (Kowalevsky, 1871). At this stage of ascidian development, haemoblasts begin to differentiate, giving rise to the blood cell types of adult forms. In *Ecteinascidia turbinata*, lymphocytes and granular leucocytes are occasionally seen and morula cells are abundant (Andrew, 1961) (see section on blood cell types, below). Morula type cells are also present in late tail bud stages of *C. picta* (Cowden, 1968).

After a brief larval period, metamorphosis occurs, transforming the larva into a juvenile adult. Following transformation, haemoblasts continue to multiply and differentiate in the pharyngeal wall around the prostigmata and migrate to other parts of the body. They become associated with the connective tissues or external gut lining in some species or with certain areas of the body wall in other species (Ermak, 1976). From these locations, the haemoblasts give rise to all other blood cell types found in the adult ascidian.

B. Haemopoietic tissues

The origin and replacement of blood cells in adult ascidians occurs in haematopoietic tissues distributed in various parts of the body. These tissues may be diffuse or organized into distinct nodules. In salps, they are located in specialized parts of the blood lacunae (Todaro, 1875; Fernandez, 1904; Brien, 1928; Pérès, 1943). In other Thaliacea, the Pyrosomidae, haematogenic sites have been identified in the connective tissues of the branchial sac and as two distinct masses along the dorsal blood sinus (Pérès, 1943; Brien, 1948). Three main areas of haematogenic activity are present in Ascidiacea; (1) in the connective tissue around the alimentary canal; (2) in the pharyngeal wall and transverse vessels of the branchial sac; (3) in discrete nodules located in the body wall (Millar, 1953; Ermak, 1976).

The distribution of haematogenic sites in several Ascidiacea have been investigated by Ermak (1976). In *C. intestinalis*, these sites are abundant in the transverse bars of the branchial sac (Fig. 2) where the haematopoietic cells are arranged in small diffuse clusters adjacent to the pharyngeal epithelium. Similar diffuse clusters are also associated with the connective tissue around the gut. Small haematogenic nodules located around the gut occur in *Chelysoma productum* and *Ascidia ceratodes*. These nodules are associated with the connective tissue and blood channels but not the external or internal gut epithelia. Nodules also frequently occur near the gonads. The colonial ascidians *Polyclinum planum* and *Euherdmania claviformis* have many small patches of haematopoietic cells in the connective tissue of the gut loop. Distinct nodules occur in the connective tissue of the body wall adjacent to the atrial epithelium in *Molgula verrucifera* and *Pyura haustor*, and frequently border on blood channels. In *Styela clava*, haematopoietic nodules occur predominantly in the pharyngeal and body walls (Figs 3, 4). They lie next to the atrial epithelium and in the connective tissue around blood channels. A few nodules also occur around the post pharyngeal gut.

The cellular organization of *S. clava* haematopoietic nodules is illustrated

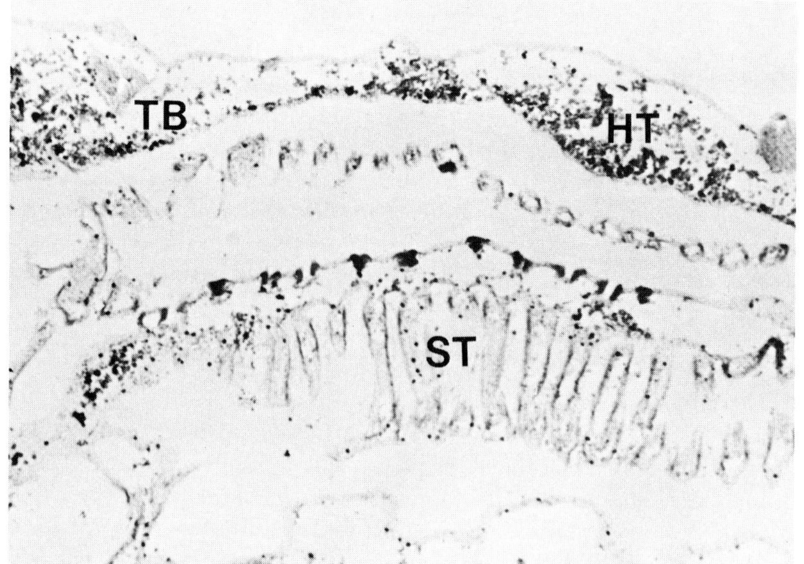

Fig. 2. Autoradiogram of longitudinal section through transverse bar (TB) and rows of stigma (ST) in pharynx of *Ciona intestinalis*. Haematogenic tissue (HT) occurs as diffuse clusters adjacent to the pharyngeal epithelium. (Reproduced with permission from Ermak, 1976.) × 100.

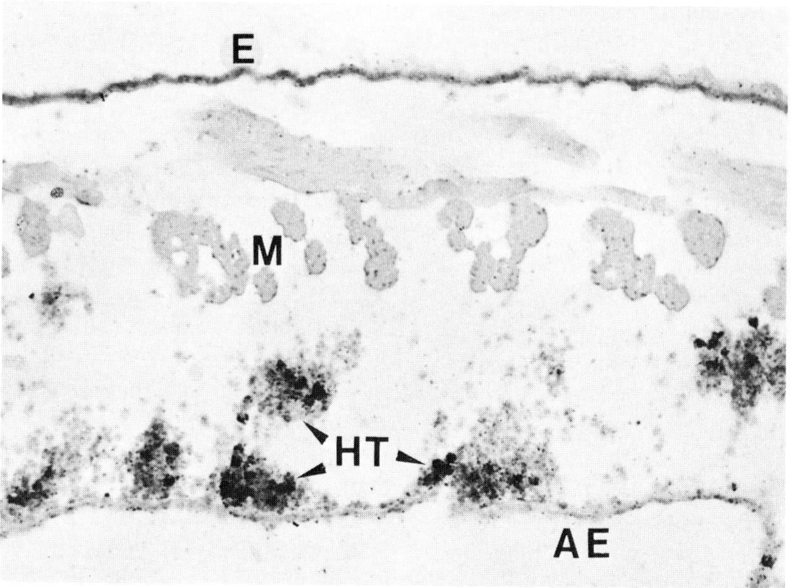

Fig. 3. Autoradiogram of cross section through body wall of *Styela clava* showing labelled haematopoietic nodules (HT) next to the atrial epithelium (AE) and in connective tissue. E, epidermis; M, muscle. (Reproduced with permission from Ermak, 1976.) × 250.

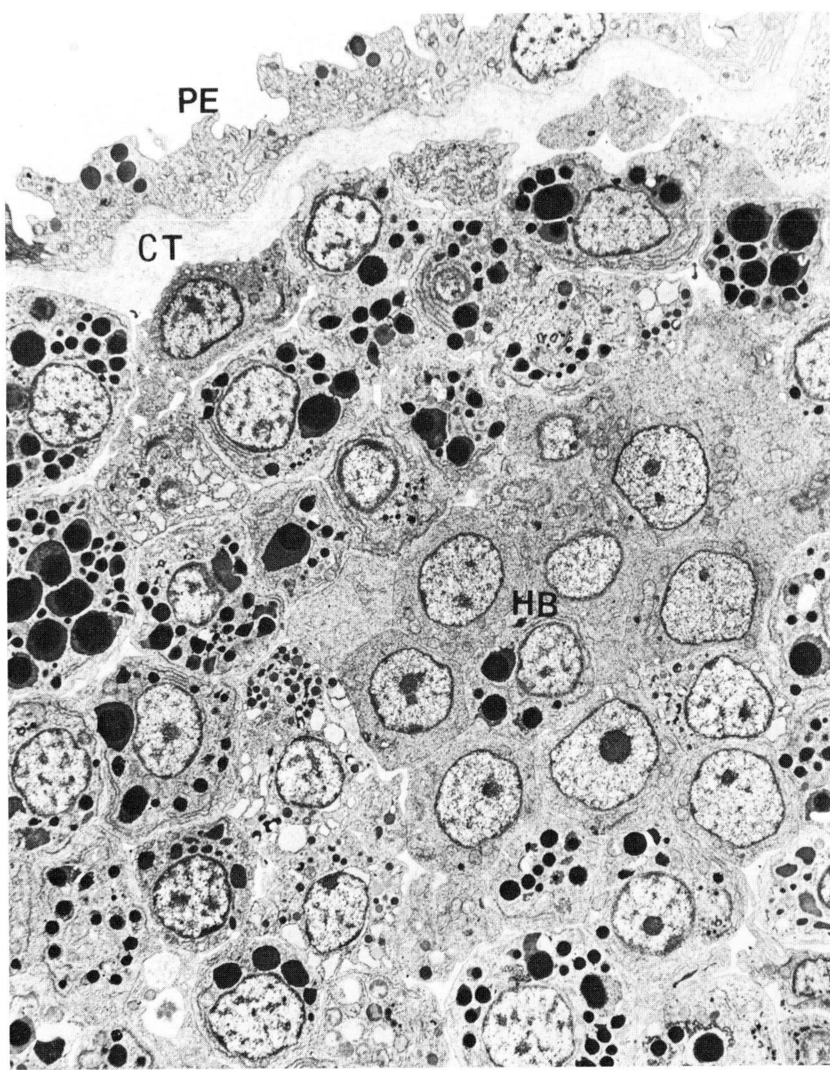

Fig. 4. Electron micrograph of haematopoietic nodule in transverse bar from pharynx of *Styela clava*. HB, haemoblasts surrounded by differentiating blood cells; CT, connective tissue fibres; PE, pharyngeal epithelium. (Reproduced with permission from Ermak, 1976.) × 10 000.

in Fig. 4. Clustered in the centre of the nodule are haemoblasts, surrounded by maturing blood cells in various stages of differentiation. Haemoblasts border directly on one another, giving them an angular outline. They have a large spherical nucleus containing one or two nucleoli and little chromatin (Fig. 5). Differentiating blood cells around these haemoblasts lose their prominent nucleolus and the amount of chromatin increases. Electron dense granules begin to appear in the cytoplasm of some cells. Away from the centre of the nodule, maturing blood cells increase in size, their granules becoming larger and more numerous. Cellular differentiation is also marked by the loss of polyribosomes, the development of elongate mitochondria, a larger Golgi apparatus and long cisternae of rough endoplasmic reticulum. Only a few of the peripheral cells appear fully matured, with complete differentiation apparently occurring in the circulating blood.

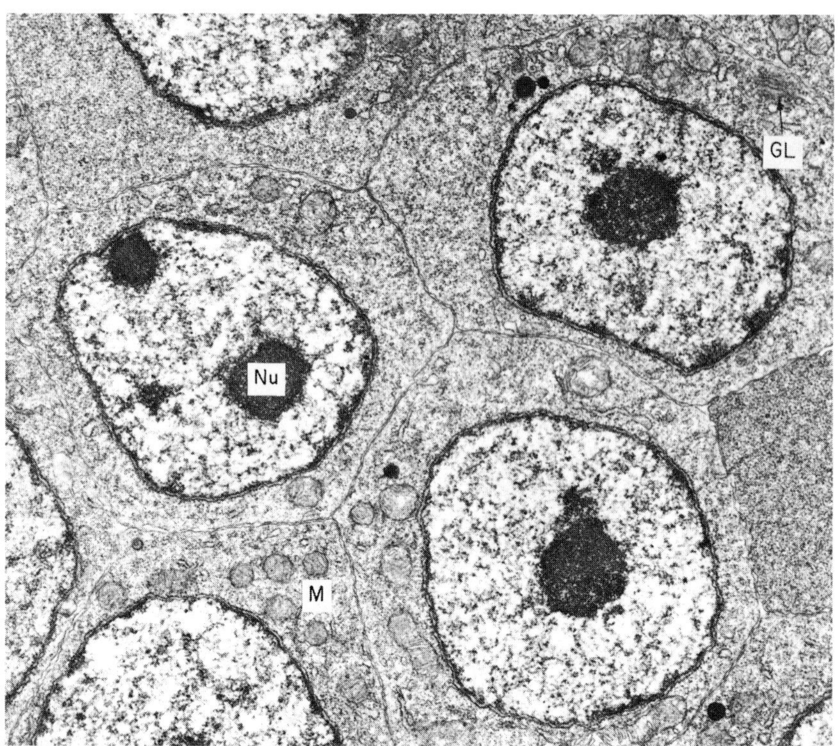

Fig. 5. Haemoblasts from centre of a blood forming nodule in the body wall of *Styela clava*. M, mitochondria; Nu, nucleolus; GL, Golgi. (Reproduced by permission from Ermak, 1976.) ×3200.

Blood cell proliferation rates have been determined in the haematopoietic nodules of *S. clava* (Ermak, 1975) using autoradiography and tritiated thymidine. Following a one hour exposure, blood cells engaged in pre-mitotic DNA synthesis were labelled in the nodules and in the blood channels. In the nodules, haemoblasts, lymphocytes and leucocytes were labelled. By day 20, most of the labelled cells were in the peripheral parts of the nodule. Cells in the interior were no longer labelled and presumably have differentiated into mature blood cells. Few lymphocytes were labelled in the circulating blood, most of the labelled cells being leucocytes and vacuolated cells. At 60 days, most of the blood cells in the nodule were unlabelled. It therefore appears that blood cells have a rapid proliferation rate and are renewed within several weeks. The presence of labelled cells in the blood channels shortly after tritiated thymidine exposure also suggests that some blood cells can divide after they are released from the nodule.

V. Structure and classification of blood cells

Ascidian blood contains 6–9 different cell types that exhibit considerable variation in different species. Blood cells have been intensively investigated in Ascidiacea and to a limited degree in Thalicacea. They appear to be absent in Larvacea (Seeliger, 1911). All blood cells are actively amoeboid and are not confined to the vascular system. Blood cells move freely throughout the animal and are highly concentrated in certain tissues.

A. Blood cell types

Blood cell morphologies have been determined from living and stained preparations by phase and light microscopy (Cuénot, 1891; Fernandez, 1904; Kollmann, 1908; Hecht, 1918; Fulton, 1920; Rapkine and Damboviceanu, 1925; George, 1926, 1930, 1939; Ohuye, 1936; Azéma, 1937; Pérès, 1943, 1944, 1945; Millar, 1953; Endean, 1955a, 1960; Andrew, 1961; Freeman, 1964; Vallee, 1967; Smith, 1970a) and by electron microscopy (Kalk, 1963b; Gansler *et al.*, 1963; Overton, 1966; Ermak, 1976; Botte and Scippa, 1977; Milanesi and Burighel, 1978). The terminology used by these investigators is not always the same. Based on a thorough study of their descriptions, it is possible to identify nine cell types that can be placed into six categories. These categories are: (1) haemoblasts; (2) lymphocytes (classified as such on morphological grounds only, no functional homology with vertebrate lymphocytes is implied); (3) leucocytes, granular and hyaline; (4) vacuolated cells, signet ring, compartment and morula; (5) pigment cells; and (6) nephrocytes.

1. Haemoblasts

Haemoblasts (Fig. 5) are found primarily in the blood forming tissues. They are undifferentiated spherical cells, 5–6 μm in diameter, with a large nucleus and a little basophilic cytoplasm. One or two nucleoli occur in the centre of the nucleus or adjacent to the nuclear membrane. Cytoplasmic organelles cluster to one side or the cell and include several round or oval mitochondria and a small Golgi apparatus. A pair of centrioles lies on the concave side of the Golgi cisternae. Most of the cytoplasm is filled with polyribosomes and a few cisternae of rough endoplasmic reticulum (Ermak, 1976; Milanesi and Burighel, 1978). Haemoblasts can also be found in the circulating blood (Pérès, 1943; Millar, 1953) and because of their morphological similarity to lymphocytes, have probably been identified as lymphocytes by some investigators.

2. Lymphocytes

Lymphocytes (Fig. 6a) are similar in morphology to haemoblasts but are smaller, measuring 3–5 μm in diameter. Several investigators (George, 1939; Andrew, 1961; Overton, 1966) state that lymphocytes have a distinct nucleolus. This may be characteristic of some species, however, recent studies (Ermak, 1976; Milanesi and Burighel, 1978) suggest that such cells may be haemoblasts. The absence of a nucleolus is considered to be characteristic of the lymphocyte (Pérès, 1943; Millar, 1953; Ermak, 1976). Within the nucleus, the chromatin occurs in patches along the nuclear membrane and in the interior of the nucleoplasm. A small ring of homogeneous, finely granular, basophilic cytoplasm contains round or oval mitochondria, polyribosomes and a few profiles of rough endoplasmic reticulum.

3. Leucocytes

Leucocytes consist of two cell types, hyaline and granular. Both are spherical in fixed preparations, varying in size from 6 to 12 μm. They assume a variety of shapes in the living state due to their amoeboid activity and pseudopod formation.

(a) Hyaline leucocytes (Figs 7a, b, c) appear to be the precursors of vacuolated cells (Kalk, 1963b). Their nucleus is round or oval and usually centrally located. The cytoplasm is homogeneous and filled with granules of uniform size. One to many vacuoles containing granular inclusions exhibiting Brownian motion are present. Under phase illumination, the cytoplasm appears reticulated or clumped (Smith, 1970a).

(b) Granular leucocytes (Figs 6b, c, 7d), frequently referred to as macrophages or phagocytes, are characterized by the presence of distinct cytoplasmic granules. These granules exhibit refractive properties under bright field illumination and appear to be associated with a reticular network by phase microscopy (Smith, 1970a). The granules do not fill the cytoplasm but leave a peripheral hyaline area. A centrally located nucleus contains clumped chromatin and no nucleolus. Ultrastructurally, they contain large numbers of oval bodies, 1–2 μm in diameter that vary in density and are embedded in masses of dense 200–300 Å particles with the characteristic appearance of glycogen (Overton, 1966). Rough endoplasmic reticulum surrounds the nucleus.

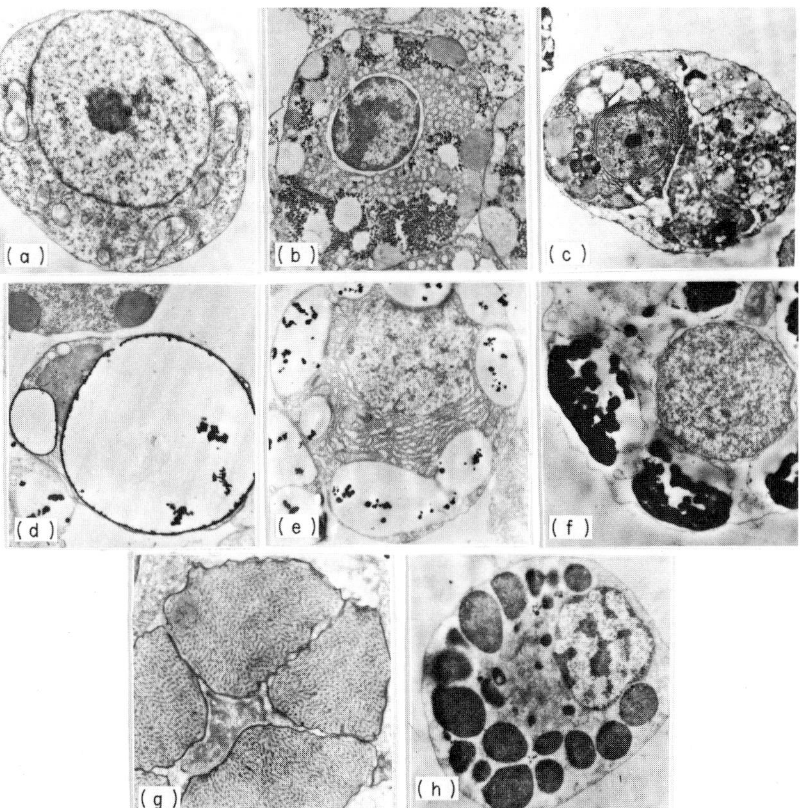

Fig. 6. Fine structure of blood cells in *Perophora viridis*. (a) Lymphocyte, ×4600; (b) granular leucocyte, ×3900; (c) granular leucocyte containing phagocytized material, ×3200; (d) signet ring cell, ×4900; (e) compartment cell, ×4100; (f) morula cell, ×5700; (g) morula cell, ×4100; (h) orange pigment cell, ×4600. (Reproduced with permission from Overton, 1966.)

4. *Vacuolated cells*

Vacuolated cells consist of three cell types, signet ring cells, compartment cells and morula cells (Figs 6d–g, 7a–d). They have a considerable size range and appearance according to their developmental stage, and characteristically contain one or more large vacuoles. Vacuolated cells appear to be interrelated, passing through a progressive cycle from signet ring to compartment to morula cell (Kalk, 1963b). These different stages and their characteristic morphologies probably reflect their physiological activities.

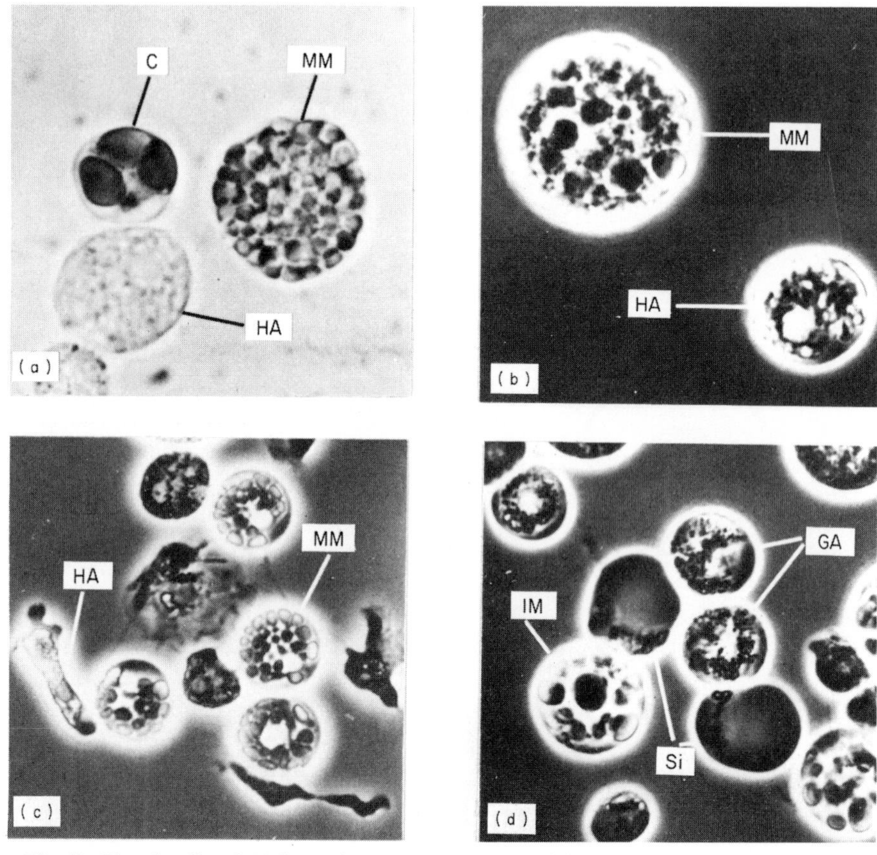

Fig. 7. Blood cells of *Halocynthia aurantium*. (a) Leishman stained smear, ×1500, (b) ×2200, (c) ×920 and (d) ×2200, living cells, phase microscopy. MM, mature morula cell; IM, immature morula cell; C, compartment cell; HA, hyaline leucocyte; GA, granular leucocyte; Si, signet ring cell. (Reproduced with permission from Smith, 1970a.)

(a) Signet ring cells (Figs 6d, 7d) are of variable size, 6–12 μm in diameter. They have a single large fluid-filled acidophilic vacuole containing granules exhibiting Brownian motion. The vacuole is lined by electron-dense material (Kalk, 1963b; Overton, 1966) and enclosed by a peripheral rim of clear structureless cytoplasm. At the periphery of the cell, the nucleus and bulk of the cytoplasm is displaced by the vacuole, forming an eccentric cresent-shaped cap. On the side nearest the vacuole, the nucleus is flattened or concave and usually devoid of a nucleolus. Greenish refractile granules occur in the cytoplasm near the nuçleus in some cells (Endean, 1960).

(b) Compartment cells (Figs 6e, 7a) are spherical with an 8–12 μm diameter. They have a variable number of large round or angular vacuoles at the periphery of the cell, giving it a compartmental appearance. Vacuoles are separated from each other by partitions of clear, non-granular cytoplasm, continuous with the perinuclear cytoplasm. Each vacuole is fluid-filled and contains electron-dense granules of variable size (Overton, 1966). In the living cell, these granules exhibit Brownian movement. The nucleus is centrally located and contains no nucleolus. It is surrounded on one side by mitochondria and numerous profiles of dense rough endoplasmic reticulum and ribosomes (Kalk, 1963b).

(c) Morula cells (Figs 6f, g, 7a–d, 8) are spherical, measuring 8–16 μm in diameter. When released from the blood and allowed to stand, they assume a berry-like or morula appearance (Fig. 7a–d). They have been referred to as green cells, colourless morula cells, vanadocytes and ferrocytes, the latter two names derived from the fact that in some species they contain vanadium whereas in other species they contain iron. Morula cells contain a variable number of tightly packed symmetrically arranged, 2–3 μm vacuoles or globules that appear wedge-shaped in some cells. Non-granular cytoplasmic extensions pass from the perinuclear cytoplasm between and around the vacuoles. In living cells, the vacuoles appear yellowish-green and have a high refractive index. Within the vacuoles are dense inclusions which may be granular or filamentous in character (Fig. 8). The nucleus is usually obscured by the vacuoles and is eccentrically located. It may be compressed into an angular mass by the vacuoles, is devoid of a nucleolus and contains scattered patches of chromatin. To one side of the nucleus is a well-developed Golgi apparatus containing irregularly-shaped masses and an endoplasmic reticulum whose cisternae enclose dense granules (Overton, 1966).

5. *Pigment cells*

Various spherical or disc-shaped coloured cells, 6–13 μm diameter, occur in the blood of some ascidians but are absent in others. The colour of these

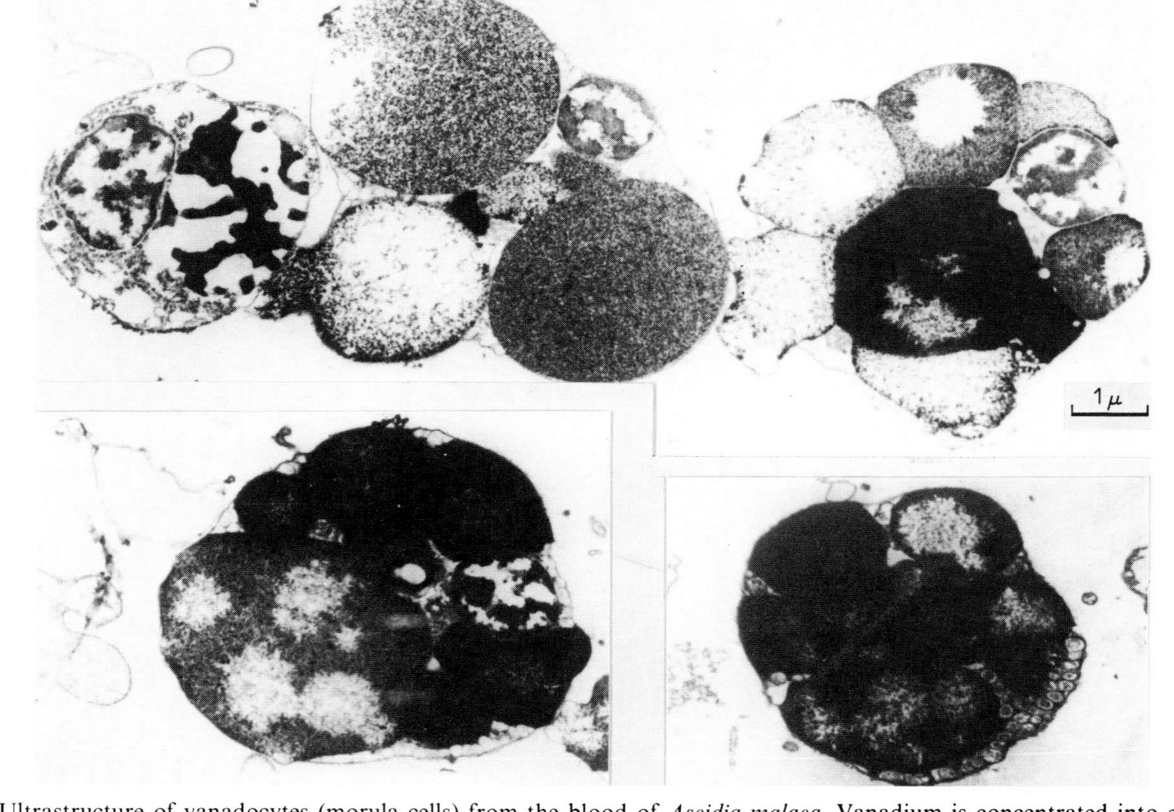

Fig. 8. Ultrastructure of vanadocytes (morula cells) from the blood of *Ascidia malaca*. Vanadium is concentrated into electron-dense cytoplasmic inclusions (vanadophores) that may be homogeneous or show a granulo-filamentous organization. (Reproduced with permission from Botte and Scippa, 1977.) × 10 200.

cells is due to the presence of granules which may be various shades of white, yellow, red, blue, brown or orange. Each species has its own type of pigment cell(s) and they are named after their colouration, i.e. blue cells, red cells, orange cells, etc. The pigments are not suspended in fluid-filled vacuoles but embedded in the cytoplasm. They occur at such high densities that the cytoplasm and nucleus are not visible. Pigments vary in size and shape, being small rounded granules, large globular bodies, fusiform granules or flat elliptical plates. Orange cells (Fig. 6h) are the most commonly encountered pigment cell. In *Perophora viridis*, they are spherical and contain a large number of round, membrane-bound, orange globules which appear to be formed in close association with the Golgi apparatus (Overton, 1966). The orange cells of *P. mammillata* are disc-shaped and the orange pigment is localized in flat, elliptical, membrane-bound plates that show strong birefrigence (Webb, 1939; Endean, 1960). The chemical nature of these pigments will be discussed later.

6. *Nephrocytes*

Nephrocytes are large spherical- or irregularly-shaped cells, up to 40 μm in diameter. They are not present in all species. Nephrocytes have little cytoplasm and a small peripheral nucleus. One or more large, fluid-filled vacuoles occupy most of the cell and contain granules that exhibit Brownian movement. At the EM level, these granules have a geometric form (Milanesi and Burighel, 1978). Instead of granules, the vacuoles may contain large concretions of calculus-like bodies that are brown by transmitted light and white or yellowish-white by reflected light (George, 1939).

B. Blood cell numbers

The number of circulating blood cells and their proportions have been investigated in only a few species (Table III). Considerable differences are present not only between species but also between individual animals of the same species. In general, lymphocytes, leucocytes and pigment cells occur in low percentages and cells of the vacuolated category predominate. The percentage, by volume, of blood occupied by blood cells is in the order of 1% in *P. stolonifera* (Endean, 1955a) to 2% in *Ascidia nigra* (Vallee, 1967). Various parameters such as animal size and physiological status can appreciably affect total and differential blood cell counts. Total cell counts increase as animal size increases in *C. intestinalis* (Wright, 1973). In *Halocynthia aurantium*, there is little change with animal size although hyaline leucocytes increase and other cell types decrease as animal size

TABLE III. Differential and total cell counts of ascidian blood cells.

Species	No. cells per mm^3 × 10^4	Lymphocytes (%)	Leucocytes Granular (%)	Hyaline (%)	Signet ring (%)	Vacuolated cells Compartment (%)	Morula (%)	Pigment cells (%)	Nephrocytes (%)	Reference
PHLEOBOBRANCHIATA										
Ascidia atra	—	<1	5	10	20	1	60	3–5		Fulton (1920)
Ascidia nigra	5·3 (3·2–7·9)	0·5	4	—	21	8	65	1·3	0·4	Vallee (1967)
Ciona intestinalis	—	17	10	17	←	43	→	0·5	12	Millar (1953)
Perophora viridis										
Regressed colony	—	5–12	47–80	—	3–9	1–4	6–16	—		Freeman (1964)
Actively growing	—	0·1–0·5	6–17	—	13–17	3–5	60–65	—		Freeman (1964)
Phallusia mammillata	6·8	rare	← 7	→	5	44	43	<1		Endean (1960)
STOLIDOBRANCHIATA										
Halocynthia aurantium	1·7	5	21	39	2	1	31	—		Smith (1970a)
Molgula manhattensis	2·1 (1·7–2·4)	3	6	—	28	17	43	—	3	Anderson (1971)
Pyura stolonifera	3·7 (1·8–6·8)	5	3	—	← 20	→	70	1	1	Endean (1955a)

increases (Smith, 1970a). Juvenile *C. intestinalis* infected with the gregarine sporozoan *Lankesteria ascidia* exhibit increased numbers of total blood cells (Wright, 1973). From these few studies, it is obvious that this is an area that deserves further attention.

C. Species distribution of blood cell types

Blood cell morphologies have been described for over 70 ascidian species, representing all families of the class Ascidiacea (Tables IV, V, VI) and some families of the class Thaliacea (Table VII). Some features of blood histology are common to all ascidians whereas others appear to be familial or generic in distribution. All ascidians have haemoblasts, lymphocytes, granular leucocytes and vacuolated cells. The major differences between families and species are the presence or absence of hyaline leucocytes, pigment cells and nephrocytes. Absence of a particular cell type may reflect a true absence as in the case for pigment cells and nephrocytes or an oversight of the investigator in recognizing a cell type. The latter may be due to the low frequency of some cell types.

D. Blood cell chemistry and histochemistry

Various methods have been used to determine the chemical composition of ascidian blood cells. Through the use of general histological and supravital stains, specific histochemical stains (Endean, 1953, 1955a, 1960; Smith, 1970b), fluorescent and electron microscopy (Kalk, 1963b; Gansler *et al.*, 1963; Overton, 1966; de Vincentis and Rüdiger, 1967; Botte and Scippa, 1977), blood cell lysate analyses (Endean, 1955a, 1960; Gilbert *et al.*, 1977) and biophysical techniques (Bielig *et al.*, 1966; Swinehart *et al.*, 1974; Kustin *et al.*, 1976), the chemical constitution of each blood cell type is beginning to be characterized. These approaches have helped to clarify some of the many functions blood cells perform since the internal milieu of each cell type reflects, to some degree, its functional capabilities.

1. Carbohydrates, lipids, nucleic acids and proteins

The histochemical composition of *P. stolonifera* (Endean, 1955a), *P. mamillata* (Endean, 1960) and *H. aurantium* (Smith, 1970b) blood cells has been studied in detail. Studies on other species are incomplete or limited to only one cell type. Differences exist not only between different cell types but also between the same blood cell type in different species.

TABLE IV. Species distribution of blood cell types in Ascidiacea, Suborder Aplousobranchiata

Family and species	Blood cell type[a]								Reference
	Haemoblast and/or lymphocyte	Leucocytes		Vacuolated cells			Pigment cells	Nephrocytes	
		Granular	Hyaline	Signet ring	Compartment	Morula			
CLAVELINIDAE									
Clavelina lepadiformis	+[b]	leukocytes à inclusion protéiques	+	cellule vacuolaire		cellule adipeuse	ochre, red	cellule à pigment purique	Azéma (1937)
Clavelina (Polycitor) nana	+	+	+	cellule vacuolaire		leukocyte adipeuse	greenish-yellow	cellule à concretion purique	Azéma (1937)
Clavelina oblonga	+	macrophage	—	+	+	colourless green cell	—	+	George (1939)
Clavelina oblongata	finely granular amoebocyte	coarsely granular amoebocyte	—	vesicular signet ring	amoeboid compartment	green cell	—	brown cell	George (1930)
Clavelina picta	+	macrophage	—	+	+	green cell; colourless green cell	—		George (1939)
	small amoebocyte	coarsely granular amoebocyte	finely granular amoebocyte	unilocular vacuolated cell	bi/trilocular vacuolated cell	green cell	—	brown cell	Andrew (1961)
Distaplia bermudensis	+	macrophage	—	+	+	colourless green cell	—	+	George (1939)
Holozoa (Distaplia) rosea	+	leucocyte granuleux		grand cellule vacuolaire		élément adipeux	brown cells	cellule à concretion purique	Azéma (1937)
Polycitor (Eudistoma) olivaceus	+	macrophage	—	+	+	green cell; colourless green cell	blue-green		George (1939)

POLYCLINIDAE									
Amaroucium areolatum	+	+	+	cellule vacuolaire		cellule adipeuse morulaire	yellow		Azéma (1937)
Amaroucium nordmani	+	leucocyte granuleux protéique	amibocyte	cellule vacuolaire		cellule adipeuse morulaire	yellow		Azéma (1937)
Aplidium (Amaroucium) bermudae	+	macrophage	—	+	+	green cell; colourless green cell	orange		George (1939)
Aplidium (Amaroucium) stellatum	+	macrophage	—	+	+	green cell; colourless green cell	—		George (1939)
Polyclinella azemai	+	amibocyte	amibocyte	cellule vacuolaire			red, grey-blue, purple		Azéma (1937)
Sydnyum (Amaroucium) punctum	+	+	+	cellule vacuolaire		cellule morulaire adipeuse	orange		Azéma (1937)
Sydnyum turbinatum	+	leucocytes granuleux	amibocyte	cellule vacuolaire		cellule vacuolaire		cellule à pigment purique	Azéma (1937)
Synocium (Morchellium) argus	+	+	+	cellule vacuolaire		cellule morulaire adipeuse	red		Azéma (1937)
DIDEMNIDAE									
Didemnum (Polysyncraton) amethyst	+	macrophage	—	+	+	green cell; colourless green cell	—		George (1939)
Didemnum maculosum	+	+	+	phagocyte univacuolaire	cellule à sphérule spéciale	cellule à sphérule spéciale			Pérès (1945)
Diplosoma gelatinosum	+	cellule à granulations		cellule vacuolaire		cellule adipeuse	—		Azéma (1937)
Diplosoma macdonaldi	+	macrophage	—	+	+	colourless green cell	—		George (1939)
Polysyncraton lacezei	+	+	+	phagocyte univacuolaire		cellule à sphérules incolores	orange		Pérès (1945)

[a] The morphological term used by each referenced investigator has been preserved. Where the terminology is the same as the heading, it is indicated by a plus (+). A dash (—) indicates that the cell type is absent. Blank spaces indicate no cell type was described that fits the heading.

[b] No attempt has been made to separate these two cell types. Some investigators have referred to haemoblasts as lymphocytes whereas others have separated them. From their descriptions, it is not possible in many cases to determine which cell type they are describing.

TABLE V. Species distribution of blood cell types in Ascidiacea. Suborder Phlebobranchiata.

	Blood cell type[a]								
	Haemoblast and/or lymphocyte	Leucocytes		Vacuolated cells					
Family and species		Granular	Hyaline	Signet ring	Compartment	Morula	Pigment cells	Nephrocytes	Reference
CIONIDAE									
Ciona intestinalis	+[b]	+	+	phagocytes univacuolaire	grand cellule reticulée a noyau achromatique	cellule à grains refringents	orange		Pérès (1943)
	+	acidophil granulocytes; phagocytes	+	vesicular cell	vesicular cell	vesicular cell	orange	+	Millar (1953)
DIAZONIDAE									
Diazona violacea	+	+		cellule vacuolaire		cellule à pigment verte			Azéma (1937)
Rhopalaea neopolitana	+	+	+	cellule vacuolaire		cellule à pigment jaune verdâtre		cellule à gros granules refringents	Azéma (1937)
	+	+	+	cellule univacuolaire		cellule à pigment jaunâtre	orange	cellule à inclusion refringents	Pérès (1943)
PEROPHORIDAE									
Ecteinascidia conklini	+	macrophages	—	+	+	green cell; colourless morula	orange	+	George (1939)
Ecteinascidia turbinata	+	macrophages; coarsely granular amoeboid	finely granular amoeboid	+	+	green cell; colourless morula	orange		George (1930, 1939)
Ecteinascidia turbinata	+ ; small amoebocyte	coarsely granular amoebocyte	finely granular amoebocyte	unilocular vacuolated cell	bi/trilocular vacuolated cell	green cell	orange	amoeboid cell with spheroids	Andrew (1961)
Perophora bermudensis	+	macrophage	—	+	+	green cell; colourless morula	orange		George (1939)
Perophora listeri	+	+	+	cellule vacuolaire vraies	cellule plurivacuolaire	cellule à pigment vert	orange		Azéma (1937)

Perophora viridis	+	granular amoeboid; macrophage	—	+	+	green cell; colourless morula	orange		George (1926, 1939)
	+	+ ; phagocyte		+	+	+ ; green cell	orange		Freeman (1964)
	+	+ ; phagocyte		+	+	+ ; green cell	orange		Overton (1966)
CORELLIDAE									
Chelyosoma siboja	hyaline amoeboid	coarsely granular amoeboid	—	vesicular amoeboid	compartmental amoeboid	green cell		brown cell	Ohuye (1936)
Corella japonica	hyaline amoeboid	coarsely granular amoeboid	finely granular amoeboid	vesicular amoeboid	compartmental amoeboid	green cell; colourless morula	orange; greyish-olive		Ohuye (1936)
Rhodosoma verecundum	+	amibocytes		amibocyte vacuolaires	amibocyte à vacuoles multiples	cellule à grains refringents	—		Pérès (1943)
ASCIDIIDAE									
Ascidia atra	A3	A2	A1	Q1; Q2	Q3; Q4	green cell	orange; blue		Fulton (1920)
Ascidia atra	+ ; small amoebocyte	coarsely granular amoebocyte	finely granular amoebocyte	unilocular vacuolated cell	bi/trilocular vacuolated cell	green cell	orange; blue		Andrew (1961)
Ascidia hygomania	+	macrophage		+	+	green cell; colourless morula	orange		George (1939)
Ascidia mentula		amibocyte typique à granulations	amibocyte typique	amibocyte de réserve à vacuoles	amibocyte de réserve à vacuoles	amibocyte à graisse	orange		Cuénot (1891)
	leucocytes hyaline stades I	leucocytes granules	leucocytes hyalins stades II	cellule vacuolaire		cellule adipeuse			Kollmann (1908)
	+		+	elements à grand vacuole		cellule adipophores	orange		Rapkine and Dambo-viceanu (1925)
	+	+	+	cellule vacuolaire vraie	cellule plurivacuolaire	cellule adipeuse	orange		Azéma (1937)

Table V.—(*continued*)

	Blood cell type[a]								
	Haemoblast and/or	Leucocytes		Vacuolated cells					
Family and species	lymphocyte	Granular	Hyaline	Signet ring	Compartment	Morula	Pigment cells	Nephrocytes	Reference
Ascidia (Phallusia) nigra	finely granular amoebocyte	coarsely granular amoebocyte	—	+	+	green cell; colourless morula	orange; blue		George (1930)
	finely granular amoebocyte	coarsely granular amoebocyte	—	+	vacuolated amoebocyte	+ ; vanadocyte	orange; blue	spherical cell	Vallee (1967)
Ascidia pygmaea	+	amoebocyte		+	+	vanadocyte			Kalk (1963b)
Ascidiella (Ascidia) aspersa	+	+	+	cellule vacuolaire	cellule plurivacuolaire	cellule adipeuse	orange		Azéma (1937)
	+	+	+			cellule à pigment jaune citron	orange		Pérès (1943)
Phallusia mammillata		amibocyte normaux à granules	amibocyte normaux	cellule vesiculaire	cellule vesiculaire	cellule graisseuse	orange		Cuénot (1891)
	leucocyte hyalin stades I	leucocyte granules	leucocyte hyalin stades II	cellule vacuolaire	cellule sphérique	cellule adipeuse	orange		Kollmann (1908)
	+	+	+	cellule vacuolaire vraie	cellule plurivacuolaire	cellule adipeuse	orange		Azéma (1937)
	+	phagocyte; amoebocyte with vacuoles	+	+	+	vanadocyte	orange	cells with reflecting discs	Endean (1960)

[a] The morphological term used by each referenced investigator has been preserved. Where the terminology is the same as the heading, it is indicated by a plus (+). A dash (—) indicates that the cell type is absent. Blank spaces indicate no cell type was described that fits the heading.

[b] No attempt has been made to separate these two cell types. Some investigators have referred to haemoblasts as lymphocytes whereas others have separated them. From their descriptions, it is not possible in many cases to determine which cell type they are describing.

Lymphocytes and hyaline leucocytes contain cytoplasmic protein and carbohydrate, but no lipid. Carbohydrate, in the form of glycogen granules, lipid droplets and large protein granules is present in the cytoplasm of granular leucocytes. Vacuolated cells contain no lipid and the contents of their vacuoles vary among the three species examined. In *P. stolonifera* and *P. mamillata*, intravacuolar contents are polysaccharides and protein while in *H. aurantium*, it is only protein. Nuclei of all cell types contain DNA and RNA and the perinuclear cytoplasm of most cell types contains RNA.

2. *Sulphuric acid*

The presence of free sulphuric acid in vacuolated (morula) cells was first observed by Henze (1911, 1912, 1913a,b) in *Ascidia mamillata* and *Ascidia mentula*. Since these initial observations, several tunicate genera (*Ascidia*, *Phallusia*, *Ascidiella*, *Chelyosoma*, *Perophora* and *Pyura*) have been shown to contain sulphuric acid (Webb, 1939; Endean, 1955a). Sulphuric acid concentrations vary from 0·30 N (1·9 %) in *P. stolonifera* (Endean, 1955a) to 1·83 N (9 %) in *A. mamillata* (Webb, 1939). Morula cells cytolyse easily and early reports on the acidity of tunicate blood plasma can be attributed to the release of their intracorpuscular sulphuric acid (Webb, 1939; Endean, 1955a).

Little is known concerning sulphate ion uptake and accumulation by morula cells. Bielig *et al.* (1961a,b) have shown that the uptake of ionic sulphate from the plasma is slow in *P. mamillata*. Intracorpuscular sulphate concentrations in *P. stolonifera* are similar to those of plasma. *P. mamillata* (Webb, 1939) and *Chelyosoma siboja* (Kobayashi, 1933, 1938), however, have intracorpuscular sulphate concentrations higher than plasma sulphate concentrations, suggesting that morula cells may actively remove sulphate from the plasma. Nothing is known about sulphuric acid synthesis within the morula cell where it appears to be bound in an organic complex with vanadium (Bielig *et al.*, 1954) or one of the other heavy metals (Endean, 1955a). Since these organometallic compounds are stable only at a low pH (Califano and Boeri, 1950), the function of sulphuric acid may be to keep the heavy metal in a reduced state (Goodbody, 1974).

3. *Heavy metals*

The first to indicate the presence of heavy metals in ascidian blood was Henze (1911, 1912) who found 42 000 parts/10^6 vanadium in *P. mamillata*. Since then, vanadium has been found in the blood and tissues of many ascidian species (Webb, 1939, 1956; Kobayashi, 1949; Bertrand, 1950; Vinogradov, 1953; Ciereszko *et al.*, 1963; Swinehart *et al.*, 1974; Danskin, 1978) at concentrations 10^5–10^6 times as great as sea water. In some species,

TABLE VI. Species distribution of blood cell types in Ascidiacea. Suborder Stolidobranchiata.

Family and species	Blood cell type[a]								Reference
	Haemoblast and/or lymphocyte	Leucocytes		Vacuolated cells			Pigment cells	Nephrocytes	
		Granular	Hyaline	Signet ring	Compartment	Morula			
STYELIDAE									
Botrylloides nigrum	+[b]	macrophage	—	+	+	green cell; colourless green cell	—	+	George (1939)
Botryllus leachi	+	+	+	cellule vacuolaire		cellule adipeuse morulaire	orange	cellule pigmentaire vacuolaire brun rouge	Azéma (1937)
Botryllus schlosseri	+	macrophage	—	+	+	green cell; colourless green cell	—	+	George (1939)
Dendrodoa (Styelopsis) grossularia	+	+		amibocyte vacuolaire		cellule adipeuse	yellow	cellule à pigment purique	Azéma (1937)
Distomus variolosus	+			cellule vacuolaire		cellule adipeuse morulaire	yellow; red	cellule vacuolaire à corps purique	Azéma (1937)
Polyandrocarpa (Eusynstyela) tincta	+	macrophage	—	+	+	green cell	carmine	+	George (1939)
Polycarpa circumarata	+	macrophage	—	+	+	colourless green cell	—		George (1939)
Polycarpa obtecta	+	macrophage	—	+	+	colourless green cell	—	+	George (1939)
Polycarpa pomaria	+	+			cellule à granulations jaune brunâtre	cellule adipeuse morulaire		cellule vacuolaire à corps puriques	Azéma (1937)
	+	+	+		cellule à noyau achromatique	cellule adipeuse morulaire	orange		Pérès (1943)

Styela clava	hyaline amoeboid	coarsely granular amoeboid	finely granular amoeboid	vesicular amoeboid	—	green cell; colourless morula	orange	brown cell	Ohuye (1936)
Styela plicata	+	macrophage	—	+	+	colourless green cell	orange		George (1939)
	+	+	+	phagocyte univacuolaire	cellule à noyau achromatique	cellule à grains refringents		cellule à cristallites biréfringents	Pérès (1943)
Symplegma viride	+ ; finely granular amoeboid	coarsely granular amoeboid; macrophage	—	+	+	green cell	orange	+	George (1930, 1939)
PYURIDAE									
Bolteniopsis prenanti	+	grand leucocyte granuleux	+	+				cellule à concretions purique	Azéma (1937)
Cynthia (Pyura) roretzi	hyaline amoeboid	coarsely granular amoeboid	finely granular amoeboid	vesicular amoeboid	compartmental amoeboid	green cell; colourless morula	orange	brown cell	Ohuye (1936)
Halocynthia aurantium	stem cell	+	+	+	+	+			Smith (1970a)
Halocynthia papillosa	+	+	+						Azéma (1937)
	+	+	+	phagocyte univacuolaire	cellule à noyau achromatique	cellule adipeuse			Pérès (1943)
Microcosmus spinosus	+	+					yellow	cellule à pigment purique	Azéma (1937)
Microcosmus sulcatus	+	+	+	phagocyte univacuolaire		cellule adipeuse	orange	cellule à grains réfringents	Pérès (1943)
Pyura stolonifera	+	macrophage		+		ferrocyte	orange	+	Endean (1955a)
Pyura vittata	+	macrophage		+	+	colourless green cell	—	+	George (1939)

TABLE VI.—(*continued*)

Family and species	Blood cell type[a]								Reference
	Haemoblast and/or lymphocyte	Leucocytes		Vacuolated cells					
		Granular	Hyaline	Signet ring	Compartment	Morula	Pigment cells	Nephrocytes	
MOLGULIDAE									
Ctenicella appendiculata		amibocyte typique à granules		amibocyte typique à vacuolaire		amibocyte à graisse			Cuénot (1891)
	+		+	grand cellule vacuolaire		cellule adipeuse	yellow	cellule excretrice	Azéma (1937)
Molgula manhattensis	+	+		grand cellule vacuolaire		cellule adipeuse	lemon		Azéma (1937)
	+	macrophage	—	+	+	green cell; colourless green cell	—		George (1939)
	+	phagocyte		+	+	vanadocyte			Anderson (1971)
Molgula occidentalis	+	macrophage	—	+	+	green cell; colourless green cell	orange		George (1939)
Molgula occulata	+	+		grand cellule vacuolaire		cellule adipeuse; cellule morulaire	red	cellule à pigment purique	Azéma (1937)
Molgula oculata	+	+		grand cellule vacuolaire		cellule morulaire; cellule à pigment vert	red	cellule à pigment purique	Azéma (1937)

[a] The morphological term used by each referenced investigator has been preserved. Where the terminology is the same as the heading, it is indicated by a plus (+). A dash (—) indicates that the cell type is absent. Blank spaces indicate no cell type was described that fits the heading.

[b] No attempt has been made to separate these two cell types. Some investigators have referred to haemoblasts as lymphocytes whereas others have separated them. From their descriptions, it is not possible in many cases to determine which cell type they are describing.

TABLE VII. Species distribution of blood cell types in Thaliacea.

Order and species	Blood cell type[a]								References
	Haemoblast and/or lymphocyte	Leucocytes		Vacuolated cells					
		Granular	Hyaline	Signet ring	Compartment	Morula	Pigment cells	Nephrocytes	
SALPIDA									
Salpa africana maxima	+[b]			+	+	green cells			Fernandez (1904)
Salpa democratica	+	+	+		leucocytes polyvacuolaire	cellule à inclusion acidophile	cellule à pigment jaune		Pérès (1943)
Salpa democratica mucronata		phagocytic cells with coarse granules				+			Dahlgrün (1901)
Salpa fusiformis	+	+	+	phagocyte univacuolaire	cellule à petite granules refringents	cellule à grand inclusion acidophile			Pérès (1943)
Salpa maxima	+	+	+	phagocyte univacuolaire	cellule à cytoplasme compartimenté	cellule à grand inclusions acidophile			Pérès (1943)
PYROSOMIDA									
Pyrosoma atlanticum	+	+	+	cellule vacuolaire	cellule à cytoplasme compartimenté				Pérès (1943)

[a] The morphological term used by each referenced investigator has been preserved. Where the terminology is the same as the heading, it is indicated by a plus (+). A dash (—) indicates that the cell type is absent. Blank spaces indicate no cell type was described that fits the heading.

[b] No attempt has been made to separate these two cell types. Some investigators have referred to haemoblasts as lymphocytes whereas others have separated them. From their descriptions, it is not possible in many cases to determine which cell type they are describing.

vanadium is not accumulated. Instead, iron (Noddack and Noddack, 1939; Endean, 1953, 1955a; Koval'skii *et al.*, 1962; Smith, 1970b; Swinehart *et al.*, 1974; Danskin, 1978), manganese (Vinogradov, 1953; Carlisle, 1968), niobium (Carlisle, 1958; Kokubu and Hidaka, 1965), titanium (Levine, 1961, 1962), zirconium (Levine, 1961, 1962; Henzlik, 1966) or tantalum (Kokubu and Hidaka, 1965) is present. It is generally agreed that vanadium and iron are concentrated within the vacuoles of the morula cell (Webb, 1939, 1956; Baltscheffsky and Baltscheffsky, 1953; Endean, 1953, 1955a, 1960; Kalk, 1963b; Koval'skii and Rezaeva, 1963; Rummel *et al.*, 1966; Smith, 1970a; Kustin *et al.*, 1976). Evidence that the other heavy metals are also concentrated by the morula cell is lacking. It is interesting, however, that in most species where vanadium is absent or in low concentrations, when looked for, one of the other heavy metals can be found.

Vanadium uptake from sea water (Goldberg *et al.*, 1951; Bayer, 1955; Bielig *et al.*, 1961a,b; Kalk, 1963a,b; Rummel *et al.*, 1966), its histogenesis and localization in morula cells (Kalk, 1963b; Gansler *et al.*, 1963; Botte and Scippa, 1977), concentration (Bertrand, 1950; Webb, 1956; Ciereszko *et al.*, 1963; Swinehart *et al.*, 1974; Danskin, 1978) and chemistry (Califano and Caselli, 1948; Califano and Boeri, 1950; Lyding, 1953; Bielig and Bayer, 1954; Bielig *et al.*, 1954; Boeri and Ehrenburg, 1954; Baltscheffsky and Mendia, 1958; Rezaeva, 1964; Koval'skii and Rezaeva, 1965; Bielig *et al.*, 1966; Swinehart *et al.*, 1974; Carlson, 1975; Kustin *et al.*, 1976; Gilbert *et al.*, 1977) have been studied in many species and recently reviewed by Goodbody (1974).

4. *Pigments*

The chemical nature of the coloured pigments present in pigment cells is uncertain. They have been identified as carotenoids (Pizon, 1899; Azéma, 1929a,b; Lederer, 1934), melanin (Pérès, 1943; Endean, 1960) and suggested to be vanadium compounds (Henze, 1913a; Hecht, 1918; George, 1926) or by-products of vanadium metabolism (Goodbody, 1974). The chromogen found in pigment cells of *Botryllus* (Pizon, 1899; Azéma, 1929a; Lederer, 1934), Polyclinidae (Azéma, 1929b), *Dendrodoa grossularia* (Lederer, 1934; Webb, 1939) and *H. papillosa* (Lederer, 1934) appears to be carotenoids. Lederer (1934) has extracted and identified the carotenoids of *H. papillosa*, *B. schlosseri* and *D. grossularia* as α- and β-carotenes, astacene esters and xanthophylls. Melanin has been identified in orange pigment cells of *P. mammillata* (Endean, 1960) and *C. intestinalis* (Pérès, 1943) and also probably occurs in *A. mentula* (Cuénot, 1891; Henze, 1913a; Webb, 1939), *A. atra* (Fulton, 1920), *Perophora viridis* (George, 1926) and *Corella japonica* (Ohuye, 1936).

No attempts have been made to identify the chemical nature of the red, blue or other coloured pigments found in other species. Vanadium inorganic compounds have a wide range of colours corresponding to different oxidation states; orange, red, green, yellow, blue. Since ascidian pigment cells exhibit a similar colour range, it has been suggested that the various chromogens present are vanadium compounds (Henze, 1913a; Hecht, 1918; George, 1926). There is however, no evidence to support this hypothesis (Webb, 1939).

5. *Nitrogenous compounds*

Nephrocyte vacuoles contain large granules or calculi in colloidal suspension. In many respects, they resemble the calculi present within the renal vesicles of some ascidians (Kupffer, 1872, 1874; Lacaze-Duthers, 1874; Roule, 1884; Herdman, 1888; Dahlgrün, 1901; Azéma, 1926, 1928). From various microchemical reactions. Azéma (1928, 1929a,b,c,d) concludes that these granules and calculi are composed of various purines. In some species of Pyuridae and Polyclinidae, they are xanthine. Botryllidae nephrocytes contain an unspecified purine and in *Ascidia pellucida*, the granules have characteristics of guanine. In addition to purines, uric acid has been identified in the nephrocyte concretions of *Botryllus schlosseri* and *Botrylloides leachi* (Sabbadin and Tondonati, 1967).

6. *Summary*

From the information presented in this section, the chemical components of each blood cell type are beginning to be characterized. Table VIII summarizes the known cytochemical components of each cell type. The diversity of substances found within them, reflects their physiological role(s) and function(s) within the ascidians.

E. Blood cell relationships

Based on cytological and cytochemical observations, various genetic relationships between the different blood cell types have been proposed (Cuénot, 1891; Kollmann, 1908; Azéma, 1929b, 1937; George, 1930, 1939; Pérès, 1943; Millar, 1953; Endean, 1960). All have assumed a monophyletic origin, deriving each cell type from the lymphocyte. The lymphocyte is regarded as an undifferentiated cell produced from the haemoblast (Pérès, 1943; Millar, 1953). Through the acquisition of granules or vacuoles, it differentiates into the other cell types. The evidence usually cited for this is the presence of morphological transition cell types between the lymphocyte and other cell types in the circulating blood. While informative, evidence based on morphological criteria alone is not conclusive.

Functional studies, the organized cellular architecture of haemopoietic tissues, and blood cell renewal kinetics suggest an alternative scheme for blood cell relationships (Fig. 9). The major difference between this scheme and others, is that the haemoblast is considered as the stem cell that gives rise to the other cell types. Haemoblasts are multipotential cells. They are radiosensitive and give rise to other blood cell types during budding (Freeman, 1964). Within the haemopoietic tissues, they are clustered at the centre of the nodule (Fig. 4) and can divide (Millar, 1953; Ermak, 1975). Surrounding them are blood cells in various differentiation stages. Lymphocytes, granular leucocytes, hyaline leucocytes and other undifferentiated cells make up the majority of the nodule cell population. Cell renewal studies (Ermak, 1975) demonstrate that after a short pulse of tritiated thymidine, nodule haemoblasts become labelled. After 20 days, the label is found primarily in the lymphocytes and leucocytes at the periphery of the nodule. Haemoblasts are no longer labelled, suggesting that they have given rise to those cells at the periphery of the nodule. Pigment cells, nephrocytes, signet ring, compartment and morula cells appear to be absent in the haematogenic tissues. Their precursors, however, are assumed to be present.

Within circulating blood, all cell types including the haemoblast, are

TABLE VIII. General cytochemical components of ascidian blood cells.

Blood cell type		Cytochemical component
Lymphocyte		protein polysaccharides
Leucocytes	granular	glycogen protein granules lipid droplets
	hyaline	protein polysaccharides
Vacuolated cells		protein polysaccharides sulphuric acid vanadium or iron (other heavy metals?)
Pigment cells		carotenes melanin
Nephrocytes		nitrogenous compounds (purines, uric acid)

present, suggesting that some blood cell development can occur outside the haematopoietic tissues. Lymphocytes and granular leucocytes appear to be released from haematogenic tissues in a mature form. Complete maturation and differentiation of the other cell types, however, probably occurs in the circulating blood. Vacuolated cells are thought to be derived from the hyaline leucocyte (Kalk, 1963b) or a cell that morphologically resembles it. Once released from the blood forming tissues, it passes through various transition stages, going from signet ring to compartment to morula cell (George, 1930; Endean, 1960; Kalk, 1963b). Stages in pigment cell and nephrocyte differentiation have not been observed. Both probably arise from one of the undifferentiated cells in the haematopoietic tissue which, upon their release, either begin to synthesize pigment or to develop vacuoles in which metabolic waste products can accumulate.

From available evidence, the postulated relationships presented in Fig. 9 are plausible and consistent with morphological and functional studies. Through appropriate experimentation and the development of *in vitro* culture conditions allowing for blood cell maturation and differentiation, blood cell relationships will be determined with more certainty.

VI. Functions of blood cells

The diversity of ascidian blood cell types reflects the various functions they perform. All cell types are amoebocytic, exhibiting varying degrees of

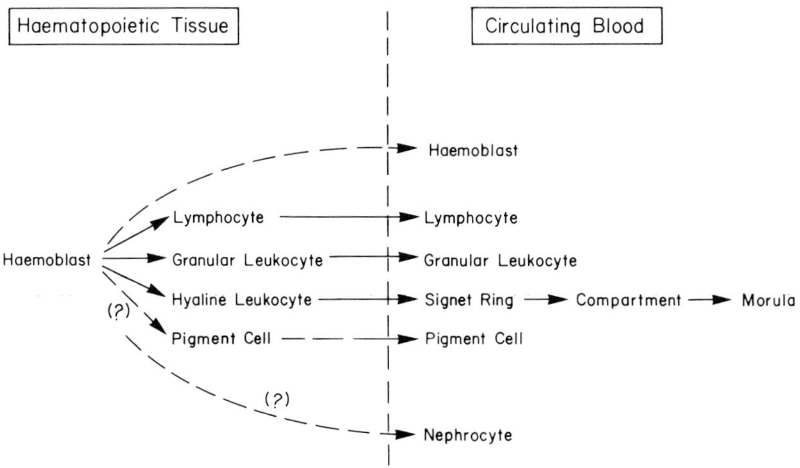

Fig. 9. Postulated relationships between the different blood cell types. See text for details.

mobility (Hecht, 1918; Fulton, 1920; Andrew, 1961). They are not confined to the circulatory system and pass freely from the blood spaces into various connective tissues. Here they can be found randomly distributed or in high concentrations. It is within the circulatory system and connective tissues that they carry out their physiological roles. Many functions can be ascribed to the blood cells, some accomplished by only one cell type, others involving several cell types. These functions include coagulation, excretion, nutrition, budding, germ cell formation, tunic formation, pigmentation and various immunological reactions.

A. Coagulation

Absence of plasma clotting factors has been demonstrated in many species (Krukenberg, 1882; Fry, 1909; Nolf, 1909; Henze, 1911; Hecht, 1918; Fulton, 1920; Huus, 1937; Webb, 1956). Haemostasis is maintained by blood cell aggregation (coagulation) (Cuénot, 1891; Fry, 1909; Henze, 1911) at the site of vascular injuries, the cells sticking together to form sheets and threads. The predominant cell type observed within these aggregates is the morula cell. Blood cells also coagulate on contact with sea water and can be made to aggregate within the vascular system by mechanical stimulation (Hecht, 1918). The process is reversible if the animal is left undisturbed. Repeated stimulation eventually leads to the loss of coagulation suggesting that it may be caused by the secretion of some substance into the blood (Hecht, 1918) by the blood cells (Fulton, 1920). In *Ascidia atra*, cytolysis of the blood cells also occurs after their initial aggregation (Fulton, 1920). This aspect has not been studied in detail or observed in other species.

The mechanism causing cell coagulation is unknown. Sulphydryl groups however, may play a role (Boolootian and Giese, 1959; Bryan *et al.*, 1964; Vallee, 1968). Vallee (1968) has investigated the effects of sulphydryl group reagents on the aggregation of *Ascidia nigra* morula cells. In the presence of cysteine, aggregation is inhibited. This can be counteracted by blocking the cysteine sulphydryl groups with iodoacetic acid. Calcium does not appear to play a role in the coagulation process. These observations suggest that morula cell membranes contain sulphydryl groups and coagulation involves the formation of disulphide linkages between adjacent cells.

B. Excretion

Ascidians are ammonotelic and uricotelic (Goodbody, 1957, 1965, 1974).

Although some tunicate species have organs or vesicles that appear to be involved in excretion, most species lack renal excretory tubule type organs (see Berrill, 1950; Goodbody, 1974). Protein and nucleic acid metabolic waste products appear to be concentrated in solid form as granular concretions in nephrocytes. The function of nephrocytes therefore is one of storage and excretion. The biosynthetic pathways used in accumulating nitrogenous wastes, their deposition into solid purine and uric acid concretions and their ultimate fate is unknown. Accumulations of nephrocytes have been observed in the connective tissues of the alimentary tract (Roule, 1884; Dahlgrün, 1901; Milanesi and Burighel, 1978) and at the tips and near the bases of the siphons (George, 1936). In these areas, it is possible that waste products are released or, the nephrocytes may be transported to the exterior, across the epithelium.

C. *Nutrition*

Many investigators have suggested that one of the functions of blood cells is to serve as storage places of nutritive materials. During circulation, they carry these nutrients to the other tissues. Blood cells containing large reserves of lipid, protein and glycogen may function in such a capacity and have been called trophocytes. The cytochemical composition of ascidian granular leucocytes (Table VIII) suggests that they may have a trophocytic function. Although this has yet to be demonstrated in solitary tunicates, there is evidence that this is one of their functions in colonial forms.

Colonial tunicates reproduce asexually by budding. The polystyelid ascidian, *Polyzoa vesiculiphora*, forms buds from the terminal ampullae of stolons. Internally, the buds are congested with blood cells and trophocytes (Fig. 10). By light and electron microscopy, the trophocytes have been identified as blood granular leucocytes (Fujimoto and Watanabe, 1976). During bud development, their numbers decline and they disappear by the time zooid formation is complete. This decrease is the result of their being specifically phagocytosed by phagocytic cells in the mesenchymal space (Fig. 11a). After their phagocytosis, they degenerate and eventually appear as myelin figures in the phagosomes of the phagocytes (Fig. 11b). Blood cells other than granular leucocytes are seldom phagocytosed. Decreases in granular leucocyte numbers have also been observed during bud development in *Perophora viridis* (Freeman, 1964) and *Clavelina lepadiformis* (Ries, 1937). These observations suggest that granular leucocytes function as trophocytes in colonial ascidians, supplying nutrients to developing bud tissues.

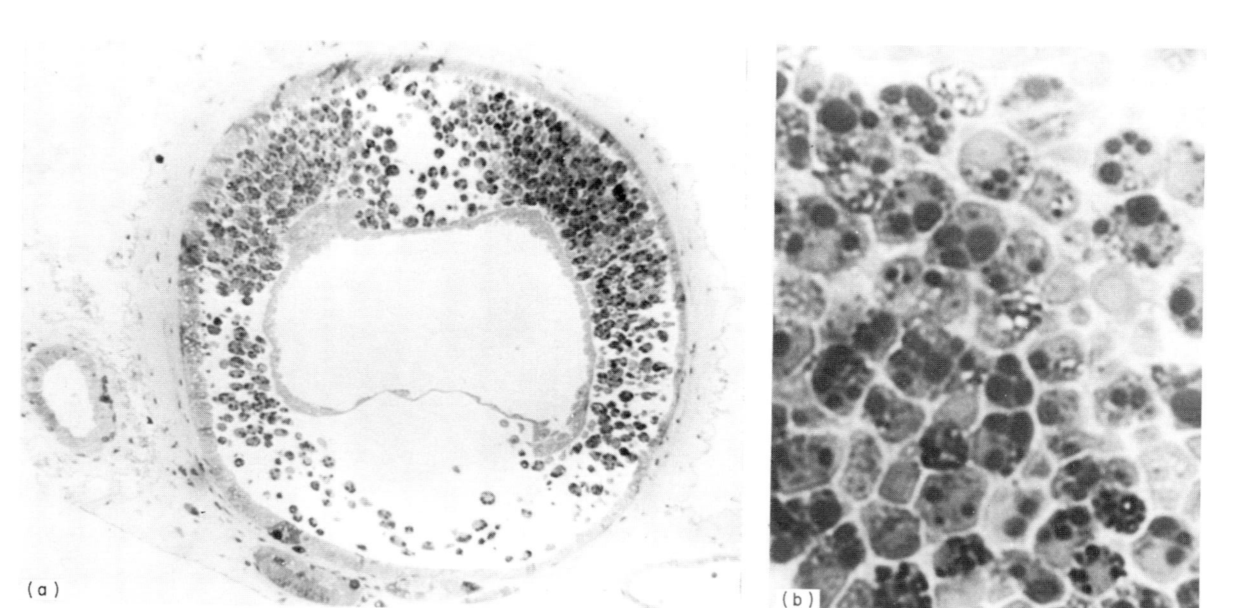

Fig. 10. Stolonic bud development in *Polyzoa vesiculiphora*. (a) Cross section of stolonic bud showing accumulation of blood cells, $\times 131$. (b) Enlargement of (a), $\times 1500$. (Reproduced with permission from Fujimoto and Watanabe, 1976.)

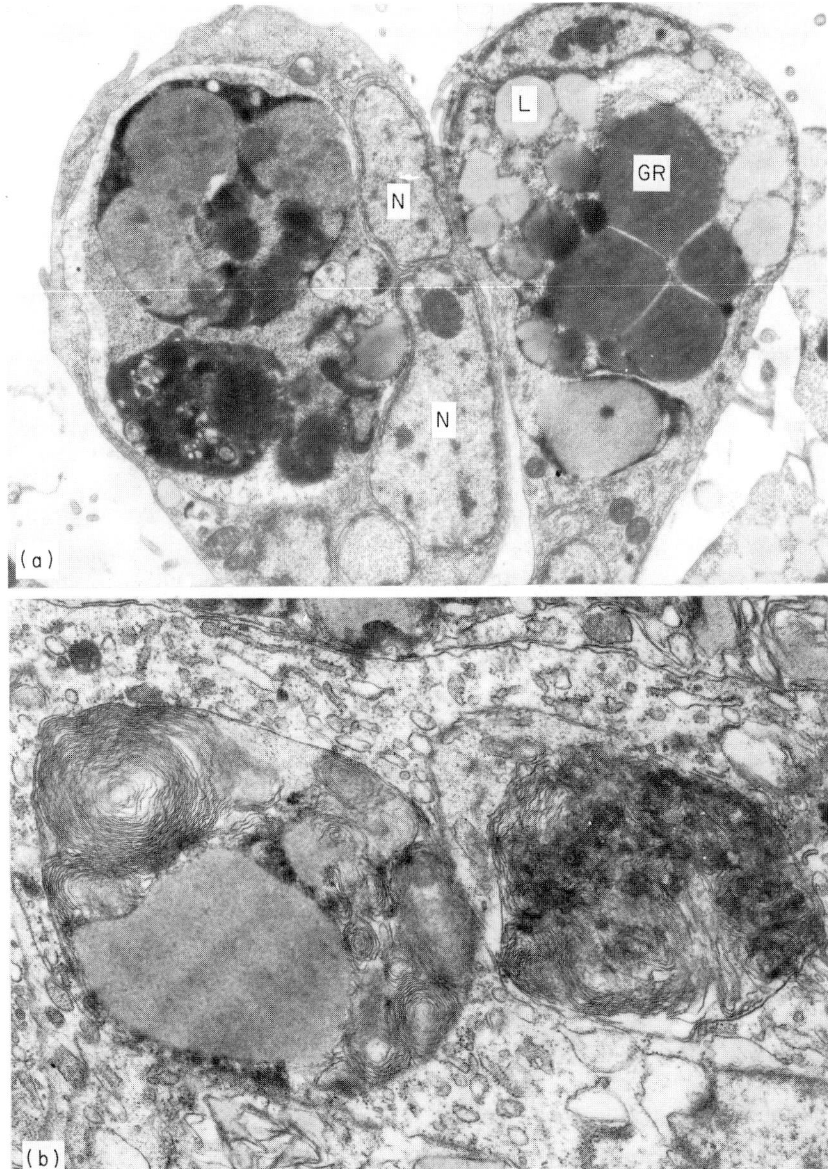

Fig. 11. (a) *Polyzoa vesiculiphora* phagocytic cells from an early stage of a prefunctional zooid phagocytosing granular amoebocytes (leucocytes). Phagosomes contain granule remnants (GR) and lipid droplets (L), characteristics of granular leucocytes. N, nucleus, $\times 7600$. (b) Myelin figures in the phagosomes of a phagocyte, $\times 12\,500$. (Reproduced with permission from Fujimoto and Watanabe, 1976.)

D. *Vascular budding*

Isolated regions of the vascular system in some colonial tunicates can produce new zooids. This mode of asexual reproduction has been termed vascular budding (Oka and Watanabe, 1957a) and occurs in the Botryllidae (Oka and Watanabe, 1957a, 1959; Milkman and Byrne, 1961), Clavelinidae (Brien, 1930) and Perophoridae (Freeman, 1964). Vascular buds appear at the bases of ampullae in *Botryllus primigenus* (Oka and Watanabe, 1957a), along the walls of old blood vessels in *Botrylloides violaceum* (Oka and Watanabe, 1959) and along the vascular stolons of *Perophora viridis* (Freeman, 1964). Their formation is initiated by the aggregation of blood cells which have been described as being lymphocytes (Oka and Watanabe, 1957a, 1959; Freeman, 1964) or haemoblasts (Sabbadin, 1955). These cells are morphologically similar to the haemoblasts found in the haematopoietic tissues and are probably haemoblasts and not lymphocytes.

The aggregation of haemoblasts is followed by their differentiation into the tissues and organs of the new zooid. In *B. primigenus* and *B. violaceum*, the aggregates initially contain approximately 15–20 haemoblasts. Through intensive mitosis, a hollow blastula-like structure forms and develops into a functional zooid. Buds in *P. viridis* form from stolon epidermal cells, septum mesenchyme cells and haemoblast aggregates from the blood. During budding, the septal mesenchyme forms a hollow endoblastic vesicle which contains the haemoblast aggregate (Fig. 12). This then differentiates into the tissues of the new zooid.

The potentiality of haemoblasts to form new zooids has been experimentally tested in *P. viridis* (Freeman, 1964, 1970a,b). *P. viridis* produces new zooids asexually at regular intervals along its stolon. When isolated sections containing a sexually immature zooid with 3–5 mm of stolon are irradiated, budding is inhibited and the preparation slowly undergoes regression and dies. If irradiated preparations are injected with blood from unirradiated zooids of the same colony, they will start to bud and produce new zooids. When the blood is fractionated into its different cell types and each cell type is injected into different irradiated preparations, only those receiving haemoblasts initiate budding. There was also a direct correlation between the number of haemoblasts injected and the time when the first buds appear. Irradiation of the haemoblasts prior to injection also inhibited budding. Haemoblasts thus appear to have the capacity to differentiate into other tissues.

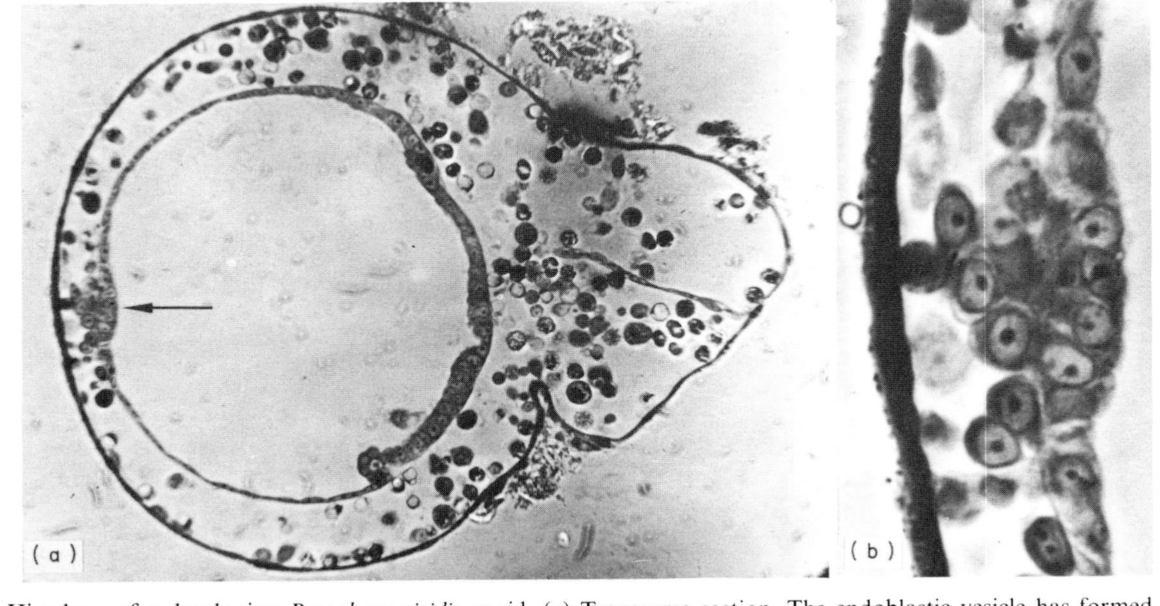

Fig. 12. Histology of a developing *Perophora viridis* zooid. (a) Transverse section. The endoblastic vesicle has formed from the mesenchymal septum. Lymphocytes (haemoblasts) have aggregated on the dorsal part of the endoblastic vesicle (arrow) to form the dorsal tube rudiment, ×320. (b) Detail of lymphocyte (haemoblast) aggregate from (a), ×1200. (Reproduced with permission from Freeman, 1964.)

E. Gonad and germ cell formation

In addition to asexual reproduction by budding, colonial ascidians also reproduce sexually. After larval metamorphosis, the developing zooid (oozooid) gives off a series of buds (blastozooids) that reproduce asexually until the gonads develop. The gonadal rudiment first appears in developing blastozooids as an aggregate of haemoblasts which lodges along the genital tract. Gonad development and germ cell formation from these haemoblast aggregates has been investigated in *Distomus variolosus* (Newberry, 1968), *Symplegma reptans* (Sugimoto and Nakauchi, 1974; Nakauchi, 1976) and *Botryllus primigenus* (Mukai and Watanabe, 1976). Irrespective of the differentiation pathways utilized by these species in gonad development and subsequent gametogenesis, all components are apparently derived from circulating haemoblasts.

Early testicular development in *D. variolosus* (Newberry, 1968) is characterized by proliferation of the haemoblast aggregate and the formation of a central cavity. Mitotic proliferation and meiotic reduction occurs, transforming the original haemoblast aggregate into a turgid sac of gametes. Ovarian development occurs in a similar manner. After formation of an ovarian cavity, scattered haemoblasts in the aggregate enlarge and eventually develop into oocytes and eggs. Others provide the ovarian matrix from which the follicular envelopes later form. Gonad formation in *S. reptans* (Sugimoto and Nakauchi, 1974; Nakauchi, 1976) appears to be similar to *D. variolosus*. The formation of gonads in *B. primigenus* however, is different since circulating haemoblasts of preceding and succeeding generations are involved in gonad formation and gametogenesis (Mukai and Watanabe, 1976).

F. Tunic formation

The outer covering of ascidians is the test or tunic. It surrounds the individual zooid of solitary tunicates and forms the matrix in which zooids of colonial species are embedded. The chemical nature and formation of the tunic has been the subject of numerous investigations and has recently been reviewed by Goodbody (1974). It appears to be produced by the epithelial cells of the blood vessels (Millar, 1953; Endean, 1961; Stiévenart, 1970), the mantle wall epithelium (Pérès, 1948a,b; Deck *et al.*, 1966; Barrington and Thorpe, 1968; Wardrop, 1970; Smith, 1970a,b; Stiévenart, 1971), or by the blood cells. All blood cell types can be found within the fibrous matrix of the tunic. The predominant cell type, however, is the morula cell. While its precise role is uncertain, available evidence suggests that the primary function of the morula cell is tunic formation. It has been suggested that they may secrete the tunic (Herdman, 1899; Ries, 1937; Endean, 1955b,c, 1960, 1961), be instrumental in the organization of the tunic (Saint-Hilaire, 1931; Das, 1936) or function in both capacities (Smith, 1970a).

Morula cells can be observed in various stages of disintegration within the tunic (Endean, 1961; Deck *et al.*, 1966; Stiévenart, 1970; Wardrop, 1970) and in association with tunic microfibrils (Endean, 1961; Stiévenart, 1970; Wardrop, 1970). Electron micrographs show that during morula cell disintegration, the vacuoles (vanadophores) break free in the test substance and are found in association with the microfibrils (Wardrop, 1970). This suggests a relationship between fibre production and morula cell disintegration. Morula cells from *P. stolonifera* have been observed to produce fibres when cytolysed *in vivo* and *in vitro* (Endean, 1955c).

More direct evidence suggesting morula cell participation in tunic formation comes from studies on tunic regeneration during wound healing (Endean, 1955c; Smith, 1970a). The initial reaction to wounding in *H. aurantium* is a massive migration of morula cells to the external edges of the tunic wound where they break down (Smith, 1970a). After several days, the matrix surrounding the wound edges becomes filled with material (Fig. 13)

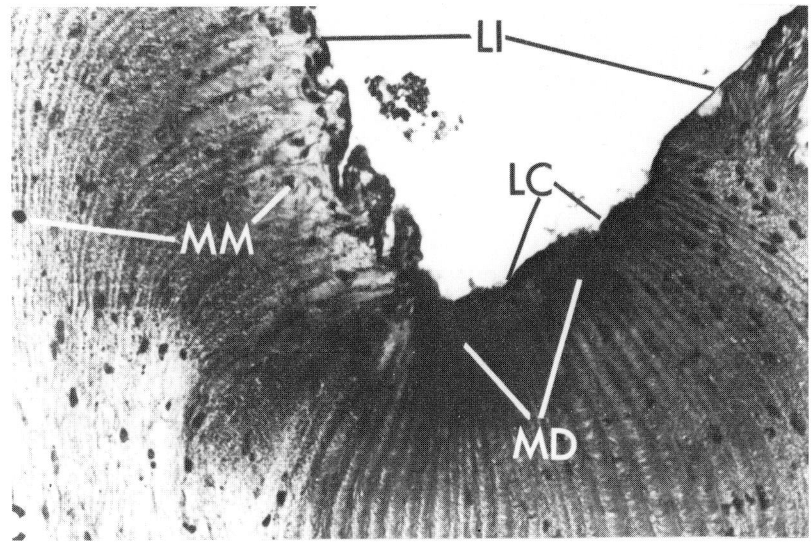

Fig. 13. Injured body wall tunic of *Hyalocynthia aurantium*. Cross section of tunic five days after injury. Mature morula cells (MM) and morula cell degradation products (MD) are present in the wound area and the laminae are constricted (LC) at the sides of the wound. LI, limits of original incision. (Reproduced with permission from Smith, 1970a.) ×85.

that has histochemical staining properties similar to the morula cell. Injury to the test of *P. stolonifera* is also followed by an influx of morula cells into the damaged region (Endean, 1955c). At the seawater interface, they cytolyse, releasing fibre-producing intraglobular material.

Since morula cells occur throughout the tunic, disintegrate there, and display aggregation and degeneration at the site of test injury, their function must be closely related to tunic formation. Most investigators agree that they migrate into the test either through the mantle wall or via the test vessels and discharge their vacuolar contents within the test matrix. The organo-metallic compound in morula cells is a strong reducing substance (Lyding, 1953; Boeri and Ehrenburg, 1954; Endean, 1955a; Rezaeva, 1964; Bielig *et al.*, 1966) maintained in a reduced state by sulphuric acid. Goodbody (1974) has suggested that when the vacuolar contents are released into the test, the chromogen is freed from the acid, its reducing properties become effective, polymerizing the test carbohydrates into the complex polysaccharides of the microfibrils.

G. Pigmentation

Ascidian pigmentation is due to the presence of various coloured blood pigment cells. The distinctive colour and colour markings of each species is a reflection of their relative number and distribution in particular regions of the zooid and the capacity of the pigment to transmit and reflect various colours. The factors responsible for their distribution and localization are unknown.

Pigment cells are particularly abundant in the mantle tissues near the siphonal tips (George, 1939) and on the branchial papillae (Andrews, 1961). Here they occur as spots or intersiphonal bands, the spots or bands exhibiting the characteristic colour of the pigment cell. It has been suggested that these pigmented areas may be specific photoreceptors for sperm release (Lambert and Brandt, 1967) or act as barriers against light wavelengths that trigger sperm release (Woollacott, 1974). The ground colour of each ascidian species is also due to the presence of blood pigment cells in the tunic matrix (George, 1939; Andrew, 1961; Mukai, 1974). Although the function of blood pigment cells in the tunic is unknown, it has been suggested that they may afford protection against ultraviolet light (Endean, 1961; Mukai, 1974; Lyerla *et al.*, 1975).

H. Immune responses

Immune reponsiveness to foreign materials (antigens, non-self tissues) lies in the ability of an animal to recognize and react against foreignness in specific ways. This recognition and reaction system is a function of the blood cells and plasma. Blood cell circulation and their ability to migrate throughout the connective tissues ensures that an effective internal defence system is present at all times. Tunicates respond to foreign materials in two ways, humoral or cellular. Humoral responses involve the natural agglutinins (Wright, 1973; Wright and Cooper, 1975) and bactericidins (Johnson and Chapman, 1970) present in the blood plasma. Cellular responses include inflammatory reactions, phagocytosis, encapsulation and histoincompatibility reactions. The cell types responsible for these reactions are the lymphocytes, hyaline and granular leucocytes, and morula cells.

1. Antigen recognition

The initial stage in an immune reaction involves antigen recognition by receptors on the cell surface. Although the chemical nature of these receptors on tunicate blood cells is unknown, their presence can be inferred from several observations. Lymphocytes from *C. intestinalis* bind sheep erythrocytes, forming rosettes (Hildemann and Reddy, 1973). Blood cells from *Ascidia mentula* have also been observed to bind bacteria in a similar fashion (Cantacuzène, 1919). *P. stolonifera* lymphocytes, granular leucocytes and vacuolated cells possess receptors for the lectins concanavalin A, wheat germ agglutinin and soybean lectin (Warr *et al.*, 1977). These receptors appear to be membrane glycoproteins since binding can be inhibited by competition with specific sugars. Unlike vertebrate lymphocytes, however, lectin binding does not induce mitosis so that it is doubtful whether tunicate lymphocytes are homologous with their vertebrate namesake.

2. Inflammatory reactions

The presence or experimental introduction of foreign substances into the tunic is followed by a pronounced blood cell infiltration into the area in and around the material (Fig. 14). Inflammatory reactions have been observed towards splinters (Metchnikoff, 1892), bacteria (Cantacuzène, 1919; Thomas, 1931a, 1932), chemical oncogens (Thomas, 1931b), carbon particles (Smith, 1970a), glass fragments (Anderson, 1971), vertebrate erythrocytes (Wright, 1973, 1974; Parrinello *et al.*, 1977), allogeneic (non-self) tissues (Anderson, 1971; Reddy *et al.*, 1975), marine hydrozoans (Anderson *et al.*, 1977) and lesions of unknown etiology (Anderson *et al.*, 1977). The sequestering and elimination of these substances, either by phagocytosis or encapsulation, is a function of their nature and size.

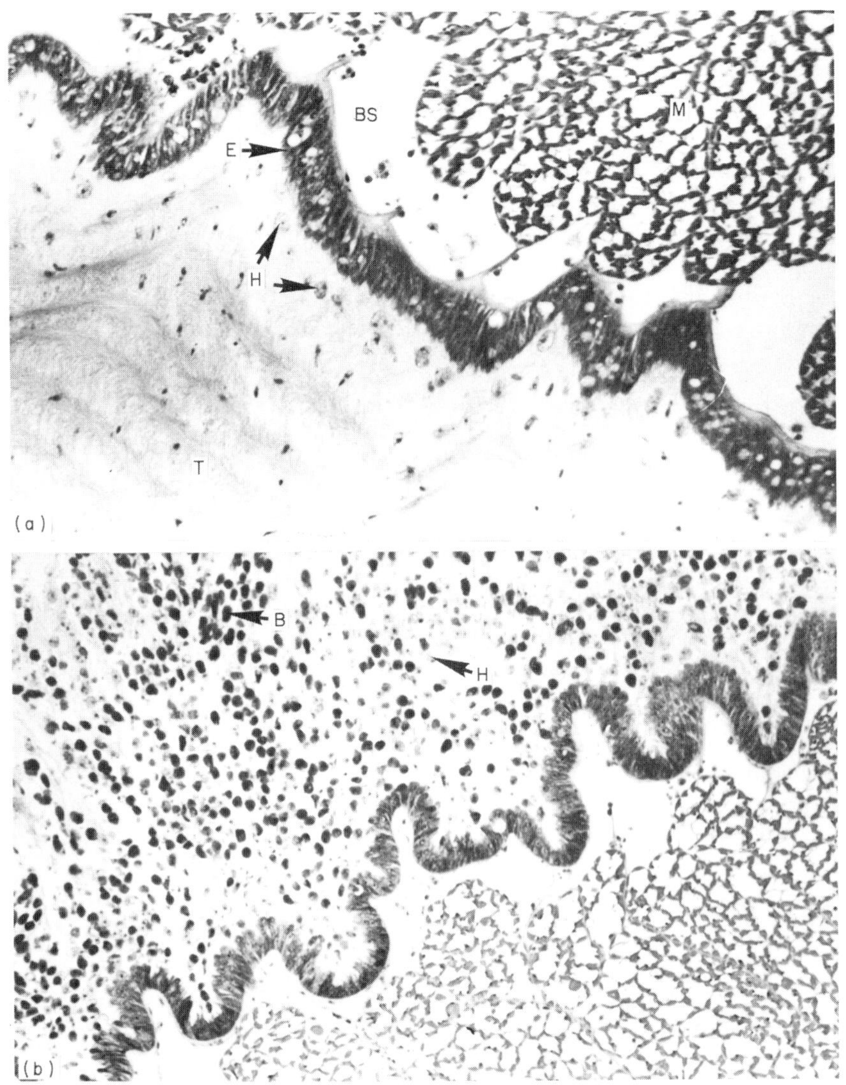

Fig. 14. Inflammatory response in the tunic of *Hyalocynthia pyriformis* to an unknown etiological agent. (a) Section of normal tunic (T) showing ordered laminae, epidermis (E), blood sinuses (BS) and muscle bundles (M). Highly staining haemocytes (H) are present in the tunic in small numbers near the blood sinuses, × 550. (b) Section of tunic in the region near lesion. The tunic is infiltrated by lightly staining eosinophilic blood cells (H) and large basophilic cells (B). Laminar tunic structure has become indistinct and disrupted, × 550. (Reproduced with permission from Anderson *et al.*, 1977).

3. *Phagocytosis*

Small particulate foreign materials introduced into the tunic or vascular system are phagocytosed by the hyaline and granular leucocytes. Vertebrate erythrocytes (Wright, 1973, 1974; Parrinello *et al.*, 1977), colloidal carbon (Smith, 1970a; Parrinello *et al.*, 1977) or bacteria (Metchnikoff, 1892; Cantacuzène, 1919; Thomas, 1931a) injected into the tunic are phagocytosed and cleared from the tunic matrix usually within 24–48 h. Similar results have been obtained with injections of carmine particles (Saint-Hilaire, 1931; Ivanova-Kazas, 1966; Anderson, 1971), trypan blue (Anderson, 1971), colloidal thorium dioxide suspensions (Brown and Davies, 1971) or vertebrate erythrocytes (Wright, 1973, 1974) into the vascular system or peritoneal cavity. Elimination of the engulfed particles depends on their chemical nature. Intracellular digestion probably occurs with erythrocytes and bacteria. Inert substances that cannot be digested appear to be transported and released to the external environment through the branchial sac (Anderson, 1971), tunic (Saint-Hilaire, 1931; Ivanova-Kazas, 1966), intestine (Brown and Davies, 1971) and neural gland (Pérès, 1943; Godeaux, 1964; Ivanova-Kazas, 1966).

4. *Encapsulation*

Foreign materials too large to be phagocytosed are encapsulated. Capsules are formed by the accumulation of blood cells around the object followed by a gradual fibrotic alteration of the cells. Blood cells responsible for encapsulation reactions are those of the vacuolated category, predominantly the morula cell. While morula cells appear to recognize foreignness, capsule formation within the tunic may represent an extension of their primary function (tunic formation) and be analogous to wound healing.

Naturally occurring encapsulation responses have been observed towards copepods which live as commensals and parasites in ascidians. *Gonophysema gullmarensis* lives in the outer wall of the peribranchial cavity of *Ascidiella aspersa* and is surrounded by a thin membrane of host tissue (Bresciana and Lützen, 1960). Within the gill cavities of *Microcosmus savignyi*, *Kystedelphys drachi* is enclosed by three or more cell layers of host tissue (Monniot, 1963). *Distaplia unigermis* however, shows no detectable responses towards the presence of parasitic copepods (Ivanova-Kazas, 1966).

Encapsulation responses have been experimentally induced by inserting splinters (Metchnikoff, 1892) and glass fragments (Anderson, 1971) or by injecting bacteria (Thomas, 1931b) and vertebrate erythrocytes (Wright, 1973, 1974; Wright and Cooper, 1975; Parrinello *et al.*, 1977) into the tunic. Injection of *Bacterium tumefaciens* into the tunic of *A. mentula* produces an initial inflammatory response followed by phagocytosis and necrosis at the injection site. The borders of the necrotic region are surrounded by concentric rings of cells, effectively walling off the inflamed area (Thomas, 1931b).

The process of encapsulation has been studied in *Molgula manhattensis* by inserting glass fragments into branchial sac tissue (Anderson, 1971). Initially, the response involves signet ring and morula cells, but only morula cells after the first two days (Fig. 15). Capsules formed are composed of multilayered structures made up of morula cells, monolayers of cells derived from the morula aggregates and strands of tunicin produced by the morula cells.

Encapsulation parameters using vertebrate erythrocytes have been determined in *C. intestinalis* (Wright, 1973, 1974; Wright and Cooper, 1975; Parrinello *et al.*, 1977). When high concentrations of human, duck, rabbit or sheep erythrocytes are injected into the tunic, they become agglutinated into a mass. Concomitant with this agglutination is a decline in plasma haemagglutinin levels (Wright, 1973, 1974). Injections that are not cleared by phagocytosis within 24 h are encapsulated by the infiltrating blood cells. Forty-eight hours after injection, a whitish halo containing granular material and vacuolated cells surrounds the agglutinated mass (Parrinello *et al.*, 1977). In some animals, the capsule assumes a light tan colour (Wright, 1974) and increases in size. Capsule formation is usually complete by 6–10 days.

Encapsulation of vertebrate erythrocytes is further characterized by the formation of a gelatinous or liquid blister within the capsule. The overlying tunic becomes thinner and ruptures, producing a wound in the tunic (Parrinello *et al.*, 1977). The capsule and its contents are then released to the exterior environment. Following capsule ejection, the tunic usually heals.

Differential responses with respect to animal age are also apparent (Wright and Cooper, 1975). Sexually immature animals exhibit fewer encapsulation responses to erythrocytes than sexually mature ones. The reasons for these differential responses are unknown but may reflect differences in blood cell populations of young and old animals. Cross immunization studies with erythrocytes from different vertebrate species have demonstrated that capsule formation is non-specific (Wright and Cooper, 1975; Parrinello *et al.*, 1977). Primary injections of non-encapsulating concentrations of duck or human erythrocytes followed 6 or 35 days later by secondary injections of either the same or opposite erythrocyte types results in capsule formation. Since capsules are formed against the secondary erythrocyte injections regardless of the primary erythrocyte type injected, the response is non-specific. Similar results have been obtained with sheep and rabbit erythrocytes (Parrinella *et al.*, 1977).

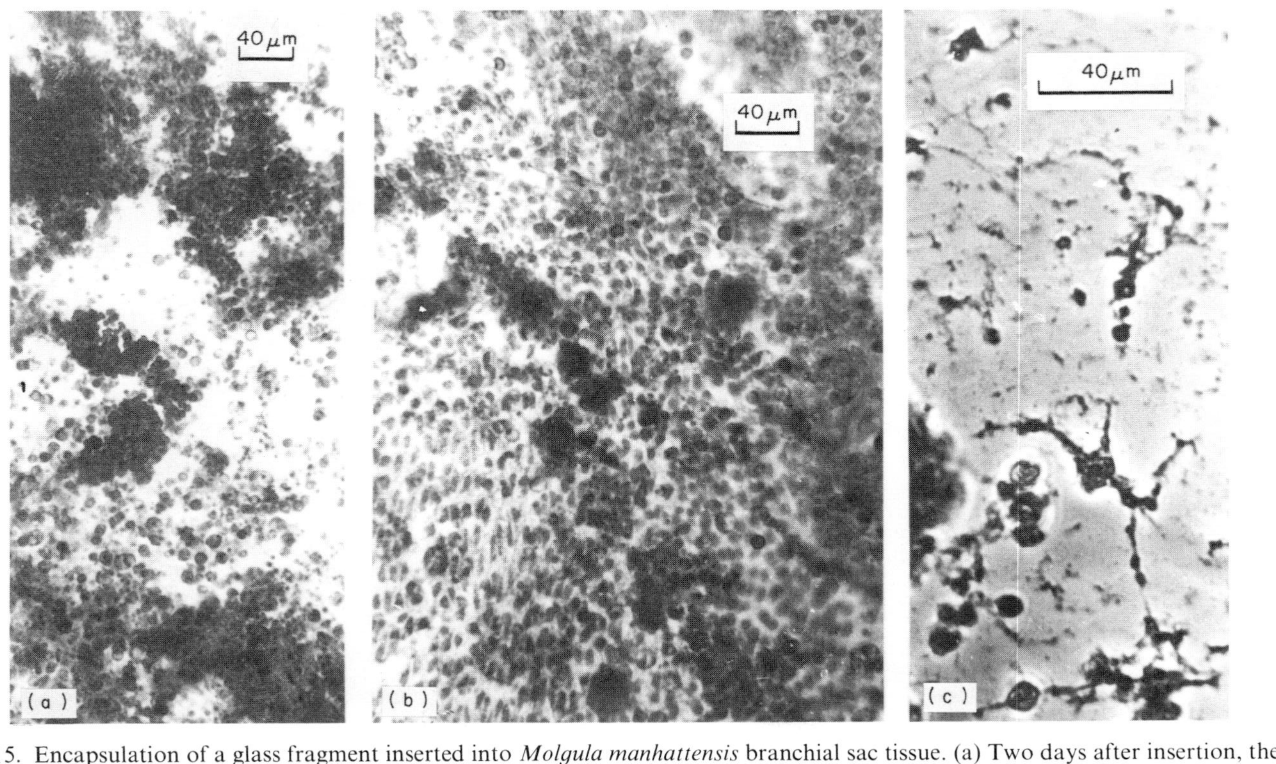

Fig. 15. Encapsulation of a glass fragment inserted into *Molgula manhattensis* branchial sac tissue. (a) Two days after insertion, the formation of multilayered vanadocyte (morula cell) aggregates can be seen in several areas. (b) Four days after insertion, formation of a cellular monolayer from a vanadocyte (morula cell) aggregate. (c) Phase contrast microscopy of vanadocytes connected to each other by strands of tunic material on a glass fragment after three days. (Reproduced with permission from Anderson, 1971.)

Secondary erythrocyte encapsulation reactions are usually stronger (heightened) than primary reactions. They occur more rapidly and in a larger number of animals (Parrinello *et al.*, 1977). Although the reasons for the heightened response are unknown, it may be due to a more rapid infiltration of cells or the fact that cells are already in the neighbouring area as a result of the primary injection. Alternatively, primary injections may have shifted blood cell type homeostasis in favour of increased morula cell production.

5. *Histoincompatibility*

Histoincompatibility implies that genetic differences existing between individuals can be recognized by cells involved in immune reactions. Two sensitive indicators of histoincompatibility are allogeneic cell interactions (mixed leucocyte cultures, MLC) and tissue graft rejection. Positive MLC reactions between allogeneic blood cells are reflected in DNA synthesis and mitosis of the responding cells. It requires that the cells be alive and antigenically disparate. Graft rejection also requires that grafted tissue be antigenically disparate from the host receiving the graft.

In vitro allogeneic interactions between blood cells have been studied only in *P. stolonifera* (Warr *et al.*, 1977). Mixed blood cell cultures from animals collected at different geographical locations were cultivated for 3–10 days and pulsed at various time intervals with ^{125}I-iododeoxyuridine (^{125}IdU). Although the cells remained viable during the culture period and incorporated ^{125}IdU, there was no significant increase in ^{125}IdU uptake over control levels. While these negative results suggest that tunicate blood cells do not proliferate in response to antigenic disparities, ideal culture conditions allowing for the full *in vitro* expression of their proliferative capacities may not have been established.

Blood cells can recognize and react to foreign tissue grafts (Anderson, 1971; Reddy *et al.*, 1975). Autogeneic and allogeneic orthotopic tunic transplants in *C. intestinalis* effectively heal to the graft bed after 5–7 days (Reddy *et al.*, 1975). Autografts remained intact with no evidence of rejection during the eight week experimental period. During the first four weeks, allografts remained viable and indistinguishable from autografts. Wrinkles together with a gradual contraction from the host tissue appeared in the grafts after 6–8 weeks. Histological sections revealed different stages of progressive allograft rejection. In contrast to autografts, large numbers of lymphocytes were found in allografts, suggesting that they may be involved in recognition and rejection. Granular leucocytes (phagocytes) were also present in increased levels in both auto- and allografts indicating the presence of a persistent, non-specific inflammatory response.

Acceptance of orthotopic branchial sac transplants, however, has not been observed in *M. manhattensis* (Anderson, 1971). Autografts and allografts did not heal and fuse with host tissue. Three days after transplantation, signet ring and morula cells began to infiltrate the grafts. By seven days, graft morphology was completely masked by morula cells. Twelve to 14 days post-grafting, the tissues were necrotic masses. Graft encapsulation, however, did not occur. Although different responses to foreign grafts have been observed in these studies, they do provide evidence that various blood cell types function in recognizing and reacting to foreign tissues. Second set grafts to determine the specificity of the response and the presence or absence of immunological memory have yet to be investigated.

In some colonial tunicates, a phenomenon known as colony specificity (or histoincompatibility) exists which is analogous to transplantation and graft rejection. Colony specificity is manifested by the fusability in nature between two colonies of the same species to form a single colony. Two pieces taken from the same colony easily fuse together, sharing a common vascular system (Figs 16a–d). Pieces from unrelated colonies, however, do not fuse (Figs 16e,f). Colony specificity was first observed by Bancroft (1903) in *Botryllus schlosseri*. Since then, it has been demonstrated in *Ecteinascidia tortugenesis*, *P. viridis*, *Perophora bermudensis* (Freeman, 1970b), *B. violaceus* (Mukai and Watanabe, 1974, 1975b), *Symplegma reptans*, *Didemnum moseleyi* (Mukai and Watanabe, 1974) and has been extensively studied in *B. schlosseri* (Sabbadin, 1962; Karakashian and Milkman, 1967) and *B. primigenus* (Oka and Watanabe, 1957b, 1960, 1967; Mukai, 1967; Tanaka, 1973; Tanaka and Watanabe, 1973; Mukai and Watanabe, 1974, 1975a). Allogeneic recognition, however, does not occur in *Botrylloides gascoi*, *Botrylloides leachi* (Bancroft, 1903), *Polycitor mutabilis* (Oka and Usui, 1944) or *Perophora orientalis* (Mukai and Watanabe, 1974). Instead, the union of two colonies is always established, either by grafting or by natural growth, regardless of their origin.

Non-fusion appears to be due to allogeneic recognition mediated by humoral factor(s) and blood cells (Tanaka and Watanabe, 1973; Tanaka, 1973, 1975). When two incompatible colonies come together, there is an initial fusion of their test matrices followed by test cell destruction and filament appearance around the disintegrated test cells in the contact area. Contraction of ampullae occurs, curring off the distal part of the ampullae, resulting in necrosis of the contact region (Figs 16e, f). Once initiated, non-fusion reactions are irreversible and progress to completion even if the incompatible colonies are separated. When two incompatible colonies are separated by a colony compatible with both of them, a rejection reaction is observed in the blood vessels of the central colony. Blood cell clusters composed of granular leucocytes appear in the blood vessels at the

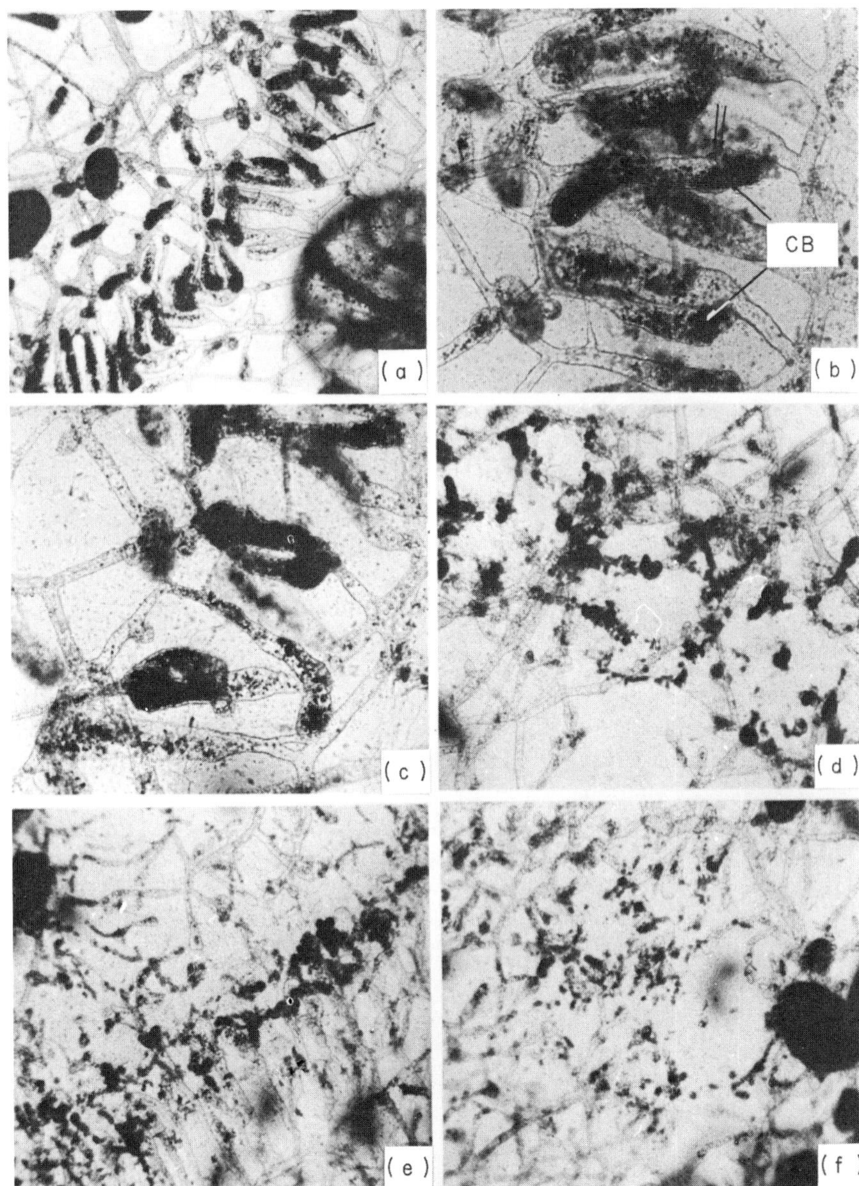

Fig. 16. Fusion and non-fusion reaction features in vascular system of *Botryllus primigenus* colonies. (a) Fusion reaction 30 min after establishing tip-to-side connection of ampullae (arrow) between compatible colonies. (b) One and one-half hours after fusion. Ampullar contraction (double arrows), and blood cell clusters (CB) are observed. (c) Four and one-half hours after fusion. Blood flow through the

interconnections of the fused colonies (Fig. 17) and the intercellular spaces become filled with filaments and granules. In the test matrix surrounding the blood vessels, test cells disintegrate with an accumulation of filaments around them similar to those observed in non-fusion reactions between two incompatible colonies. Two types of factors thus appear to mediate non-fusion reactions. One, found in the test matrix and blood, causes the disintegration of test cells and granular leucocytes. The second factor appears to be released by the disintegrating test or blood cells, causing ampullar or blood vessel constriction, resulting in necrosis of the contact area.

I. Summary

The physiological role(s) and function(s) of ascidian blood cells are as diverse as the various blood cell types. Although all cell types are found in most ascidians, extrapolation of the function(s) observed in one species or family to all species should be done with caution. Table IX summarizes blood cell functions observed and described in this section. While the functional role(s) of some cell types appear to be well established, others are only suggestive. Further studies utilizing histochemical procedures, *in vitro* cell cultivation and modern biochemical techniques should resolve many of these uncertainties.

VII. Summary and concluding remarks

Over the past 145 years, significant progress and insight into the morphology and function of the ascidian circulatory system, blood and blood cells has been accomplished. The vascular system is a haemocoel, with no muscular arteries, valvular veins or dilatable capillaries. Blood, composed of plasma and cells, is pumped through a system of connective tissue lacunae by peristaltic contractions of a tubular heart enclosed in a pericardium. The heart contains no valves and is composed of a single layer of myoepithelial cells that are devoid of innervation. Blood plasma does not clot, is

---

connections between colonies is at a standstill. (d) Twenty hours after fusion. Complete fusion by newly established connections between colonies. (e) Non-fusion reaction between incompatible colonies is evidenced by the formation of a necrotic zone. (f) Partial destruction of vascular system in the central colony. (a), (d–f), ×15; (b) and (c), ×45. (Reproduced with permission from Tanaka, 1973.)

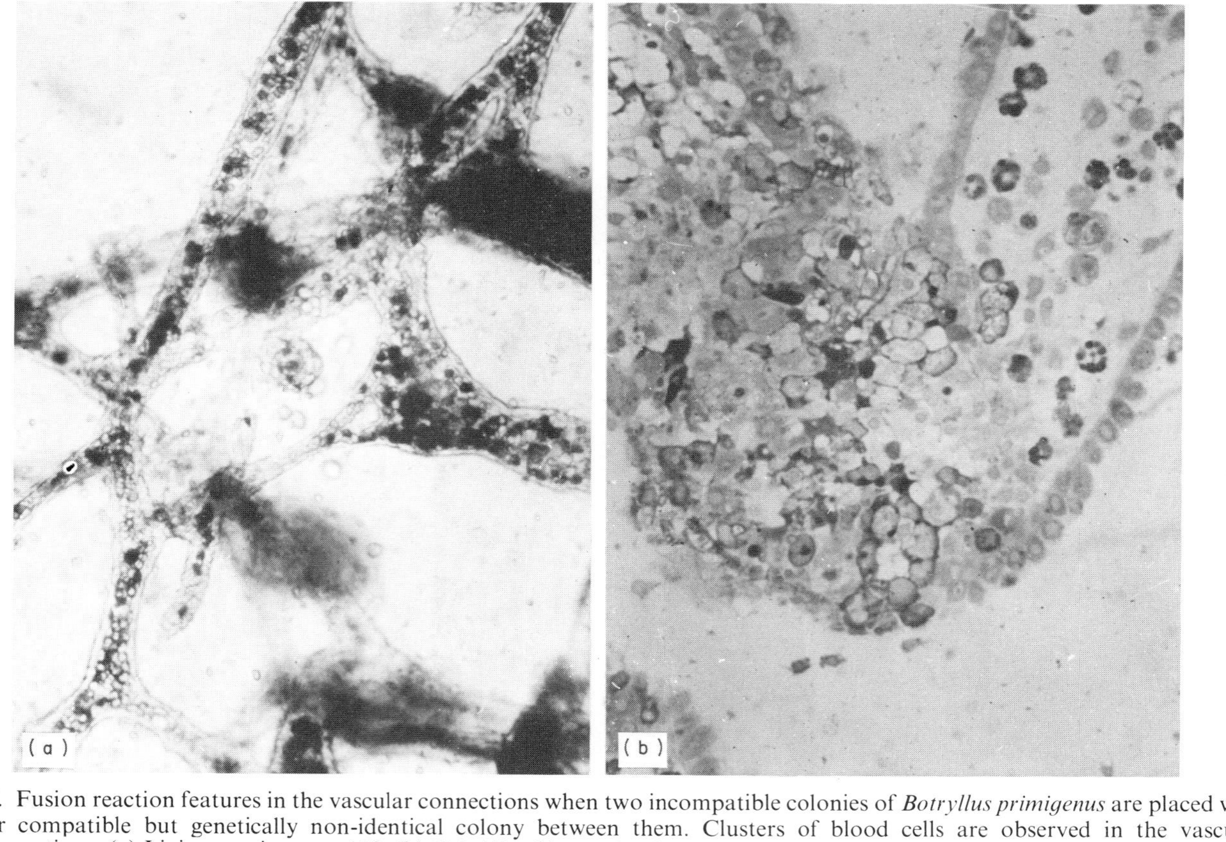

Fig. 17. Fusion reaction features in the vascular connections when two incompatible colonies of *Botryllus primigenus* are placed with another compatible but genetically non-identical colony between them. Clusters of blood cells are observed in the vascular interconnections. (a) Living specimen, $\times 113$. (b) Toluidine blue stained section showing blood cells clustered in blood vessel at the interconnection of two fused colonies, $\times 640$. (Reproduced with permission from Tanaka, 1973.)

colourless, iso-osmotic with sea water, slightly alkaline and has a low carbon dioxide capacity. Respiratory proteins are absent and oxygen concentrations are similar to those of sea water. Plasma proteins do not have an osmotic function and appear to be involved in immune responses.

Ascidian blood contains a variety of cells that originate from haematopoietic tissues located in the pharyngeal wall, gut connective tissue and body wall. Blood cells have a rapid proliferation rate and are renewed within several weeks. They are actively amoeboid and occur in high concentrations in some body tissues. Blood cell morphologies have been described for over 70 species. Nine cell types have been identified which can be placed into six categories: (1) haemoblasts; (2) lymphocytes; (3) leucocytes, granular and hyaline; (4) vacuolated cells, signet ring, compartment and morula; (5) pigment cells; and (6) nephrocytes.

The diversity of cytochemical components within each cell type reflects their physiological role(s) and function(s). Lymphocytes and hyaline leucocytes contain cytoplasmic protein and carbohydrate but no lipid. Cytoplasmic glycogen granules, lipid droplets and large protein granules are present in granular leucocytes. Vacuolated cells contain no lipid and their intravacuolar contents have been identified as polysaccharides, proteins,

TABLE IX. Summary of tunicate blood cell functions.

Cell type	Function
Haemoblast	stem cell for other blood cell types, all species bud formation, some colonial ascidians gonad formation in synstyelid ascidians
Lymphocyte	immune responses (antigen recognition (?), agglutinin production (?), graft rejection (?))
Granular leucocyte	trophocytic, nutrition, immune responses, phagocytosis
Hyaline leucocyte	immune responses, phagocytosis, progenitor of vacuolated cells (?)
Vacuolated cells	tunic formation, wound healing, immune responses, encapsulation coagulation
Pigment cells	pigmentation, phototrophic (protection from light) (?)
Nephrocyte	excretion

sulphuric acid and organo-metallic compounds of vanadium or iron. The chemical nature of the cytoplasmic coloured pigments in pigment cells is uncertain, but believed to be various carotenoids or melanin. Nephrocytes contain large intravacuolar purine or uric acid granules and calculi in colloidal suspension.

Blood cells perform many different functions. Haemoblasts are stem cells for the other blood cells, produce new zooids through vascular budding in some colonial tunicates and form the gonads in synstyelid ascidians. The function of lymphocytes is unclear, but they appear to be involved in immune responses. Granular leucocytes are trophocytic and remove foreign materials by phagocytosis. Phagocytosis is also observed in hyaline leucocytes which are also believed to be the progenitors of vacuolated cells. A variety of functions are executed by the vacuolated cells. They are involved in tunic formation and wound healing, encapsulate foreign materials too large to be phagocytosed and coagulate at the site of vascular injuries. Pigment cells are responsible for the distinctive colour and colour markings of each species. Their function is unknown but they may afford protection against ultraviolet light. Protein and nucleic acid metabolic waste products are concentrated in solid form as granular concretions by nephrocytes. Their function is thus one of storage and excretion.

While much is known about ascidian blood and blood cells, it is apparent that numerous areas with unanswered questions exist. Many of them have been mentioned in the text. Blood chemistry studies are totally lacking and the origin, nature and function of the plasma proteins unknown. Nothing is known about the distribution and localization of intracellular enzymes nor the biosynthetic pathways nephrocytes use in accumulating nitrogenous wastes or how they dispose of them. The chemical nature, synthesis and function of the various pigments in pigment cells have yet to be determined. Synthesis, molecular structure and function of the organo-metallic compounds of vacuolated cells and their relationship to tunic formation need to be elucidated. Finally, the mechanism(s) by which the various blood cells recognize and respond to foreign materials need to be ascertained.

Ascidians are the most advanced group of invertebrates and are generally considered to be the ancestors of vertebrates (Berrill, 1950). While no attempt has been made to compare ascidian blood cells with vertebrate blood cells, there are many similarities between them (Wright, 1976). Most notable is the origin and location of the haematopoietic tissues. The participation of granular leucocytes (macrophage-like cells) and possibly lymphocyte-like cells in cellular immune reactions and the recent observation that ascidian plasma proteins may be similar to vertebrate immunoglobulins (Marchalonis and Warr, 1978), suggests that the origins of vertebrate humoral and cellular immune responses may be found in the ascidians. With further study and continued experimentation, many of the questions posed will be answered and a more fuller understanding of urochordate blood cells achieved.

Acknowledgements

I wish to thank Dr Elizabeth A. Stein for her many helpful comments and criticisms during the preparation of the manuscript. I am deeply indebted to and graciously acknowledge Drs Robert S. Anderson, Lucio Botte, Thomas H. Ermak, Gary Freeman, Hirokazu Fujimoto, Jane Overton, Michael J. Smith and Kunio Tanaka who provided the figures which made this chapter clearer and more complete. I thank Academic Press, Birkhauser Verlag, Elsevier/North-Holland Biomedical Press, Wistar Institute Press and Woods Hole Marine Biological Laboratory for permission to publish these figures. My sincere thanks to Miss Patricia H. Byrnes and Mrs Lois Treichler-Gehringer for their typing and technical assistance and to Mr Bobbie McAllister for preparing the line figure. Supported by USPHS Grant HD 09333 from the National Institute of Child Health and Human Development.

References

Anderson, R. S. (1971). *Biol. Bull., Woods Hole* **141**, 91–98.
Anderson, R. S. and Good, R. A. (1975). *Biol. Bull., Woods Hole* **148**, 357–369.
Anderson, R. S., Jordan, L. A. and Harshbarger, J. C. (1977). *J. Invertebr. Pathol.* **30**, 160–168.
Andrew, W. (1961). *Quart. Jl. Microsc. Sci.* **102**, 89–105.
Azéma, M. (1926). *C. r. hebd. Séanc. Acad. Sci., Paris* **183**, 1299–1301.
Azéma, M. (1928). *C. r. Ass. Anat.* **23**, 14–25.
Azéma, M. (1929a). *C. r. Séanc. Soc. Biol.* **102**, 823–825.
Azéma, M. (1929b). *C. r. Séanc. Soc. Biol.* **102**, 918–920.
Azéma, M. (1929c). *Bull. Soc. zool. Fr.* **54**, 13–20.
Azéma, M. (1929d). *Bull. Soc. zool. Fr.* **54**, 617–619.
Azéma, M. (1937). *Annls. Inst. océanogr., Monaco* **17**, 1–150.
Baltscheffsky, H. and Baltscheffsky, M. (1953). *Pubbl. Staz. zool. Napoli* **24**, 447–451.
Baltscheffsky, H. and Mendia, L. (1958). *Pubbl. Staz. zool. Napoli* **30**, 9–15.
Bancroft, F. W. (1903). *Proc. Calif. Acad. Sci.* **3**, 137–186.
Barrington, E. J. W. and Thorpe, A. (1968). *Proc. R. Soc., Series B* **171**, 91–109.
Bayer, E. (1955). *Experientia* **12**, 365–368.
Benham, W. B. (1894). *Quart. Jl. Microsc. Sci.* **35**, 97–118.
Berrill, N. J. (1950). "The Tunicata With An Account of the British Species". Ray Society, London.
Bertrand, D. (1950). *Bull. Am. Mus. nat. Hist.* **94**, 403–456.

Bialaszewicz, K. (1933). *Arch. Int. Physiol.* **36**, 41–53.
Bielig, H. J. and Bayer, E. (1954). *Experientia* **10**, 300–302.
Bielig, H. J., Bayer, E., Califano, L. and Wirth, L. (1954). *Pubbl. Staz. zool. Napoli* **25**, 26–66.
Bielig, H. J., Joste, E., Pfleger, K., Rummel, W. and Seifen, E. (1961a). *Hoppe-Seyler's Z. physiol. Chem.* **325,** 122–131.
Bielig, H. J., Joste, W., Pfleger, K. and Rummel, W. (1961b). *Hoppe-Seyler's Z. physiol. Chem.* **325**, 132–145.
Bielig, H. J., Bayer, E., Dell, H. D., Robins, G., Möllinger, H. and Rüdiger, W. (1966). *Prot. Biol. Fluids* **14**, 197–204.
Boeri, E. and Ehrenberg, A. (1954). *Archs Biochem. Biophys.* **50**, 404–416.
Boolootian, R. A. and Giese, A. G. (1959). *J. exp. Zool.* **140**, 207–229.
Botte, L. and Scippa, S. (1977). *Experientia* **33**, 80–81.
Brescianai, J. and Lützen, J. (1960). *Cah. Biol. mar.* **1**, 157–184.
Bretting, H. and Renwrantz, L. (1973). *Z. ImmunForsch.* **145**, 242–249.
Brien, P. (1928). *Recl. Inst. zool. Torley-Rousseau* **2**, 5–116.
Brien, P. (1930). *Annls. Soc. r. zool. Belg.* **61**, 19–112.
Brien, P. (1948). *In* "Traité de Zoologie" (P. Grassé, Ed.), Tome XI, pp. 553–751. Masson et Cie, Paris.
Brien, P. and Blanjean, F. (1939). *Annls. Soc. r. zool. Belg.* **69**, 247–271.
Brown, A. C. and Davies, A. B. (1971). *J. Invertebr. Pathol.* **18**, 267–279.
Bryan, F. T., Robinson Jr., C. W., Gilbert, C. P. and Langdell, R. R. (1964). *Science* **144**, 1147–1148.
Burighel, P. and Brunetti, R. (1971). *Boll. Zool.* **38**, 273–289.
Califano, L. and Caselli, P. (1948). *Pubbl. Staz. zool. Napoli* **21**, 261–271.
Califano, L. and Boeri, E. (1950). *J. exp. Zool.* **27**, 253–256.
Cantacuzène, J. (1919). *C. r. Séanc. Soc. Biol.* **82**, 1019–1022.
Carlisle, D. B. (1958). *Nature, Lond.* **181**, 933.
Carlisle, D. B. (1968). *Proc. R. Soc., Series B* **171**, 31–42.
Carlson, R. M. K. (1975). *Proc. Nat. Acad. Sci., U.S.A.* **72**, 2217–2221.
Ciereszko, L. S., Ciereszko, E. M., Harris, E. R. and Lane, C. A. (1963). *Comp. Biochem. Physiol.* **9**, 137–140.
Cowden, R. R. (1968). *Trans. Amer. Microsc. Soc.* **87**, 521–524.
Cuénot, L. (1891). *Archs. Zool. exp. gén.* **9**, 13–90.
Dahlgrün, W. (1901). *Arch. mikrosk. Anat. EntwMech.* **58**, 608–640.
Danskin, G. P. (1978). *Can. J. Zool.* **56**, 547–551.
Das, S. M. (1936). *J. Morphol.* **59**, 586–601.
Deck, J. D., Hay, E. D. and Revel, J. P. (1966). *J. Morphol.* **120**, 267–280.
de Vicentis, M. and Rüdiger, W. (1967). *Experientia* **23**, 245–246.
Ebara, A. (1971). *Comp. Biochem. Physiol.* **39A**, 795–805.
Endean, R. (1953). *Nature, Lond.* **172**, 123.
Endean, R. (1955a). *Aust. J. mar. Freshwat. Res.* **6**, 35–59.
Endean, R. (1955b). *Aust. J. mar. Freshwat. Res.* **6**, 139–156.
Endean, R. (1955c). *Aust. J. mar. Freshwat. Res.* **6**, 157–164.
Endean, R. (1960). *Quart. Jl. Microsc. Sci.* **101**, 177–197.
Endean, R. (1961). *Quart. Jl. Microsc. Sci.* **102**, 107–117.
Ermak, T. H. (1975). *Experientia* **31**, 837–839.
Ermak, T. H. (1976). *In* "Phylogeny of Thymus and Bone Marrow-Bursa Cells" (R. K. Wright and E. L. Cooper, Eds), pp. 45–56. Elsevier/North-Holland, Amsterdam.

Fernandez, M. (1904). *Jena. Z. Naturw.* **32**, 323–422.
Form, D. M., Warr, G. W. and Marchalonis, J. J. (1979). *Fedn Proc. Fedn Am. Socs. exp. Biol.* **38**, 934.
Franz, V. (1927). *Ergebn. Anat. Entwickl. Gesch.* **27**, 464–568.
Freeman, G. (1964). *J. exp. Zool.* **156**, 157–183.
Freeman, G. (1970a). *J. reticuloendoth. Soc.* **7**, 183–194.
Freeman, G. (1970b). *Transplantation* **2**, 236–239.
Fry, H. J. B. (1909). *Folia haemat.* **8**, 467.
Fujimoto, H. and Watanabe, H. (1976). *J. Morphol.* **150**, 623–638.
Fuke, M. T. and Sugai, T. (1972). *Biol. Bull., Woods Hole* **143**, 140–149.
Fulton, J. F. (1920). *Acta zool., Stockh.* **1**, 381–431.
Gansler, H., Pfleger, K., Seifen, E. and Bielig, H. J. (1963). *Experientia* **19**, 232–234.
George, W. C. (1926). *J. Morph. Physiol.* **41**, 311–331.
George, W. C. (1930). *J. Morph. Physiol.* **49**, 385–413.
George, W. C. (1936). *Biol. Bull., Woods Hole* **71**, 249–254.
George, W. C. (1939). *Quart. Jl. Microsc. Sci.* **81**, 391–431.
Gilbert, K., Kustin, K. and McLeod, G. C. (1977). *J. Cell Physiol.* **93**, 309–312.
Godeaux, J. (1964). *Sonderdr. Stud. Gen., Jahrg* **17**, 176–190.
Goldberg, E. D., McBlair, W. and Taylor, K. M. (1951). *Biol. Bull., Woods Hole* **101**, 84–94.
Goodbody, I. (1957). *J. exp. Biol.* **34**, 297–305.
Goodbody, I. (1965). *J. exp. Biol.* **42**, 299–305.
Goodbody, I. (1974). *Adv. mar. Biol.* **12**, 1–149.
Hecht, S. (1918). *Am. J. Physiol.* **45**, 157–187.
Henze, M. (1911). *Hoppe-Seyler's Z. physiol. Chem.* **72**, 494–501.
Henze, M. (1912). *Hoppe-Seyler's Z. physiol. Chem.* **79**, 215–228.
Henze, M. (1913a). *Hoppe-Seyler's Z. physiol. Chem.* **86**, 340–344.
Henze, M. (1913b). *Hoppe-Seyler's Z. physiol. Chem.* **86**, 345–346.
Henzlik, R. E. (1966). *Proc. Indiana Acad. Sci.* **75**, 284.
Herdman, W. A. (1888). *Zool. Challenger Exped. Lond.* **27**, 1–166.
Herdman, W. A. (1899). "Ascidia. L.M.B.C. Memoirs on Typical British Marine Plants and Animals", 1, 1–60.
Hildemann, W. H. and Reddy, A. L. (1973). *Fedn Proc. Fedn Am. Socs. exp. Biol.* **32**, 2188–2194.
Huus, J. (1937). *In* "Handbuch der Zoologie" (W. Kukenthal, Ed.), Vol. V, Part 2, pp. 614–616. De Gruyter, Berlin.
Ichikawa, A. (1966). *In* "6th International Congress for Electron Microscopy" (R. Vyeda, Ed.), Vol. II, pp. 695–696. Maruzen, Tokyo.
Ivanova-Kazas, O. M. (1966). *Arkh. Anat. Gistol. Embriol.* **51**, 48–56.
Johnson, P. T. and Chapman, F. A. (1970). J. Invertebr. Pathol. **16**, 259–267.
Kalk, M. (1963a). *Nature, Lond.* **198**, 1010–1011.
Kalk, M. (1963b). *Quart. Jl. Microsc. Sci.* **104**, 483–493.
Kalk, M. (1970). *Tissue and Cell* **2**, 99–118.
Karakashian, S. and Milkman, R. (1967). *Biol. Bull., Woods Hole* **133**, 473.
Katow, H. and Watanabe, H. (1978). *J. Ultrastruct. Res.* **64**, 23–34.
Kawaguti, S. and Ikemoto, N. (1958). *Biol. J. Okayama Univ.* **4**, 93–101.
Kobayashi, S. (1933). *Sci. Rep. Tôhoku Univ.* **8**, 277–285.
Kobayashi, S. (1938). *Sci. Rep. Tôhoku Univ.* **13**, 25–35.
Kobayashi, S. (1949). *Sci. Rep. Tôhoku Univ.* **18**, 185–193.
Kokubu, N. and Hidaka, T. (1965). *Nature, Lond.* **205**, 1028–1029.

Kollmann, M. (1908). *Annls Sci. nat.* **8**, 1–240.
Koval'skii, V. V. and Rezaeva, L. T. (1963). *Dokl. Akad. Nauk SSSR* **148**, 238–240.
Koval'skii, V. V. and Rezaeva, L. T. (1965). *Usp. sovrem. Biol.* **60**, 45–61.
Koval'skii, V. V., Rezaeva, L. T. and Kol'tsov, G. V. (1962). *Dokl. Akad. Nauk SSSR* **147**, 1215–1217.
Kowalevsky, A. O. (1867). *Mém Acad. Sci., St. Pétersburg* **10**, 1–19.
Kowalevsky, A. O. (1871). *Arch. mikrosk. Anat. EntwMech.* **7**, 101–130.
Kriebel, M. E. (1968). *J. gen. Physiol.* **52**, 46–59.
Krijgsman, B. J. (1956). *Biol. Rev.* **31**, 288–312.
Krukenberg, C. F. W. (1882). *In* "Vergleichend-Physiologische Studien", Part 1, pp. 87–138. C. Winter, Heidelberg.
Kupffer, C. W. von (1872). *Arch. mikrosk. Anat. EntwMech.* **8**, 358–396.
Kupffer, C. W. von (1874). "Tunicata". Die zweite Deutsche NordpolFahrt, Bd. II, Leipzig.
Kustin, K., Levine, D. S., McLeod, G. S. and Curby, W. A. (1976). *Biol. Bull., Woods Hole* **150**, 426–441.
Lacaze-Duthiers, H. (1874). *Archs Zool. exp. gén.* **3**, 257–330.
Lambert, C. C. and Brandt, C. L. (1967). *Biol. Bull., Woods Hole* **132**, 222–228.
Lankester, E. R. (1889). *Quart. Jl. Microsc. Sci.* **29**, 365–402.
Lederer, E. (1934). *C. r. Séanc. Soc. Biol.* **117**, 1086–1088.
Levine, E. P. (1961). *Science* **133**, 1352–1353.
Levine, E. P. (1962). *J. Morphol.* **111**, 105–137.
Lister, J. J. (1834). *Phil. Trans. R. Soc.* **124**, 365–388.
Lorber, V. and Rayns, D. G. (1972). *J. Cell Sci.* **10**, 211–227.
Lorber, V. and Rayns, D. G. (1977). *Cell Tiss. Res.* **179**, 169–175.
Lyding, S. (1953). *Ark. Kemi* **6**, 261–269.
Lyerla, T. A., Lyerla, J. H. and Fisher, M. (1975). *Biol. Bull., Woods Hole* **149**, 178–185.
Macara, I. G., McLeod, G. C. and Kustin, K. (1979). *Comp. Biochem. Physiol.* **62A**, 821–826.
Marchalonis, J. J. and Warr, G. (1978). *Dev. Comp. Immunol.* **2**, 443–460.
Metchnikoff, E. (1892). "Leçons sur la Pathologie Comparée de l'Inflammation". Masson et Cie, Paris.
Milanesi, C. and Burighel, P. (1978). *Acta zool., Stockh.* **59**, 135–147.
Milkman, R. (1967). *Biol. Bull., Woods Hole* **132**, 229–243.
Milkman, R. and Byrne, S. (1961). *Biol. Bull., Woods Hole* **121**, 376.
Millar, R. H. (1953). "Ciona. L.M.B.C. Memoirs on Typical British Marine Plants and Animals", 35, 1–123.
Milne-Edwards, H. (1842). *Mem. Acad. Sci., Paris* **18**, 217–326.
Moller, P. C. and Philpott, C. W. (1973). *J. Morphol.* **139**, 389–406.
Monniot, C. (1963). *Vie Milieu* **14**, 263–273.
Mukai, H. (1967). *Sci. Rep. Tôhoku Univ.* **13**, 51–73.
Mukai, H. (1974). *Annotnes zool. jap.* **47**, 43–47.
Mukai, H. and Watanabe, H. (1974). *Biol. Bull., Woods Hole* **147**, 411–421.
Mukai, H. and Watanabe, H. (1975a). *Proc. Japan Acad.* **51**, 44–47.
Mukai, H. and Watanabe, H. (1975b). *Proc. Japan Acad.* **51**, 48–50.
Mukai, H. and Watanabe, H. (1976). *J. Morphol.* **148**, 337–362.
Mukai, H., Sugimoto, K. and Taneda, Y. (1978). *J. Morphol.* **157**, 49–78.
Nakauchi, M. (1976). *In* "The Laboratory Animal in the Study of Reproduction" (Th. Antikatzides, S. Erichsen and A. Spiegel, Eds), pp. 89–98. Gustav Fischer Verlag, Stuttgart.

Newberry, A. T. (1968). *J. Morphol.* **126**, 123–162.
Noddack, I. and Noddack, W. (1939). Ark. Zool. **32**, 1–35.
Nolf, P. (1909). *Arch. Int. Physiol.* **7**, 280–301.
Ohuye, T. (1936). *Sci. Rep. Tôhoku Univ.* **11**, 191–206.
Oka, H. and Usui, M. (1944). *Sci. Rep. Tokyo Bunrika Daig., Series B* **7**, 23–53.
Oka, H. and Watanabe, H. (1957a). *Biol. Bull., Woods Hole* **112**, 225–240.
Oka, H. and Watanabe, H. (1957b). *Proc. Japan Acad.* **33**, 657–659.
Oka, H. and Watanabe, H. (1959). *Biol. Bull., Woods Hole* **117**, 340–346.
Oka, H. and Watanabe, H. (1960). *Bull. biol. Stn Asamushi* **10**, 153–155.
Oka, H. and Watanabe, H. (1967). *Kagaku, Tokyo* **37**, 307–313.
Oliphant, L. W. and Cloney, R. A. (1972). *Z. Zellforsch. mikrosk. Anat.* **129**, 395–412.
Overton, J. (1966). *J. Morphol.* **119**, 305–326.
Parrinello, N. and Patricolo, E. (1975). *Experientia* **31**, 1092–1093.
Parrinello, N., Patricolo, E. and Canicatti, C. (1977). *Boll. Zool.* **44**, 373–381.
Pérès, J. M. (1943). *Annls Inst. océanog., Monaco* **21**, 229–359.
Pérès, J. M. (1944). *Bull. Inst. océanogr., Monaco* **857**, 1–8.
Pérès, J. M. (1945). *Bull. Inst. océanogr., Monaco* **882**, 1–18.
Pérès, J. M. (1948a). *Arch. Anat. microsc. Morph. exp.* **37**, 230–260.
Pérès, J. M. (1948b). *Bull. Inst. océanogr., Monaco* **936**, 923–941.
Pizon, A. (1899). *C. r. hebd. Séanc. Acad. Sci., Paris* **129**, 395–398.
Rapkine, L. and Damboviceanu, A. (1925). *C. r. Séanc. Soc. Biol.* **93**, 1427–1429.
Reddy, A. L., Bryan, B. and Hildemann, W. H. (1975). *Immunogenetics* **1**, 584–590.
Renwrantz, L. and Uhlenbruck, G. (1974). *Vox Sang.* **26**, 385–391.
Rezaeva, L. T. (1964). *Zh. obshch. Biol.* **25**, 347–356.
Ries, E. (1937). *Wilhelm Roux Arch. EntwMech. Org.* **137**, 363–371.
Robertson, J. D. (1954). *J. exp. Biol.* **31**, 424–442.
Roule, L. (1884). *Annls. Mus. Hist. nat. Marseille* **2**, 1–270.
Rummel, W., Bielig, H. J., Forth, W., Pfleger, K., Rüdiger, W. and Seifen, E. (1966). *Prot. Biol. Fluids* **14**, 205–210.
Sabbadin. A. (1955). *Archo ital. Anat. Embriol.* **60**, 33–67.
Sabbadin, A. (1962). *Rend. Accad. Naz. Lincei* **32**, 1031–1035.
Sabbadin, A. and Tondonati, A. (1967). *Monitore zool. ital.* **1**, 185–190.
Saint-Hilaire, K. (1931). *Zool. Jahrbuch. Abt. Anat. Ontog.* **54**, 455–608.
Schulze, W. (1964). *Experientia* **20**, 265–266.
Seeliger, O. (1911). *In* "Klassen und Ordnungen des Tier-Reichs". Bd. III, Suppl. Tunicata I. Abt. Die Appendicularian und Ascidian (H. G. Bronn, Ed.), pp. 84–154. C. F. Winter'sche Verlagshandung, Leipzig.
Selys-Longchamps, M. de (1901). *Archs Biol.* **17**, 499–542.
Smith, M. J. (1970a). *Biol. Bull., Woods Hole* **138**, 354–378.
Smith, M. J. (1970b). *Biol. Bull., Woods Hole* **138**, 379–388.
Smith, M. J. and Dehnel, P. A. (1970). *Comp. Biochem. Physiol.* **40B**, 615–622.
Stiévenart, J. (1970). *Annls Soc. r. zool. Belg.* **100**, 139–157.
Stiévenart, J. (1971). *Annls Soc. r. zool. Belg.* **101**, 25–56.
Sugimoto, K. and Nakauchi, M. (1974). *Biol. Bull., Woods Hole* **147**, 213–226.
Swinehart, J. H., Biggs, W. R., Halko, D. J. and Schroeder, N. C. (1974). *Biol. Bull., Woods Hole* **146**, 302–312.
Tanaka, K. (1973). *Cell. Immunol.* **7**, 427–443.
Tanaka, K. (1975). *Adv. exp. med. Biol.* **64**, 115–124.
Tanaka, K. and Watanabe, H. (1973). *Cell. Immunol.* **64**, 115–124.
Thomas, J. A. (1931a). *C. r. Séanc. Soc. Biol.* **108**, 694–696.

Thomas, J. A. (1931b). *C. r. Séanc. Soc. Biol.* **108**, 667–669.
Thomas, J. A. (1932). *Annls Inst. Pasteur, Paris* **49**, 234–274.
Todaro, F. (1875). *Atti Accad. naz. Lincei Memorie* **2**, 720–792.
Vallee, J. A. (1967). *Bull. S. Calif. Acad. Sci.* **66**, 23–28.
Vallee, J. A. (1968). *Bull. S. Calif. Acad. Sci.* **67**, 89–95.
Van Beneden, E. and Julin, Ch. (1885). *Archs Biol.* **6**, 237–476.
Van Beneden, P. J. (1847). *Nouv. Mém. Acad. Roy. Belg.* **20**, 1–66.
Vinogradov, A. P. (1953). "The Elementary Chemical Composition of Marine Organisms". Sears Foundation for Marine Research, Yale University, New Haven.
von Skramlik, E. (1929). *Z. vergl. Physiol.* **9**, 553–563.
von Skramlik, E. (1938). *Ergebn. Biol.* **15**, 166–308.
Wardrop, A. B. (1970). *Protoplasma* **70**, 73–86.
Warr, G. W., Decker, J. M., Mandel, T. E., Deluca, D., Hudson, R. and Marchalonis, J. J. (1977). *Aust. J. exp. biol. med. Sci.* **55**, 151–164.
Webb, D. A. (1939). *J. exp. Biol.* **16**, 499–523.
Webb, D. A. (1956). *Pubbl. Staz. zool. Napoli* **28**, 273–288.
Weiss, J. and Morad, M. (1974). *Science* **186**, 750–752.
Weiss, J., Goldman, Y. and Morad, M. (1976). *J. gen. Physiol.* **68**, 503–518.
Woollacott, R. M. (1974). *Devl. Biol.* **40**, 186–195.
Wright, R. K. (1973). Ph.D. Dissertation, University California at Santa Barbara.
Wright, R. K. (1974). *J. Invertebr. Pathol.* **24**, 29–36.
Wright, R. K. (1976). *In* "Phylogeny of Thymus and Bone Marrow-Bursa Cells" (R. K. Wright and E. L. Cooper, Eds), pp. 57–70. Elsevier/North-Holland, Amsterdam.
Wright, R. K. and Cooper, E. L. (1975). *Amer. Zool.* **15**, 21–27.

Section IX

Comparative Aspects of the Structure and Function of Invertebrate and Vertebrate Leucocytes

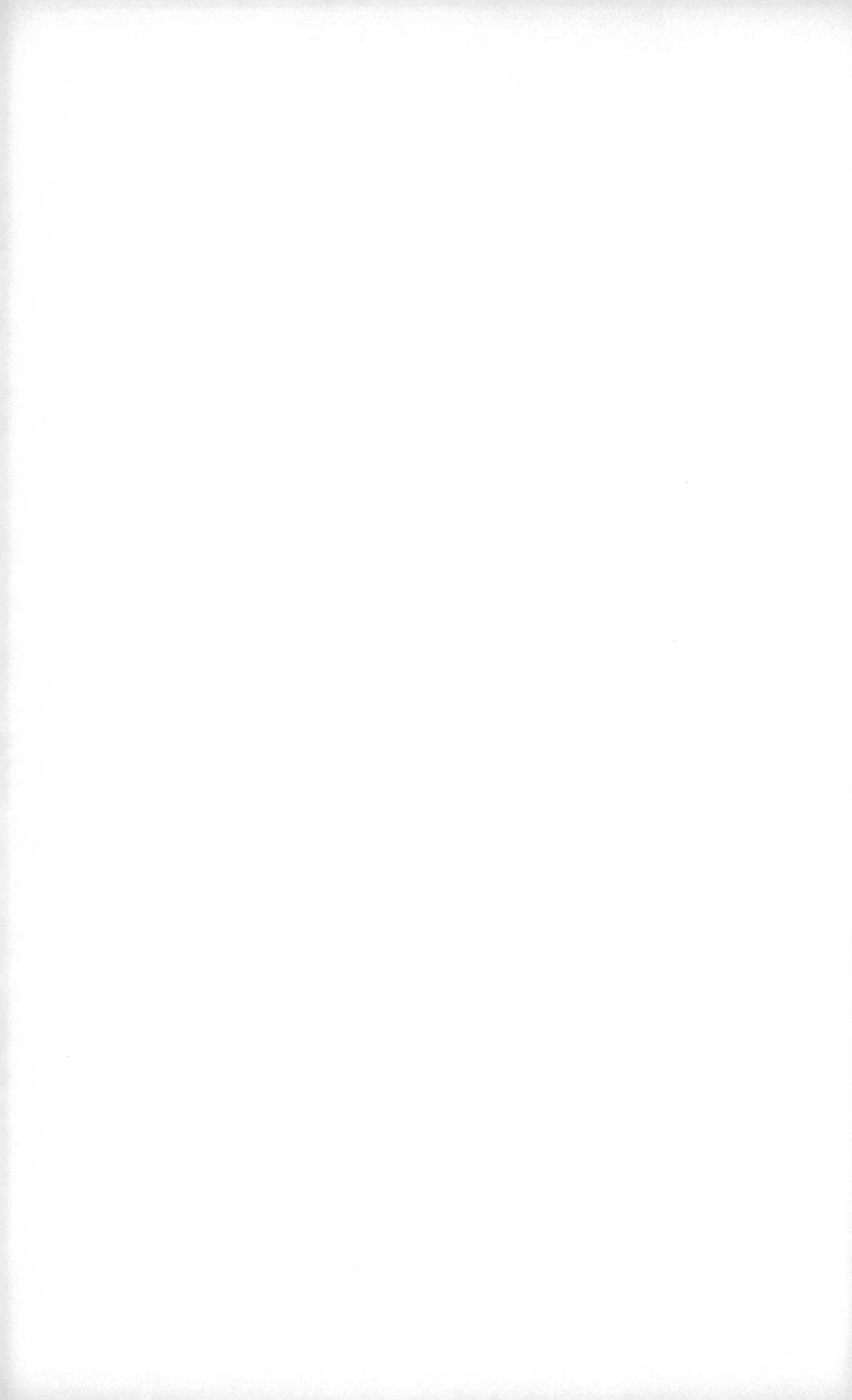

17. Comparative aspects of the structure and function of invertebrate and vertebrate leucocytes

R. S. ANDERSON

Sloan-Kettering Institute for Cancer Research, Donald S. Walker Laboratory, 145 Boston Post Road, Rye, New York 10580, U.S.A.

CONTENTS

I. Introduction

Current evidence suggests that the leucocytes of all animals have evolved for a common purpose, namely, to defend the host organism against foreign invaders. The ability of these cells to respond to non-self extends to recognition of microorganisms, parasites, exogenous proteins, erythrocytes, malignant cells, etc. Leucocytes mediate two major defence mechanisms: phagocytosis (and/or encapsulation) and elaboration of various effector substances.

Vertebrate haematopoietic progenitor cells differentiate into lymphoid stem cells and into stem cells which ultimately give rise to erythrocytes, magakaryocytes, granulocytes, monocytes or macrophages. Some invertebrate blood cells morphologically resemble one or more of these cell types, however, functional capacities of these cells may be quite different. Although caution should be exercised in trying to establish homology between leucocyte classes in phylogenetically diverse organisms, it is helpful to look for analogous properties. Such comparison is necessary if immunologists studying invertebrate animals hope to describe phenomana using terms developed by workers studying similar reactions in vertebrates. The terms used in vertebrate immunology are precisely defined and their use is preferable to developing specialized invertebrate semantics, which would be poorly understood by other workers in the field. The various properties of invertebrate leucocytes have already been covered in detail in this volume; therefore, I will cite only a few examples of their reactivities and compare these to comparable mammalian situations. In my attempt to present an ordered overview of this subject, rather than making a comprehensive review of the literature basic concepts will be stressed.

II. Enzyme content of vertebrate and invertebrate leucocytes

In higher animals, granule-containing blood cells, particularly neutrophils, are active in phagocytosing and destroying infective microbes. Many invertebrates have granular haemocytes morphologically similar to myelocytes or band forms of immature polymorphonuclear cells (PMNs). Primary granules appear in the cytoplasm early in the development of PMNs; these contain many enzymes including myeloperoxidase, lysozyme, bactericidal cationic proteins, acid phosphatase, β-galactosidase, β-glucuronidase, esterase and other hydrolytic enzymes (Baggiolini, 1972). Myeloperoxidase (MPO) is located exclusively in the primary granules of PMNs and is the best enzymatic marker of this cell population (Bainton and Farquhar, 1968a,b). As the PMNs mature, secondary (specific) granules appear in the cytoplasm; these soon outnumber the primary granules as the cells continue to differentiate. Secondary granules are rich in alkaline phosphatase, lysozyme and aminopeptidase.

The monocyte-macrophage series of vertebrate leucocytes also possesses cytoplasmic granules containing hydrolytic enzymes. The granule-related enzymatic contents of these cells increase with maturation, particularly when the cells are activated, as in certain infections. In vertebrates, bone marrow promonocytes give rise to blood monocytes, which are the precursors of macrophages seen in tissues and in the pleural, peritoneal and alveolar spaces. The accepted pathway of monocyte differentiation into macrophages, multinucleated giant cells, and epithelioid cells was described by *in vitro* observations of Lewis (1925) and *in vivo* by Ebert and Florey (1939), and by many subsequent investigators. Blood monocytes have centrally located nuclei which are often kidney- or horseshoe-shaped. Granules which stain with neutral red or Janus green are often seen in the perinuclear region. The characteristics of macrophages differ considerably, depending on their location in the body; as will be detailed later, the biochemistry of alveolar macrophages differs from other macrophages. All macrophages are thigmotactic (attach to glass), phagocytic, and contain a host of enzymes including β-glucuronidase, β-galactosidase, myeloperoxidase (only in macrophage precursor cells), esterases, lipases, acid phosphatase, aryl sulphatase and lysozyme (particularly in alveolar macrophages).

Many hydrolytic enzymes are also found in invertebrate haemocytes and in serum, presumably as a result of degranulation reactions. Examples of cell-associated enzymes in molluscs are β-glucuronidase, acid phosphatase, alkaline phosphatase, amylase, lipase and lysozyme (Cheng and Rodrick, 1975), *N*-acetyl-β-glucosaminidase and indoxyl esterase (Moore and Lowe, 1977) and non-specific esterase (Feng *et al.*, 1971). The presence of lysosomes, suggested by non-specific esterase and acid phosphatase activity, and by supravital staining of the granules by neutral red, was confirmed by electron microscopy and cytochemistry (Yoshino and Cheng, 1976). Considerable work has been done on inverbebrate lysozyme because it may play a role in controlling bacterial infection. Lysozyme-like activity has been measured not only in molluscs (McDade and Tripp, 1967), but also in *Asterias rubens* (Jollès and Jollès, 1975) and insects (Powning and Davidson, 1973). Anderson and Cook (1979), demonstrated basal levels of lysozyme activity in the haemocytes and serum of larval *Spodoptera eridania*, and studied the induction of this activity by various agents. The blood cells released lysozyme *in vitro* and were thus implicated as major contributors to serum levels of the enzyme.

Therefore, the data suggest that invertebrate blood phagocytes have characteristic lysosomal enzymes which can degrade ingested materials. The *in vivo* and *in vitro* destruction of bacteria and other biological materials has been described in many invertebrate species. Furthermore, enzymes released during degranulation reactions probably also serve as mediators in protective mechanisms. It would be difficult to differentiate invertebrate haemocytes from mammalian PMNs or macrophages based on lysosomal hydrolases; however, studies of myeloperoxidase content are more revealing. As was noted previously, this enzyme is readily shown in PMNs and, to a lesser extent, in immature macrophage precursors. Myeloperoxidase is virtually absent in invertebrate haemocytes (Anderson *et al.*, 1973b; Cheng, 1976), suggesting a closer relationship to macrophages than PMNs.

III. Cell surface receptors

First, we should consider what is known about the binding and phagocytosis of erythrocytes by human monocytes; binding and uptake of erythrocytes by haemocytes is one of the most commonly studied immunological reactions of invertebrates. In man, senescent or damaged erythrocytes are coated with immunoglobulin G (IgG) molecules via the Fab portion of the antibody. Monocytes bear surface receptors for the Fc fragment of certain IgG classes which mediates the binding of opsonized erythrocytes (LoBuglio *et al.*, 1967). In the same way, macrophages recognize IgG-coated microorganisms. The surface receptors bind IgG antigen complexes more avidly than unreacted IgG, permitting the macrophage to selectively identify immune complexes. Human monocytes do not have receptors for IgM or IgA, but may have receptors for some complement components bound to IgM or IgA (Huber and Fudenberg, 1968; Kaplan *et al.*, 1972). IgG receptors are also found on neutrophils and B-lymphocytes.

In addition to antibody or complement-mediated binding of erythrocytes to leucocytes is a process of non-immune erythrocyte binding, a characteristic of T-lymphocytes (Jondal *et al.*, 1972).

There are numerous reports of the formation of mammalian and avian erythrocyte rosettes around invertebrate haemocytes. Presumably, this represents a primitive type of recognition reaction against antigens found on many kinds of membranes. Frequently, the intensity of the reaction may be modified by chemical alteration of the erythrocytes, such as treatment with formaldehyde. Renwrantz and Cheng (1977) reported that the haemocytes of the gastropod, *Helix pomatia*, were capable of directly binding various kinds of red cells, and that non-native agglutinins of plant and animal origin could serve as linking agents in haemocyte-rbc reactions. The coelomocytes of earthworms can also form spontaneous rosettes with sheep red blood cells (Toupin and Lamoureux, 1976). The rosette-forming coelomocyte population was composed of nonadhering, nongranular cells, morphologically resembling vertebrate T-lymphocytes, which characteristically form similar rosettes. The authors suggest that these cells might be the evolutionary precursors or analogues of T-cells. It must be remembered, however, that the spontaneous production of non-immune rosettes is also a property of mammalian macrophages. Anderson (1977), showed that insect macrophages (plasmatocytes, see Chapter 13) possess membrane receptors for unmodified avian and mammalian erythrocytes. In this case, adhering hyaline haemocytes were the only rosette-forming blood cell subpopulation. It was shown that neuraminidase treatment of either insect blood cells or the target erythrocytes had little effect on binding; the enhanced binding of neuraminidase-treated erythrocytes is thought to be a specific property of human T-cells (Baxley *et al.*, 1973). Insect macrophages, like their mammalian counterparts, form rosettes in the absence of humoral agents, such as haemagglutinins. The binding of erythrocytes to insect and mammalian leucocytes involves normal microfilament function, as shown by the reversible inhibition of rosetting by cytochalasin B, and is independent of microtubules (Anderson, 1977).

Whereas binding of red cells to insect blood cells has been shown not to require serum factors (Scott, 1971b; Anderson *et al.*, 1973a), other invertebrates apparently may require opsonins to promote binding of foreign particles. For example, Prowse and Tait (1969) reported that serum factors were required for the uptake of formalin-treated yeast by the haemocytes of *Helix aspersa*. In the oyster *Crassostrea virginica*, erythrocytes could be phagocytosed in the absence of serum factors, but uptake was stimulated by the presence of a native haemagglutinin (Tripp and Kent, 1967).

Evidence for the presence of circulating red cell opsonins has also been presented in the case of the sea hare, *Aplysia californica* (Pauley *et al.*, 1971) and the octopus *Eledone cirrosa* (Stuart, 1968). Anderson and Good (1976) studied *in vitro* phagocytosis of yeast, red cells, and bacteria by the haemocytes of the gastropod mollusc, *Otala lactea*, which lacks serum haemagglutinins. Uptake of fresh or formalin-treated bacteria was variable and not affected by serum factors. Untreated yeast or red blood cells were not extensively phagocytosed; formalin treatment enhanced phagocytosis of these particles. The presence of haemolymph stimulated the uptake of formalized yeast but not formalized red cells. It was interesting that haemagglutinin-containing extracts of *O. lactea* albumin gland were shown to opsonize formalized red cells.

It may be seen that, although all invertebrate cells can react to foreign material, the requirements for binding and phagocytosis differ considerably. Probably at least some binding of particulates can occur independently of humoral factors. However, serum components, particularly agglutinins, will often facilitate haemocyte-particle interaction. Clearly, factors other than agglutinins can also augment binding and phagocytosis.

Receptors for native serum components may be expressed on invertebrate haemocytes but there is no evidence of receptors for mammalian antibodies. No increased binding of sheep red blood cells (SRBC), after sensitization with rabbit anti-SRBC, was seen in several insect species (Rabinovitch and De Stefano, 1970; Scott, 1971a; Anderson, 1976). Similar results were obtained by Stuart (1968) using haemocytes of the lesser octopus, *Eledone cirrosa*.

Receptors for complement components are present on human PMNs, macrophages and B-lymphocytes. These receptors function in binding complement-containing immune complexes and in complement-mediated chemotactic responses. While invertebrates do not possess direct acting haemolytic complement, it has been suggested that they might have the terminal components which comprise the alternate pathway of complement activation (Day *et al.*, 1970). Anderson *et al.* (1972) also showed that insect haemolymph contained a factor which, when reacted with cobra venom factor, could lyse sheep erythrocytes via activation of frog terminal complement components. This indicated the presence of a humoral molecule similar to the complement component three proactivator found in human serum. Despite this indirect evidence of a complement system akin to the properdin system, no complement receptors have yet been shown on invertebrate blood cells. In preliminary studies, erythrocyte rosette formation around insect haemocytes was unchanged by sensitization with antibody and complement (Anderson, 1976).

IV. Invertebrate lymphocytes

The question of the existence of lymphocytes in invertebrates is still debated. There is no doubt that cells which resemble vertebrate lymphocytes are found in certain invertebrates. Many authors choose to refer to these cells as lymphocytes. In fact, these cells are probably haemocyte progenitor cells. Traces of rudimentary lymphoid systems are rarely seen in animals lower than primitive vertebrates. For example, in the lamprey a primitive thymus is present as clusters of lymphoid cells are found from the second to the fifth pharyngeal pouches. Clusters of lymphoid cells are also seen in the lamprey's spleen and lymphocytes are present in its blood. This animal can produce antibody, develop delayed hypersensitivity reactions and reject skin homografts (Finstad *et al.*, 1964; Papermaster *et al.*, 1964).

The B-cell category of lymphocyte does not exist in invertebrates; classical antibody has never been demonstrated in an invertebrate. Certain T-cell functions are carried out by invertebrate haemocytes, particularly those involved in graft rejection. However, with a few notable exceptions, specificity and immunological memory characteristically found in higher animals having well-developed lymphoid systems is hard to demonstrate in invertebrates.

Lymphocytes are effector cells of central importance in the immune responses of higher animals. Although many lymphocyte-like functions may be mediated by invertebrate haemocytes, there is little evidence to support the idea that these functions are carried out by lymphocyte-like cells. It is probable that the majority of invertebrate cellular immune responses are carried out by more mature blood cells, which usually far outnumber the prohaemocytes or "lymphocytes".

There are some very interesting recent studies of tunicate haemocytes and haematopoiesis which provide insight into possible phylogenetic origins of vertebrate lymphocytes and lymphoid tissue. Tunicates are thought to occupy a phylogenetic niche between invertebrates and vertebrates (Berrill, 1955). These organisms have a diverse array of blood cell types (George, 1939; Endean, 1960) including lymphocytes, vanadocytes, signet ring cells, amoebocytes and compartment cells (see Chapter 16). Amoebocytes are involved in phagocytosis of foreign materials and vanadocytes are active in encapsulation reactions and cellular responses to injury (Anderson, 1971). Lymphocytes are reported to participate in allograft rejection (Reddy *et al.*, 1975), sheep erythrocyte rosetting (Hildemann and Reddy, 1973), and mitogen responsiveness (Hildemann and Uhlenbruck, 1974; see, however, Warr *et al.*, 1977). Haemopoietic tissue is found in the pharyngeal and gut walls of primitive adult tunicates; in more advanced ascidians this tissue is organized into distinct lymph nodules in connective tissue underlying epithelia or blood sinuses (Ermak, 1976). Mitotically active haemocytoblasts are found in clusters in the centre of these nodules, surrounded by maturing blood cells. The so-called "lymphocytes" in tunicate blood are most likely haemocytoblasts or stem cells, comprising 5–15% of the circulating blood cells.

Although tunicata lymphocytes resemble vertebrate lymphocytes and have some functional properties in common, many of these characteristics are shared by non-lymphoid leucocytes. Also, the fact that invertebrate "lymphocytes" give rise to other blood cell types clearly separates them from typical lymphocytes of higher animals. Vertebrate lymphoid cell, red cell, granulocyte, and macrophage precursors may arise from a common pluripotent stem cell; however, early in haematopoiesis precursor cells are committed to either lymphoid cell lines or to the erythroid, granulocytic, megakaryocytic pathway and lymphocytes and their immediate precursors do not differentiate into other blood cell types.

V. Metabolism of leucocytes during phagocytosis

Although PMNs and platelets account for the bulk of oxygen utilization of whole blood, PMNs are quite able to move about and phagocytose in the absence of oxygen. However, the process of bacterial killing is dependent on the presence of oxygen. Particle ingestion is characteristically accompanied by a marked increase in respiration and the generation of hydrogen peroxide. The increased oxygen uptake is not mediated via the usual mitochondrial pathway, as shown by the failure of cyanide to poison the process (Karnovsky, 1962). Carbohydrate metabolism of PMNs is characterized by considerable anaerobic glycolysis, dependence on glycolysis for production of energy for phagocytosis, and greatly increased glucose oxidation via the hexose monophosphate (HMP) shunt during particle ingestion.

It is now possible to correlate certain biochemical changes with the various stages of phagocytosis by PMNs. Adhesion of foreign particles to cell membrane receptors does not require metabolic energy; glycolysis and RNA synthesis is stimulated by ingestion; increases in HMP shunt activity, O_2 consumption, and H_2O_2 production accompany degranulation; killing is effected by H_2O_2, myeloperoxidase (MPO), and cationic proteins; digestion is accomplished by granule-derived hydrolytic enzymes.

The metabolic events accompanying phagocytosis by monocytes and peritoneal macrophages are similar to those seen in neutrophils. The biochemistry of alveolar macrophage is unique. Apparently the metabolism of mononuclear leucocytes is strikingly influenced by their microenvironment, particularly regarding the partial pressure of oxygen. Human alveolar macrophages do not operate well at low oxygen levels, whereas monocytes and macrophages can function under anaerobic conditions (Cohen and Cline, 1971). Alveolar macrophages also lack the typical respiratory burst accompanying phagocytosis in other macrophages, monocytes and PMNs. The energy for phagocytosis in the alveolar macrophage is derived from oxidative phosphorylation (Karnovsky, 1962) rather than from glycolysis as is the case for other blood phagocytes. Human monocytes, other than alveolar macrophage, show a post-phagocytic increment in respiration, H_2O_2 generation, and HMP shunt stimulation (Cline and Lehrer, 1968).

Surprisingly few studies have been made of the comparative biochemistry of invertebrate blood phagocytic cells. No attempt has been made to study the metabolism of haemocyte coelomocyte subpopulations. Anderson *et al.* (1973b) studied various aspects of the metabolism of insect leucocytes; a similar study was carried out on molluscan blood cells by Cheng (1976). The conclusions of both of these papers were essentially the same; therefore, in the following discussion I will present these data as characteristic of invertebrate haemocytes. This may be a dangerous assumption; hopefully, more detailed metabolic studies of leucocytes from other invertebrate species will be forthcoming.

Phagocytosis by invertebrate haemocytes was accompanied by little or no increase in oxygen consumption. This lack of a respiratory burst was not typical of vertebrate blood phagocytes other than alveolar macrophages. Particle ingestion stimulated glycogen breakdown, glucose consumption and lactate production. It was shown that glycolysis provided the energy for phagocytosis by invertebrate cells, as was the case for mammalian leucocytes, including PMNs and peritoneal macrophages. The respiratory chain inhibitor KCN had little effect on the respiratory burst associated with phagocytosis and subsequent killing of bacteria by PMNs and macrophages. Bacterial killing by invertebrate cells was also cyanide-insensitive. However, various glycolytic inhibitors reduced the bactericidal capacity of insect haemocytes; this effect resulted from impaired phagocytosis of bacteria. These inhibotor studies reinforced the concept that glycolysis provided the major energy sources for phagocytosis by invertebrate cells. An indication of oxidative glucose metabolism by haemocytes was gained by quantifying the production of labelled CO_2 by resting and phagocytically stimulated insect haemocytes incubated with ^{14}C-glucose or ^{14}C-trehalose (the usual blood sugar of insects). The average increase in $^{14}CO_2$ production during phagocytosis was about 20%. This represented the sum of the activities of the HMP shunt and tricarboxylic acid cycle, and was low compared to the increase observed in mammalian cells.

Phagocytosis by mammalian leucocytes induces a marked increase in CO_2 production from the first carbon of glucose relative to the sixth carbon. This reflects stimulated metabolism of glucose via the HMP shunt rather than the tricarboxylic acid cycle and glycolysis. Studies of the metabolism of specifically labelled glucose by insect haemocytes during phagocytosis showed increased ultilization of glucose-1-^{14}C relative to glucose-6-^{14}C. It was concluded that direct oxidation of glucose was not stimulated by phagocytosis.

It appears that the metabolic events accompanying phagocytosis by invertebrate blood cells are fundamentally different from those characteristic of PMNs and most macrophages. However, as was mentioned, subpopulations of mammalian macrophages differ substantially from each other in their phagocytic metabolism. One could speculate that invertebrate haemocytes are closer to phylogenetic precursors of macrophages than PMNs. At this very preliminary stage of knowledge in this area, any generalizations based on biochemical similarities are probably premature.

VI. Mechanisms of bacterial killing by leucocytes

Both PMNs and macrophages of vertebrates are thought to utilize H_2O_2, a by-product of HMP activity, as an antimicrobial compound. The ability of human macrophages to kill is impaired in the absence of oxygen (Cline, 1970a). Killing is enhanced by H_2O_2 production (Cline, 1970b) and reduced in disease conditions in which H_2O_2 production is impaired (Rodey *et al.*, 1969). Reduction of nitroblue tetrazolium (NBT) has been shown to be associated with the increment in respiration and H_2O_2 production in leucocytes. Insect haemocytes phagocytosed zymosan particles and NBT, but there was no NBT reduction, as indicated by the absence of the deep blue formazan-containing vacuoles characteristically seen in human leucocytes (Anderson *et al.*, 1973b).

A potent antimicrobial system has been described in PMNs involving H_2O_2—MPO, and a halide (Klebanoff, 1968). A MPO-H_2O_2-Cl^- complex is formed *in vivo*, which reacts with bacterial amino acids to form unstable amino acid chloramines which are spontaneously decarboxylated and deaminated to yield antimicrobial aldehydes (Sbarra *et al.*, 1972). Although the NBT method suggested that H_2O_2 was not produced during phagocytosis, we decided to look for other components of this system in insect haemocytes. Using the method of Kaplow (1965), insect haemocyte granules were shown to be positive for MPO in only 1–2% of the cells. Myeloperoxidase may play some role in killing by macrophage precursors, but killing by macrophages is not dependent on the presence of the enzyme (Lehrer and Cline, 1969). If human leucocytes are placed in medium containing Na ^{125}I and stimulated with zymosan particles, they will iodinate the particles by the action of MPO and H_2O_2 (Pincus and Klebanoff, 1971). Our attempts to measure iodination in insect haemocytes were unsuccessful. Mammalian PMNs also have granule-associated antibacterial cationic proteins (Zeya and Spitznagel, 1966a,b). In preliminary studies we have been unable to isolate by electrophoresis comparable bactericidal proteins from insect haemocytes.

Based on information now available, invertebrate haemocytes do not use oxygen-dependent antimicrobial systems typical of mammalian PMNs. Like macrophages, they seem to lack MPO and bactericidal cationic proteins. There is no evidence that invertebrate haemocytes possess an H_2O_2-generating system similar to that seen in PMNs and macrophages. Several oxygen-independent bactericidal systems are present in haemocytes. The acidity of phagosomes is probably toxic to many bacterial species. Lysozyme and other haemocytic enzymes have antimicrobial activity. The exact mechanisms by which invertebrate cells and macrophages in higher animals kill bacteria remain largely unknown. The extent to which these processes prove to be similar will be of great interest in future considerations of comparative haematology.

VII. Macrophage activation

The phenomenon of macrophage activation is well known in higher animals. Briefly, this activation causes the cells to become larger than usual, to have increased hydrolase activity, to be more phagocytically active, and to be more effective in bacterial killing. It is important to note that this activation is non-specific, in that activated macrophages show increased reactivity against both the activating agent and other material.

Although it is by no means a common phenomenon, augmented cellular immune responsiveness can be induced in certain invertebrate species. The data of McKay and Jenkin (1970) may provide an example of invertebrate macrophage activation. Crayfish (*Parachaeraps bicarinatus*) lack natural or induced bacterial opsonins or bactericidal factors. However, injection of bacterial vaccines produced increased protection against subsequent bacterial infection. Haemocytes from immunized animals were more phagocytically active than cells from control animals, as measured by *in vitro* phagocytosis of erythrocytes. Hence, induced resistance to infection could probably be correlated with enhanced phagocytic and/or bacterial capacity of haemocytes.

VIII. Concluding remarks

The blood cells of all animals are capable of recognizing foreign materials. The specificity of this response is highest in animals with well-developed lymphoid systems and immunoglobulins. It is not surprising that invertebrate immune responses generally lack specificity and memory components because they lack organized lymphoid tissue and antibodies. They often possess cells which morphologically resemble vertebrate lymphocytes; however, these cells are thought to be progenitors of other blood cell types. Furthermore, there is little evidence that these cells are actually involved in immune reactions of any kind. Since the term "lymphocyte" has more immunological than morphological connotations, it probably should be avoided in discussions of invertebrate haematology.

Current concepts in phylogenetic relationships indicate that protochordates represent the line which leads directly to the vertebrates. If any invertebrate group might be expected to have lymphocytes, the tunicates would be the most likely candidates. However, Warr *et al.* (1977) could not induce blastogenic transformation of tunicate "lymphocytes" in response to mitogens or allogeneic cells. These *in vitro* responses are considered to be classical functional properties of vertebrate lymphocytes. The only clearly defined function of tunicate "lymphocytes" is that of haemocyte stem cells, as shown by cell reconstitution experiments in X-irradiated tunicates (Freeman, 1970).

The more mature granulocytes and hyalinocytes of invertebrates are effector cells in various cellular immune reactions including phagocytosis, encapsulation, defence against microbial infection, graft rejection, etc. These cells more closely resemble granulocytes and macrophages of higher animals than lymphocytes. Based on the limited information available, invertebrate haemocytes seem to be more closely related to the monocyte-macrophage series than to PMNs.

References

Anderson, R. S. (1971). *Biol. Bull., Woods Hole* **141**, 91–98.

Anderson, R. S. (1976). *In* "Phylogeny of Thymus and Bone Marrow-Bursa Cells" (R. K. Wright and E. L. Cooper, Eds), pp. 27–34. Elsevier/North-Holland Biomedical Press, Amsterdam.

Anderson, R. S. (1977). *Cell Immunol.* **29**, 331–336.

Anderson, R. S. and Cook, M. L. (1979). *J. Invertebr. Pathol.* **33**, 197–203.

Anderson, R. S. and Good, R. A. (1976). *J. Invertebr. Pathol.* **27**, 57–64.

Anderson, R. S., Day, N. K. B. and Good, R. A. (1972). *Infect. Immun.* **5**, 55–59.

Anderson, R. S., Holmes, B. and Good, R. A. (1973a). *J. Invertebr. Pathol.* **22**, 127–135.

Anderson, R. S., Holmes, B. and Good, R. A. (1973b). *Comp. Biochem. Physiol.* **46B**, 595–603.

Baggiolini, M. (1972). *Enzyme* **13**, 132–160.

Bainton, D. F. and Farquhar, M. G. (1968a). *J. Cell Biol.* **39**, 286–298.

Bainton, D. F. and Farquhar, M. G. (1968b). *J. Cell Biol.* **39**, 299–317.

Baxley, G., Bishop, G. B., Cooper, A. G. and Wortis, H. H. (1973). *Clin. Exp. Immunol.* **15**, 385–392.

Berrill, N. J. (1955). "The Origin of Vertebrates." Oxford University Press, London.

Cheng, T. C. (1976). *J. Invertebr. Pathol.* **27**, 263–268.

Cheng, T. C. and Rodrick, G. E. (1975). *Comp. Biochem. Physiol.* **52B**, 443–447.

Cline, M. J. (1970a). *Infect. Immun.* **2**, 156–161.

Cline, M. J. (1970b). *Infect. Immun.* **2**, 601–605.

Cline, M. J. and Lehrer, R. I. (1968). *Blood* **32**, 423–435.

Cohen, A. B. and Cline, M. J. (1971). *J. Clin. Invest.* **50**, 1390–1398.

Day, N. K. B., Gewurz, H., Johannsen, R., Finstad, J. and Good, R. A. (1970). *J. exp. Med.* **132**, 941–950.

Ebert, R. H. and Florey, H. W. (1939). *Br. J. Exp. Pathol.* **20**, 342–356.

Endean, R. (1960). *Quart. Jl. Microsc. Sci.* **101**, 177–197.

Ermak, T. H. (1976). *In* "Phylogeny of Thymus and Bone Marrow-Bursa Cells" (R. K. Wright and E. L. Cooper, Eds), pp. 45–56. Elsevier/North Holland Biomedical Press, Amsterdam.

Feng, S. Y., Feng, J. S., Burke, C. N. and Khairallah, L. M. (1971). *Z. Zellforsch. mikrosk. Anat.* **120**, 222–245.

Finstad, J., Papermaster, B. W. and Good, R. A. (1964). *Lab. Invest.* **13**, 490–512.

Freeman, G. (1970). *J. Reticuloendothel. Soc.* **7**, 183–194.
George, W. C. (1939). *Quart. Jl. Microsc. Sci.* **81**, 391–427.
Hildemann, W. H. and Reddy, A. L. (1973). *Fed. Proc.* **32**, 2188–2194.
Hildemann, W. H. and Uhlenbruck, G. (1974). *In* "Progress in Immunology" (L. Brent and J. Holborow, Eds), Vol. 2, pp. 292–296. North-Holland, Amsterdam.
Huber, H. and Fudenberg, H. H. (1968). *Int. Arch. Allergy* **34**, 18–31.
Jollès, J. and Jollès, P. (1975). *Eur. J. Biochem.* **54**, 19–23.
Jondal, M., Holm, G. and Wigzell, H. (1972). *J. exp. Med.* **136**, 207–215.
Kaplan, M. E., Dalmasso, A. P. and Woodson, M. (1972). *J. Immunol.* **108**, 275–278.
Kaplow, L. S. (1965). *Blood* **26**, 214–219.
Karnovsky, M. L. (1962). *Physiol. Rev.* **42**, 143–168.
Klebanoff, S. J. (1968). *J. Bacteriol.* **95**, 2131–2138.
Lehrer, R. I. and Cline, M. J. (1969). *J. Clin. Invest.* **48**, 1478–1488.
Lewis, M. R. (1925). *Am. J. Pathol.* **1**, 91–100.
LoBuglio, A. F., Cotran, R. S. and Jandl, J. H. (1967). *Science* **158**, 1582–1585.
McDade, J. E. and Tripp, M. R. (1967). *J. Invertebr. Pathol.* **9**, 531–535.
McKay, D. and Jenkin, C. R. (1970). *Aust. J. exp. biol. med. Sci.* **48**, 609–617.
Moore, M. N. and Lowe, D. M. (1977). *J. Invertebr. Pathol.* **29**, 18–30.
Papermaster, B. W., Condic, R. M., Finstad, J. and Good, R. A. (1964). *J. exp. Med.* **119**, 105–130.
Pauley, G. B., Granger, G. A. and Krassner, S. M. (1971). *J. Invertebr. Pathol.* **18**, 207–218.
Pincus, S. H. and Klebanoff, S. J. (1971). *N. Engl. J. Med.* **284**, 744–750.
Powning, R. F. and Davidson, W. J. (1973). *Comp. Biochem. Physiol.* **45B**, 669–686.
Prowse, R. H. and Tait, N. N. (1969). *Immunology* **17**, 437–443.
Rabinovitch, M. and DeStefano, M. (1970). *Exp. Cell Res.* **59**, 272–282.
Reddy, A. L., Bryan, B. and Hildemann, W. H. (1975). *Immunogenetics* **1**, 584–590.
Renwrantz, L. R. and Cheng, T. C. (1977). *J. Invertebr. Pathol.* **29**, 97–100.
Rodey, G. E., Park, B. H., Windhorst, D. B., Holmes, B. and Good, R. A. (1969). *Blood* **33**, 813–820.
Sbarra, A. J., Paul, B. B., Jacobs, A. A., Strauss, R. R. and Mitchell, G. W. (1972). *J. Reticuloendothel. Soc.* **12**, 109–126.
Scott, M. T. (1971a). *Archs. Zool. exp. gén.* **112**, 73–80.
Scott, M. T. (1971b). *Immunology* **21**, 817–828.
Stuart, A. E. (1968). *J. Pathol. Bacteriol.* **96**, 401–412.
Toupin, J. and Lamoureux, G. (1976). *Cell. Immunol.* **26**, 127–132.
Tripp, M. R. and Kent, V. E. (1967). *In Vitro* **3**, 129–135.
Warr, G. W., Decker, J. M., Mandel, T. E., DeLuca, D., Hudson, R. and Marchalonis, J. J. (1977). *Aust. J. exp. biol. med. Sci.* **55**, 151–164.
Yoshino, T. P. and Cheng, T. C. (1976). *Trans. Amer. Microsc. Soc.* **95**, 215–220.
Zeya, H. I. and Spitznagel, J. K. (1966a). *J. Bacteriol.* **91**, 750–754.
Zeya, H. I. and Spitznagel, J. K. (1966b). *J. Bacteriol.* **91**, 755–762.

Taxonomic Index

D

H

I

J

K

L

M

V

Z

Subject Index

B

H

I

K

L